Contemporary Issues in Reproductive Health

Contemporary Issues in Reproductive Health

Edited by Sidney Alvarado

hayle
medical

New York

Hayle Medical,
750 Third Avenue, 9th Floor,
New York, NY 10017, USA

Visit us on the World Wide Web at:
www.haylemedical.com

ISBN: 978-1-63241-760-2

Cataloging-in-Publication Data

Contemporary issues in reproductive health / edited by Sidney Alvarado.
    p. cm.
Includes bibliographical references and index.
ISBN 978-1-63241-760-2
1. Reproductive health. 2. Fertility, Human. 3. Human reproduction. I. Alvarado, Sidney.
RG133 .C66 2019
618.178--dc23

Table of Contents

Preface

Reproductive health is concerned with the sexual and reproductive health of a human being. It focuses on enabling individuals to lead a satisfying, responsible, and safer sexual life, in which they are able to reproduce according to their own will. Reproductive health is also concerned with the awareness among people regarding affordable, safe and effective methods of birth control. The methods or devices used to prevent pregnancy are known as birth control or contraception. Some of the commonly used birth control methods include the use of oral pills, vaginal rings, condoms, intrauterine devices, tubectomy and vasectomy. This book elucidates the concepts and innovative models around prospective developments with respect to reproductive health. It strives to provide a fair idea about this discipline and to help develop a better understanding of the latest advances within this field. As this field is emerging at a rapid pace, the contents of this book will help the readers understand the modern concepts and applications of the subject.

This book is a comprehensive compilation of works of different researchers from varied parts of the world. It includes valuable experiences of the researchers with the sole objective of providing the readers (learners) with a proper knowledge of the concerned field. This book will be beneficial in evoking inspiration and enhancing the knowledge of the interested readers.

In the end, I would like to extend my heartiest thanks to the authors who worked with great determination on their chapters. I also appreciate the publisher's support in the course of the book. I would also like to deeply acknowledge my family who stood by me as a source of inspiration during the project.

Editor

Sex composition and its impact on future childbearing

Sowmya Rajan[1*], Priya Nanda[2], Lisa M. Calhoun[3] and Ilene S. Speizer[3,4]

Abstract

Background: The sex composition of existing children has been shown to influence childbearing decision-making and behaviors of women and couples. One aspect of this influence is the preference for sons. In India, where son preference is deeply entrenched, research has normally focused on rural areas using cross-sectional data. However, urban areas in India are rapidly changing, with profound implications for childbearing patterns. Yet, evidence on the effect of the sex composition of current children on subsequent childbearing intentions and behavior in urban areas is scant. In this study, we analyze the impact of sex composition of children on subsequent (1) parity progression, (2) contraceptive use, and (3) desire for another child.

Methods: We analyze prospective data from women over a four year period in urban Uttar Pradesh using discrete-time event history logistic regression models to analyze parity progression from the first to second parity, second to third parity, and third to fourth parity. We also use logistic regression models to analyze contraceptive use and desire for another child.

Results: Relative to women with no daughters, women with no sons had significantly higher odds of progressing to the next birth (parity 1 – aOR: 1.31; CI: 1.04–1.66; parity 2 – aOR: 4.65; CI: 3.11–6.93; parity 3 – aOR:3.45; CI: 1.83–6. 52), as well as reduced odds of using contraception (parity 2 – aOR:.58; CI: .44–.76; parity 3 – aOR: .58; CI: .35–.98). Relative to women with two or more sons, women with two or more daughters had significantly higher odds of wanting to have another child (parity 1 – aOR: 1.33; CI: 1.06–1.67; parity 2 – aOR: 3.96; CI: 2.45–6.41; parity 3–4.89; CI: 2.22–10.77).

Conclusions: Our study demonstrates the pervasiveness of son preference in urban areas of Uttar Pradesh. We discuss these findings for future programmatic strategies to mitigate son preference in urban settings.

Keywords: Son preference, Sex composition, India, Parity progression, Contraceptive use, Fertility desires

Plain English summary

In India, son preference is prevalent, and has been shown to influence parental reproductive decision making and behavior. When parents have a strong son preference but do not have their desired number of sons, they are more likely to want to continue childbearing, less likely to use contraception, and more likely to have more children. In this study, we use longitudinal data from urban Uttar Pradesh to examine how the sex composition of current children influences future reproductive intentions and behavior. Specifically, we examine if the sex composition of children is associated with parity progression, modern contraceptive use, and desire for an additional child.

We use baseline and endline data from the Measurement, Learning, & Evaluation Project in urban Uttar Pradesh. Our findings show that at parities one, two, and three, women continue to have children if they have no son or only one son at baseline. Having no sons (or only daughters) at baseline is also associated with lower odds of using modern contraception, and higher odds of wanting another child at endline.

* Correspondence: Sowmya.vrajan@gmail.com
[1]Global Health Innovations Center, Duke University, Durham, NC 27701, USA
Full list of author information is available at the end of the article

This study shows that the sex composition of children is associated with women's future reproductive decision-making and behavior, including greater desire for additional children, more births, and less modern contraceptive use. Interventions to mitigate the negative effects of son preference must emphasize both the intrinsic value of girls, and the deleterious consequences of high-parity births and low contraceptive use.

Background

A strong preference for sons over daughters has been documented in India for much of the last century [1–5]. Termed "son preference," this phenomenon is also prevalent in several countries in South and East Asia, such as Bangladesh, Nepal, China, and Vietnam [1, 4]. Parents value sons over daughters for various social, economic, and religious reasons [2, 3, 6]. For instance, daughters are considered a burden because of large dowry and marriage expenses, their exclusion and discrimination in inheritance laws, and lower value as agricultural labor [6]. These and other reasons have normalized a strong preference for sons in several regions of India, and consequent discrimination against daughters in childhood health, nutrition, and mortality [1]. However, even in countries with a strong preference for sons, many parents also want to have at least one daughter [6]. This has been true in India as well, where Hindu parents earn merit for giving away a daughter in marriage without expecting anything in return (*kanya daan*) [6].

Parents pursue different strategies to implement their preference for sons over daughters [5]. Over the last three decades, a commonly used strategy to achieve the desired number/ proportion of sons has been sex-selective abortion [5]. The widespread availability and use of sex selection technologies (such as ultrasound and amniocentesis) in India and East Asian countries such as South Korea and Taiwan has contributed to severely distorted sex ratios at birth (over 1.10 boys to girls) [5, 7, 8].

Another strategy that parents employ is adopting different stopping or contraception rules for childbearing depending on the sex composition of their existing children [5, 9]. In other words, parents continue having children until they achieve their desired number (or proportion) of sons [5, 6]. Continuing to bear children until parents reach their desired number of sons would not only increase the number of unwanted daughters within families, but also unwanted and total fertility in the aggregate [3]. In India, studies have shown that couples who do not have their desired number of sons are less likely to use contraception, more likely to have shorter birth intervals, more likely to want additional children, and more likely to progress to higher parities [6, 10–14].

The current approach to studying son preference in families is by examining the association between the sex composition of children and various outcomes by using cross-sectional data; many of these studies focus on rural areas or national samples [1, 3, 6, 9, 14–16]. Our study contributes to existing literature by using longitudinal data from urban areas of Uttar Pradesh. Specifically, we hypothesize that the sex composition of current children influences subsequent childbearing intentions and behaviors over a four year study period in urban Uttar Pradesh. We approached our analyses with the following hypotheses among women at the first, second, and third parities:

1. Parity progression (to second, third, and fourth parities) will be higher among women with a daughter-dominant sex composition of current children.
2. Modern contraceptive use will be lower among women whose children have a daughter-dominant sex composition.
3. Desire for additional children will be greater among women whose children have a daughter-dominant sex composition.

Study context

Uttar Pradesh, situated in the North of India, is the most populous state with nearly 200 million individuals, according to the 2011 Census [17]. The state has a poor record in health and human development and suffers from weak public health infrastructure, in regards to quality of service delivery and capacity of trained providers [18]. It also ranks high in infant and child mortality, and low in modern contraceptive use and women's education [19]. Further, Uttar Pradesh has consistently had among the highest total fertility rates (TFR) in the country [20]: while TFR has been declining in India for the previous two decades with about 2.6 children per woman in 2008, it was 3.8 children per woman in Uttar Pradesh in the same year [21]. However, data from the 2015 to 16 National Family Health Surveys show that TFR is now steadily declining in Uttar Pradesh as well, with 2.7 children per woman in the state, and 2.1 children per woman in its urban areas [19].

Methods

In 2009, the Bill & Melinda Gates Foundation launched the Urban Reproductive Health Initiative (URHI) in select cities in four countries – India, Kenya, Nigeria and Senegal –with a particular focus on the urban poor. The goal of the program was to improve access to and use of family planning and reproductive health services in urban areas. At the same time, the Measurement, Learning & Evaluation (MLE) Project, led by the

Carolina Population Center at the University of North Carolina at Chapel Hill, was funded to perform rigorous impact evaluation of the URHI programs in all four countries. In India, the URHI project was called the Urban Health Initiative (UHI), and fielded in urban sites of the state of Uttar Pradesh (UP) in late 2010. The program was deployed and evaluated in six cities– Agra, Aligarh, and Moradabad from western UP, and Allahabad, Gorakhpur, and Varanasi from eastern UP [22]. These cities were selected by UHI in conjunction with the Government of Uttar Pradesh and the Government of India, based on criteria such as their population size, geographic and regional diversity, large slum populations, and low contraceptive prevalence [13, 22]. Estimates from the provisional population totals from the 2011 Census show that these six cities contributed to 18% (or 8.0 million people) of the total 44.5 million urban residents in the state [17].

The MLE Project undertook longitudinal surveys across three periods to collect baseline, midterm, and endline data. MLE used a multi-stage sampling design to collect baseline data in 2010 from a representative sample of households and women in each city. An important component of the sampling strategy was the oversampling of slums in each city to evaluate and examine program activities targeted towards the urban poor [22]. Prior to selection of primary sampling units, all cities were mapped to identify the location and boundaries of registered slums from the government's list. In a second step, to identify additional slums, densely populated areas with poor access to water and sanitation services were mapped during the process of ground truthing[1] the registered slums [23, 24]. In each city, half of selected primary sampling units were slum areas and the other half were non-slum areas; this permitted obtaining an over sample of the urban poor. In each selected primary sampling unit, a random sample of 30 households was selected for a detailed household interview with the head of the household as well as interviews with all currently married women ages 15–49 years. Among the topics covered in the women's survey were basic sociodemographic characteristics, reproductive preferences and behavior, maternal and child health services, contraceptive knowledge and use, media use and gender relations. In 2014, the endline survey was conducted in which field teams sought to find all women who were usual residents at baseline, including those that were no longer married and were outside the age range of 15–49 years, and still residing in a study city in order to measure program exposure and changes in contraceptive use and fertility behaviors. The response rate for the endline survey was 83.6% [24]. In order to make the sample truly representative of the population, we use endline weights in the descriptive

analyses reported in this study. All MLE surveys and study procedures were approved by the Institutional Review Board Committees of the University of North Carolina at Chapel Hill, ICRW and Mamta-Health Institute for Mother and Child in India.

A total of 14,043 women had complete interviews at baseline and endline. While nonresponse and attrition from baseline to endline could be a source of bias, with a response rate of 83.6%, we believe that this bias will not affect our study findings substantially [15]. Additionally, by weighting all analyses, we hope to also adjust for nonresponse bias. For the analyses described in this study, we focus on the sample of women who had at least one birth, but not more than three births at baseline, were not sterilized, menopausal, infecund or pregnant at baseline, and were re-interviewed at endline. The focus on this sub-sample relates to our interest in how sex composition of previous children influence parity progression, contraceptive use, and subsequent fertility intentions which means we need to restrict our sample to women who had at least one birth. Further, because over 75% of births at baseline were in parities 1 to 3, we also restrict our analyses to these critical parities. Last, because fertility intentions are recorded only for women who were fecund (not sterilized and menopausal), and not pregnant at the time of baseline interview, we include the sample of women who had valid reports of fertility intentions at baseline.

We analyzed three outcome variables for this study. The first outcome of interest is whether each respondent progressed from parities one, two, and three to parities two, three, and four respectively between baseline and endline. These variables are coded as binary variables for each parity transition. The second outcome relates to contraceptive use to examine if respondents used modern contraception at endline (use of modern method vs. no or traditional method). The last outcome examines desire for another child at endline: want another child (soon or later) vs. want no more children.

The key predictor variable is the sex composition of living children at parities one, two, and three at the time of the baseline interview. At parity one, the two possible categories for sex composition of existing children are: (1) one son (reference) and (2) one daughter. At parity two, the categories of sex composition of existing children are: (1) two sons (reference), (2) one son and one daughter, and (3) two daughters. At parity three, the categories of sex composition of children are: (1) three sons(reference), (2) two sons, one daughter, (3) two daughters, one son, and (4) three daughters. We chose the reference categories to indicate the son-dominant category within each parity, where applicable. The son-dominant category at parity one is one son; at parity two, it is two sons; and at parity three, it is three sons.

For all three models, controls include standard demographic variables that affect the outcomes. These include age at baseline (15–24 years, 25–34 years, and over 35 years), education (no education, primary, secondary, and more than secondary), religion (Hindu, and other religion), household wealth quintile (poorest, poor, medium, rich, and richest), city (Agra, Aligarh, Allahabad, Gorakhpur, Moradabad, and Varanasi), and slum residence (slum, non-slum). Household wealth quintiles were constructed similar to the Demographic and Health Surveys and as described by Filmer and Pritchett [25]. To elaborate, wealth indices were constructed using data on the ownership of consumer goods, assets, and materials used to construct the house/ dwelling, at the household level, comprising 27 different variables. This information was used to conduct principal components analysis and estimate a factor (or wealth) score for each household. Households were then placed in quintiles, ranging from lowest (poorest) to highest (richest). We also include baseline fertility intentions for another child (want another child, and want no more children), as well as any contraceptive use at baseline (yes/ no).

Because all our outcome variables are binary, we use logistic regressions for all multivariate analyses. First, for parity progression, we use a series of discrete-time logistic regressions predicting whether the respondent had a second, third, or fourth birth since the time of their first, second, or third birth respectively. Second, we use logistic regression to estimate modern method use at endline (modern method vs. no/ traditional method). Next, we use logistic regressions to predict endline fertility intentions (want another child vs. want no more). For all outcomes, we show the adjusted estimates controlling for baseline sociodemographic characteristics, fertility intentions and FP use. We present results from the logistic regression models as odds ratios, which can be interpreted as follows: if the odds ratio is greater than 1.0, the association of the particular independent variable with the outcome is positive; if the odds ratio is less than 1.0, the association of the particular independent variable with the outcome is negative. All models control for clustering in the data using the svy commands in Stata statistical software.

Results
Sociodemographic characteristics
Table 1 presents key descriptive statistics showing the characteristics of mothers with one, two or three children at baseline who were not pregnant or infecund (menopausal, hysterectomy, sterilized) at the time of the baseline interview, and followed up at endline four years later ($N = 5761$). More than half of the women in our sample were between 25 and 34 years old at baseline (51.73%); and more than a quarter of them were 35 years

and older (27.63%). Nearly a fifth of the women in this sample had no education (19.21%), a third had more than secondary school education (33.66%), and nearly 40% had completed secondary school education (39.41%). The majority of this sample was Hindu (80.39%), and resided in non-slums (84.10%). Over half of the sample was from households in the two highest quintiles – rich and richest (55.15%).

In this study sample, over 40% had two children (44.41%), nearly a third had one child (30.80%), and a quarter had three children (24.79%). Among these women, just over a fifth had no sons (22.96%), whereas nearly a third had no daughter (32.22%). More than half of the sample had one son (52.18%), whereas a little under half of the sample had one daughter (48.40%). Nearly two thirds of the women wanted no more children at baseline (66.91%), but less than half were using a modern contraceptive method (47.63%) at baseline.

Sex composition and parity progression
Table 2 shows the results of the multivariate logistic regression analyses of the sex of previous child(ren) on women's parity progression from the first, second, and third births between baseline and endline. Although not presented in the multivariate tables, we controlled for baseline sociodemographic characteristics, fertility intentions, and contraceptive use in all models. Our findings show patterns of association between the sex composition of previous children and subsequent childbearing that are consistent with a preference for sons. Model 1 shows that in the transition from first to second birth, women with one daughter had significantly higher odds of progressing to a second birth (aOR: 1.31; 95% CI: 1.04–1.66) compared to women with one son. Model 2 shows the association between sex of previous children in the transition to the third birth. The adjusted coefficients show that relative to women whose two children were both sons, those who had one son and one daughter had increased odds of progressing to a third birth (aOR: 1.65; 95% CI: 1.21–2.26). Women whose two children were both daughters had more than four times higher odds of progressing to a third birth (aOR: 4.65; 95% CI: 3.11–6.93). Model 3 shows the association of sex composition in the transition to the fourth birth. Relative to women with three sons, those with three daughters had over three times higher odds of progressing to a fourth birth (aOR: 3.45; 95% CI: 1.83–6.52).

Sociodemographic variables, fertility intentions, and parity progression (not shown)
Fertility intentions reported at baseline were also strong predictors of subsequent childbearing for the progression to second and third births. Relative to women who want another child, those who want no more children

Table 1 Baseline characteristics of married, non-pregnant, fecund mothers with one, two or three children at baseline (and followed up endline)

Characteristic	Percent	N = 5761
Age (years)		
15–24	20.65	1189
25–34	51.73	2980
Over 35 years	27.63	1592
Education		
None	19.21	1106
Primary	7.73	446
Secondary	39.41	2270
More than secondary	33.66	1939
Religion		
Hindu	80.39	4630
Other	19.61	1131
Wealth quintile		
Poorest	11.17	643
Poor	14.25	821
Medium	19.43	1120
Rich	25.97	1496
Richest	29.18	1681
Slum residence		
Slum	15.90	915
Non slum	84.10	4846
City		
Agra	23.10	1331
Aligarh	12.78	736
Allahabad	20.48	1180
Gorakhpur	15.79	910
Moradabad	9.70	558
Varanasi	18.15	1046
Number of children		
1	30.80	1775
2	44.41	2558
3	24.79	1428
Number of sons		
0	22.96	1323
1	52.18	3006
2	21.80	1256
3	3.06	176
Number of daughters		
0	32.22	1857
1	48.40	2789
2	17.50	1009
3	1.87	108

Table 1 Baseline characteristics of married, non-pregnant, fecund mothers with one, two or three children at baseline (and followed up endline) *(Continued)*

Characteristic	Percent	N = 5761
Fertility intentions		
Want soon/ want later	33.09	1906
Want no more	66.91	3855
Contraceptive use		
No method	27.01	1556
Modern method	47.63	2744
Traditional method	25.36	1461

Note: Endline weights used for percentages and number of observations

had significantly lower odds of progressing to the next birth. Among the other variables, age has a curvilinear relationship with childbearing: younger women in the prime reproductive years have greater odds of progressing to the next parity, whereas the oldest women have reduced odds of transitioning to the next parity. Women from wealthier households have lower odds of

Table 2 Odds Ratios from Logit Regression of Baseline Sex Composition on Having Second, Third, and Fourth Child After Baseline

Sex composition of previous children at baseline	Odds ratios (95%CI)	P
Model 1		
Parity 1 (N = 1661)	*(parity 1 - > parity 2)*	
1 son (ref)	1.00	–
0 sons, 1 daughter	1.31	.022
	(1.04–1.66)	
Model 2		
Parity 2 (N = 2490)	*(parity 2 - > parity 3)*	
2 sons (ref)	1.00	–
1 son, 1 daughter	1.65	.002
	(1.21–2.26)	
0 sons, 2 daughters	4.65	.000
	(3.11–6.93)	
Model 3		
Parity 3 (N = 1610)	*(parity 3 - > parity 4)*	
3 sons (ref)	1.00	–
2 sons, 1 daughter	.74	.269
	(.44–1.25)	
1 son, 2 daughters	1.51	.100
	(.92–2.48)	
0 sons, 3 daughters	3.45	.000
	(1.83–6.52)	

Note: All models adjust for respondent's baseline age, education, religion, household wealth, slum and city residence, fertility intentions, and contraceptive use progressing to a subsequent birth. Education, religion, city of residence, and slum residence were not consistently associated with progressing to the next birth.

Sex composition and modern contraceptive use

In Table 3, we present odds ratios and 95% confidence intervals of the association between sex composition at baseline and modern method use at endline by parity, net of baseline sociodemographic characteristics and fertility intentions. Model 4 shows that among women with one child at baseline, there was no significant association between the sex of that child and the odds of using modern contraception at endline. Model 5 provides evidence that among women with two children, modern method use was associated with the sex of previous children. Specifically, at parity two, relative to women who had two sons, women who had one son and one daughter at baseline had lower odds of using modern contraception at endline (aOR: 0.82; 95% CI: .67–.99). Women who had two daughters relative to two sons had significantly lower odds of using modern contraception (aOR: 0.58; 95% CI: .44–.76). Model 6 shows that women who

had three daughters at baseline had significantly lower odds of using modern contraception, relative to women with three sons (aOR: 0.58; 95% CI: .35–.98).

Sociodemographic variables, fertility intentions and contraceptive use (not shown)

Women who did not want more children at baseline had substantially increased odds of using modern contraception in every parity. At every parity, younger women had higher odds of using modern contraception. Women who had completed at least secondary schooling were significantly more likely to use modern contraception at all parities. Wealth and religion were not significantly associated with modern method use across parity.

Sex composition and desire for another child

Table 4 presents the results of the association between sex composition of children at baseline and desire for an additional child at endline, net of sociodemographic characteristics and fertility intentions. Model 7 in Table 4 shows that the association between baseline sex composition and desire for another child at endline is positive and significant among women with one child at baseline. Specifically, at parity one, women who had one daughter rather than one son at baseline had significantly higher odds of wanting another child at the endline interview (aOR: 1.33; 95% CI: 1.06–1.67). In Model 8, relative to women

Table 3 Odds Ratios from Logit Regression of Baseline Sex Composition on Modern Contraceptive Use at Endline

Sex composition of previous children at baseline	Odds ratios (95%CI)	P
Model 4		
Parity 1 (N = 1661)		
1 son (ref)	1.00	–
0 sons, 1 daughter	1.04	.723
	(.84–1.29)	
Model 5		
Parity 2 (N = 2490)		
2 sons (ref)	1.00	–
1 son, 1 daughter	.82	.045
	(.67–.99)	
0 sons, 2 daughters	.58	.000
	(.44–.76)	
Model 6		
Parity 3 (N = 1610)		
3 sons (ref)	1.00	–
2 sons, 1 daughter	.83	.314
	(.58–1.19)	
1 son, 2 daughters	.76	.144
	(.53–1.09)	
0 sons, 3 daughters	.58	.043
	(.35–.98)	

Note: All models adjust for respondent's baseline age, education, religion, household wealth, slum and city residence, fertility intentions, and contraceptive use

Table 4 Odds ratios from Logit Regression of Baseline Sex Composition on Desire for another Child at Endline

Sex composition of previous children at baseline	Odds ratios (95%CI)	P
Model 7		
Parity 1 (N = 1661)		
1 son (ref)	1.00	–
1 daughter	1.33	.013
	(1.06–1.67)	
Model 8		
Parity 2 (2490)		
2 sons (ref)	1.00	–
1 son, 1 daughter	.68	.082
	(.44–1.05)	
0 sons, 2 daughters	3.96	.000
	(2.45–6.41)	
Model 9		
Parity 3 (1610)		
2 or more sons (ref)	1.00	–
2 or more daughters	4.89	.000
	(2.22–10.77)	

Note: All models adjust for respondent's baseline age, education, religion, household wealth, slum and city residence, fertility intentions, and contraceptive use with two sons, those with two daughters had nearly four times the odds of wanting another child at endline, among women with two children (aOR: 3.96; 95% CI: 2.45–6.41). At parity 3, we combine the categories of women who had three sons, and those with two sons and a daughter, because of the very small cell size of women with three sons who wanted another child ($n = 5$). Similarly, we combine the categories of women who had three daughters and those with two daughters and a son because of the relatively small cell size of women with three daughters and who wanted another child ($n = 42$). Relative to women with two or more sons, those with two or more daughters at baseline had nearly five times the odds of wanting another child (aOR: 4.89; 95% CI: 2.22–10.77).

Sociodemographic variables, fertility intentions and desire for another child (not shown)

Baseline desire for another child is a strong predictor of desire for another child at endline: women who did not want another child at baseline had significantly lower odds of wanting another child at endline. Desire for another child declined with age in the third parity: it was highest at young ages and gradually declined as women age. Neither wealth nor education was associated with the desire for another child at endline. Women who were not Hindu were less likely to want another child at endline.

Discussion

Urban areas of Uttar Pradesh, a state in Northern India, provide an opportune site to examine the evolution of reproductive behavior in the context of strong son preference. Our study shows that the sex composition of a woman's child(ren) is related to her subsequent fertility trajectory. Using prospective data, we found that the sex of a woman's previous children strongly influences whether she desires another child, will use contraception, and has a subsequent birth.

We highlight three main findings from our study. First, in line with our first hypothesis, women in this urban Uttar Pradesh sample prefer to have a sex composition for their children that is son-dominant, and this desire is manifested in their childbearing behavior. Our findings suggest that at every parity, women who have a sex composition that is daughter-dominant are more likely to progress to the next parity. These associations are substantial and significant, and suggest that women who do not have a son-dominant sex composition are more likely to continue childbearing.

Second, we find modest and inconsistent support for our second hypothesis. Women with a daughter-dominant sex composition base their decision to use modern contraception only after the first parity. In the first parity, the sex of the child has no association with women's use of modern contraception, suggesting a desire for two children. At parity two, both women with no sons and women with one son are less likely to use modern contraception, relative to those with two sons (son-dominant sex composition). Parity three presents a different picture: we find that women with one, two, or three sons are not significantly different from each other in their use of modern contraception. It is only when women in the third parity have no sons (daughter-dominant sex composition) that they are significantly less likely to use modern contraception.

Last, consistent with our third hypothesis, we find that women with a daughter-dominant sex composition of their children at baseline are more likely to want to have another child at endline. This association is evident in all three parities.

Our findings are consistent with earlier studies from India that show an association between sex composition of previous children and reproductive outcomes such as parity progression, desire for an additional child, and contraceptive use [3, 6, 9, 10, 13, 26]. In general, using cross-sectional data, these studies show that women with fewer sons than daughters (or daughter-dominant sex composition) are more likely to desire another child, more likely to continue to have children, and less likely to use effective contraception [3, 6, 9, 10, 13, 26]. For instance, using baseline MLE data, Calhoun et al. [13] find that son-dominant sex composition is associated with desire for another child: women with more sons than daughters are more likely to want no more children, relative to those with more daughters than sons. Other studies show that regardless of the number of daughters, couples have at least one or two sons before they begin to use contraception [26]. In the same vein, Jayaraman et al. [3] show that the desire for an additional child decreases with the number of sons in the family. In contrast, some studies note a preference for at least one daughter [6, 13, 27]– a finding that is not evident in the parity progression models of this study.

Our findings extend the breadth of earlier studies by examining these outcomes over a four year follow-up period, and by accounting for women's baseline fertility intentions, contraceptive use, and a variety of sociodemographic controls in predicting future childbearing intentions behavior. Almost all the studies that examine son preference use cross-sectional surveys. Although cross-sectional studies serve many useful purposes, a main drawback is that they do not allow us a sequential understanding of women's reproductive behavior. However, reproductive decision-making follows an inherently sequential pattern [26, 28], and childbearing decisions are usually made based on current familial circumstances that relate to the composition of children already present in the family [26, 28].

Our study has unique strengths and limitations. First, with baseline and endline data and retrospective birth histories, we are able to use event history analytical techniques to estimate parity progression among fecund women conditional on sex composition. Second, most studies of son preference focus on rural areas or on nationally representative samples. Our study however, uses data from a large sample of women from six cities in Uttar Pradesh. Using data from urban areas allows us to analyze reproductive behavior and son preference in areas where the spread of modernization and changing values over family size and composition ideals is already under way. To elaborate, urban areas have value systems that are markedly different from their rural counterparts which have been found to be influential in women's decisions regarding their family [29]. While this modern outlook might reduce parental preference for sons [11, 29], others show that son preference is intensified in urban areas [2]. Our analysis confirms the latter view: son preference is strong in this urban context which makes having only daughters less desirable.

Our study also has its limitations. First, our sample is restricted to women who were not sterilized, menopausal or pregnant at baseline. We use this restricted sample in order to use valid fertility intentions in our analysis of the relationship between sex composition and fertility. However, we acknowledge that we lose information about the sex composition and son preference of women who were already sterilized at baseline. Second, this study could also be strengthened if we had dynamic measures of fertility intentions. As is well-known, intentions measured at a particular time point could be unreliable as fertility intentions are fluid [30]. Lastly, our study does not attempt to demonstrate the influence of sex-selective abortions on women's reproductive behavior. While this is a pervasive practice in much of northern India, we are unable to examine its role on women's fertility in our analysis.

Conclusions

Our study highlights that son preference is a pervasive phenomenon in India that is not restricted to rural areas. While enabling women to meet their reproductive preferences should be an intrinsic social welfare goal, policies need to be in place that help parents appreciate the value of a daughter. Many such laws are already in place in India, such as the Preconception and Prenatal Diagnostic Techniques Act of 1994 that prohibits the use of sex-selection technologies to abort a female fetus. Programs that work explicitly to enhance the value of girls can also alleviate the perceived burden of daughters to parents. Over time as these types of programs are rolled out, there will be a need to undertake similar analyses to the ones presented here to determine whether policies and programs lead to changes in son-preference in urban (and rural) India.

Abbreviations
ICRW: International Center for Research on Women; MLE Project: Measurement, Learning & Evaluation Project; TFR: Total fertility rate; UHI: Urban Health Initiative; URHI: Urban Reproductive Health Initiative

Acknowledgements
This manuscript was made possible by support from the Bill & Melinda Gates Foundation (BMGF) under terms of the Measurement, Learning & Evaluation (MLE) for the Urban Reproductive Health Initiative, and the Carolina Population Center. The authors are grateful for general support from the Carolina Population Center and its NIH Center grant (P2C HD050924). The authors' views expressed in this publication do not necessarily reflect the views of BMGF. An earlier version of this paper was presented at the Annual Meetings of the Population Association of America in Washington D.C. in March 2016.

Funding
This project was made possible with funding from The Bill & Melinda Gates Foundation, under terms for the Measurement, Learning & Evaluation (MLE) Project. All views, analysis, and interpretation in this manuscript are the authors' and do not reflect those of any funding agency listed earlier.

Authors' contributions
SR performed all analyses and wrote the manuscript. All authors read, edited, and approved the manuscript.

Competing interests
The authors declare that they have no competing interests.

Author details
[1]Global Health Innovations Center, Duke University, Durham, NC 27701, USA. [2]Bill & Melinda Gates Foundation, New Delhi, India. [3]Carolina Population Center, University of North Carolina at Chapel Hill, Chapel Hill, USA. [4]Gillings School of Global Public Health, University of North Carolina at Chapel Hill, Chapel Hill, USA.

References
1. Dasgupta M. Selective discrimination against female children in rural Punjab, India. Popul Dev Rev. 1987;13(1):77–100.
2. Guilmoto C. The sex ratio transition in Asia. Popul Dev Rev. 2009;35:519–49. https://doi.org/10.1111/j.1728-4457.2009.00295.x
3. Jayaraman A, Mishra V, Arnold F. The relationship of family size and composition to fertility desires, contraceptive adoption and method choice in South Asia. Int Perspect Sex Reprod Health. 2009;3:29–38.

4. Leone T, Matthews Z, Dalla ZG. Impact and determinants of sex preference in Nepal. Int Fam Plan Perspect. 2003;29:69–75. https://doi.org/10.2307/3181060

5. Bongaarts J. The implementation of preferences for male offspring. Popul Dev Rev. 2013;39:185–208. https://doi.org/10.1111/j.1728-4457.2013.00588.x.

6. Arnold F, Choe MK, Roy TK. Son preference, the family-building process and child mortality in India. Popul Stud. 1998;52:301–15. https://doi.org/10.1080/0032472031000150486

7. Park CB, Cho N-H. Consequences of son preference in a low-fertility society: imbalance of the sex ratio at birth in Korea. Popul Dev Rev. 1995;21:59–84. https://doi.org/10.2307/2137413

8. Chung W, Dasgupta M. The decline of son preference in South Korea: the roles of development and public policy. Popul Dev Rev. 2007;33:757–83. https://doi.org/10.1111/j.1728-4457.2007.00196.x

9. Chaudhuri S. The desire for sons and excess fertility: a household-level analysis of parity progression in India. Int Perspect Sex Reprod Health. 2012;38:178–86.

10. Clark S. Son preference and sex composition of children: evidence from India. Demography. 2000;37:95–108. https://doi.org/10.2307/2648099

11. Bhat PM, Zavier A. Fertility decline and gender bias in northern India. Demography. 2003;40:637–57. https://doi.org/10.2307/1515201

12. Dyson T, Moore M. On kinship structure, female autonomy, and demographic behavior in India. Popul Dev Rev. 1983;9:35–60. https://doi.org/10.2307/1972894

13. Calhoun LM, Nanda P, Speizer IS, Jain M. The effect of family sex composition on fertility desires and family planning behaviors in urban Uttar Pradesh, India. Reprod Health. 2013;10:48. https://doi.org/10.1186/1742-4755-10-48

14. Rajaretnam T, Deshpande RV. The effect of sex preference on contraceptive use and fertility in rural South India. Int Fam Plan Perspect. 1994;20:88–95. https://doi.org/10.2307/2133510

15. Bulatao RA. Values and disvalues of children in successive childbearing decisions. Demography. 1981;18:1–25. https://doi.org/10.2307/2061046

16. Pande RP. Selective gender differences in childhood nutrition and immunization in rural India: the role o siblings. Demography. 2003;40:395–418. https://doi.org/10.1353/dem.2003.0029

17. Census of India. 2011. Accessed 03 Nov 2017. http://censusindia.gov.in/2011-prov-results/paper2/data_files/UP/7-pop-12-22.pdf.

18. United Nations Development Programme. Human development report 2016: human development for everyone. New York, NY; 2016. Accessed 03 Nov 2017. http://hdr.undp.org/sites/default/files/2016_human_development_report.pdf

19. International Institute of Population Sciences. State Fact Sheets – 2015-16. National Family Health Survey (NFHS-4). 2016. Accessed 03 Nov 2017. https://dhsprogram.com/pubs/pdf/OF31/OF31.UP.pdf.

20. International Institute for Population Sciences - IIPS/India and Macro International. India National Family Health Survey (NFHS-3) 2005–06. Volume 1. Mumbai, India: IIPS and Macro International; 2007.

21. Government of India. Accessed 03 Nov 2017. http://niti.gov.in/content/total-fertility-rate-tfr-birth-woman.

22. Speizer IS, Nanda P, Achyut P, Pillai G, Guilkey D. Family planning use among urban poor women from six cities of Uttar Pradesh, India. J Urban Health. 2012;89:639–58. https://doi.org/10.1007/s11524-011-9667-1

23. Achyut PMA, Montana L, Sengupta R, Calhoun LM, Nanda P. Integration of family planning with maternal health services: an opportunity to increase postpartum modern contraceptive use in urban Uttar Pradesh, India. J Fam Plann Reprod Health Care. 2016;42 https://doi.org/10.1136/jfprhc-2015-101271

24. Montana LLP, Mankoff C, Speizer IS, Guilkey D. Using satellite data to delineate slum and non-slum sample domains for an urban population survey in Uttar Pradesh, India. Spat Demogr. 2016;4:1–16. https://doi.org/10.1007/s40980-015-0007-z

25. Achyut PBA, Calhoun LM, Corroon M, Guilkey DK, Kebede E, Lance PM, Mishra A, Nanda P, O'Hara R, Sengupta R, Speizer IS, Stewart JS, Winston J. Impact evaluation of the urban health initiative in urban Uttar Pradesh, India. Contraception. 2016;93:519–25. https://doi.org/10.1016/j.contraception.2016.02.031

26. Speizer IS, Calhoun LM, Hoke T, Sengupta R. Measurement of unmet need for family planning: longitudinal analysis of the impact of fertility desires on subsequent childbearing behaviors among urban women from Uttar Pradesh, India. Contraception. 2013;88:553–60. https://doi.org/10.1016/j.contraception.2013.04.006

27. Filmer D, Pritchett LH. Estimating wealth effects without expenditure data—or tears: an application to educational enrollments in states of India. Demography. 2001;38 https://doi.org/10.1353/dem.2001.0003

28. Raley S BS. Sons, daughters, and family processes: Does gender of children matter? Annu Rev Sociol 2006, 32:401–421. https://doi.org/10.1146/annurev.soc.32.061604.123106.

29. Edmeades J, Pande R, Macquarrie K, Falle T, Malhotra A. Two sons and a daughter: sex composition and women's reproductive behaviour in Madhya Pradesh, India. J Biosoc Sci. 2012;44:749–64. https://doi.org/10.1017/s0021932012000119

30. Das GM. Family systems, political systems and Asia's 'missing girls': the construction of son preference and its unraveling. Asian Population Stud. 2010;6:123–52. https://doi.org/10.1080/17441730.2010.494437

Community approval required for periconceptional adolescent adherence to weekly iron and/or folic acid supplementation

Adélaïde Compaoré[1], Sabine Gies[2,3], Bernard Brabin[4], Halidou Tinto[1] and Loretta Brabin[5*] (iD)

Abstract

Background: Iron deficiency remains a prevalent adolescent health problem in low income countries. Iron supplementation is recommended but improvement of iron status requires good adherence.

Objectives: We explored factors affecting adolescent adherence to weekly iron and/or folic acid supplements in a setting of low secondary school attendance.

Methods: Taped in-depth interviews were conducted with participants in a randomised, controlled, periconceptional iron supplementation trial for young nulliparous women living in a rural, malaria endemic region of Burkina Faso. Participants with good, medium or poor adherence were selected. Interviews were transcribed and analysed thematically.

Results: Thirty-nine interviews were conducted. The community initially thought supplements were contraceptives. The potential benefits of giving iron supplementation to unmarried "girls" ahead of pregnancy were not recognised. Trial participation, which required parental consent, remained high but was not openly admitted because iron supplements were thought to be contraceptives. Unmarried non-school attenders, being mobile, were often sent to provide domestic labour in varied locations. This interrupted adherence - as did movement of school girls during vacations and at marriage. Field workers tracked participants and trial provision of free treatment encouraged adherence. Most interviewees did not identify health benefits from taking supplements.

Conclusions: For success, communities must be convinced of the value of an adolescent intervention. During this safety trial, benefits not routinely available in iron supplementation programmes were important to this low income community, ensuring adolescent participation. Nevertheless, adolescents were obliged to fulfil cultural duties and roles that interfered with regular adherence to the iron supplementation regime.

Keywords: Iron supplementation, Adolescents, Adherence, Burkina Faso, Qualitative, Non-pregnant, Pregnant

* Correspondence: loretta.brabin@manchester.ac.uk
[5]Division of Cancer Sciences, Faculty of Biology, Medicine and Health, University of Manchester, Manchester, UK
Full list of author information is available at the end of the article

Background

The nutritional status of adolescents is frequently sub-optimal [1] with a high prevalence of iron deficiency and anaemia [2]. In high prevalence areas, daily iron and folic acid is offered routinely to pregnant women, with intermittent iron supplementation recommended for menstruating women [3]. Achieving high coverage for routine daily iron supplementation in pregnancy has proved difficult and it is uncertain whether, even with intermittent (ie less frequent) dosing, high coverage of non-pregnant women is achievable [4]. Sub-optimal adherence is attributed to side effects which might be reduced by intermittent dosing [5] as well as to operational factors [6]. Reaching unmarried adolescents is challenging as they do not regularly present at health services [7], consequently most adolescent iron intervention studies have been conducted among school attenders [8–11]. Evidence for the effectiveness of iron/folic acid supplementation from community-based studies is weak because of underpowered studies [12]. Without good adherence to the recommended supplementation regime, expected improvements in iron status will not be achieved.

A Cochrane review on iron supplementation (all ages) found inadequate reporting on adherence [13]. Direct observation, the most reliable method, was implemented in a periconceptional, randomised controlled trial (RCT) in Burkina Faso of iron supplementation of never pregnant young women aged 15–24 years, 93% of whom were adolescents (< 20 years) at recruitment [14]. Periconceptional supplementation can provide iron and folic acid in early gestation and prolong the period available for repletion of iron stores before delivery [15]. This was the first periconceptional RCT to recruit nulliparous, mainly adolescent participants, as a high pregnancy rate is more easily achieved by recruiting older, parous women [16]. In our study, field workers (FW) visited homes weekly to deliver weekly iron and folic acid (intervention) or folic acid alone (control). Field records showed varied adherence patterns, with some adolescents periodically absent for "travel," and others regularly not at home for the arranged weekly visit. The purpose of this qualitative study was to interview participants with varied adherence characteristics in order to better understand factors affecting regular consumption of supplements and encourage adherence.

Plain English summary

Non-pregnant adolescent girls were followed in an iron and folic acid supplementation trial in rural Burkina Faso, aiming to improve iron stores of young women before their first pregnancy. Families were reliant on subsistence activities, school attendance was low and nutritional status poor. Taking iron supplements regularly is important for improving iron status, but girls were often absent from home at weekly visits when tablets were given. This qualitative study was done to establish why tablets were being missed and to try to encourage adherence. We interviewed 39 young women, with good, medium and poor adherence levels, some of whom had become pregnant during the 18 month supplementation period. Adolescents required approval from male relatives to join the study. Interviews established that many families thought girls were receiving contraceptive pills, which would be generally unacceptable for cultural reasons. Since free treatment was available in the trial, approvals were largely given although most were not allowed to admit they were taking part. Families relied on adolescent domestic labour, and unmarried girls could be sent to work outside the study area, interrupting the iron schedule for indefinite periods. If becoming pregnant before marriage they were also sent away in disgrace. Once married, husbands wanted wives to become pregnant quickly and often stopped the supplements. Adolescents did not relate to the health message that taking iron would benefit a future pregnancy. Maintaining adherence to iron supplements, especially among non-school attenders is operationally challenging and dependent on communities realising benefits from adolescent health interventions.

Methods
Background

As giving iron potentially increases malaria and risk of other infections, the RCT assessed the safety and efficacy of iron supplementation of nulliparous women living in a malaria endemic area. In Burkina Faso 52% of young women are married by the age of 18 and 27% have given birth [17]. The population was rural, traditional, predominantly of Mossi tribal origin and reliant on subsistence farming and cattle husbandry. The literacy rate was low in both men and women (~ 23%). Recruitment took place between April 2011 and June 2012 in 30 study villages in the Districts of Nanoro and Yako belonging to the Health and Demographic Surveillance System [18], situated 85 km from Ouagadougou, the capital city. Health care was provided by twelve peripheral health centres and one referral hospital. All healthy, non-pregnant women aged 15–24 years living in these villages were invited to participate. Age and nulliparity were determined at the pre-screening stage. Women with predefined medical conditions were excluded at recruitment by the medical team, as were women with obvious pregnancies, or no menses in the previous three months. Participants ($n = 1959$) were allocated to receive weekly either 60 mg iron and 2.8 mg folic acid (intervention arm) or 2.8 mg folic acid (control arm). Women who remained non-pregnant continued to receive supplements at weekly visits from field workers for18 months, ie up to end assessment. Those who became pregnant continued weekly supplements until their first scheduled antenatal visit (trial primary endpoint at 13–18 weeks gestation), after which routine daily iron and folic acid was provided. In Burkina Faso antenatal care is free. Women attended a second study visit at 33–36 weeks gestation and were followed until delivery. As a safety trial, it was considered unethical to provide no treatment for illness reported at weekly visits and free treatment was made available.

The National Institutes of Health (NIH) funded this trial as part of a competitive grant call on safety of iron supplementation. NIH played no roles in the conduct or analysis of the study. The research was approved by the national Ethical Committee for Health Research and the Institutional Ethical Committee of Centre Muraz in Burkina Faso, and the Ethical Committees of the Liverpool School of Tropical Medicine, United Kingdom, the University of Antwerp, Belgium and the University of Manchester.

Prior to enrolment the study team visited each village to inform elders and obtain agreement for young women to take part. Thereafter FWs went to each eligible compound to answer questions, emphasising benefits of iron and folic acid for a future pregnancy. At enrolment written consent was given for unmarried participants by parents/guardian or nominated senior women. Individuals also gave their own written consent (or thumb mark) and indicated willingness to be contacted for a future interview. Mean age of participants was 16.8 ± 1.7 years. Median adherence (number of directly observed treatments as a percentage of the number of weeks participating) was 79% (Interquartile range 58%–90%, $n = 1954$), with no difference by trial arm [14].

Qualitative interviews

Selection was based on adherence level, calculated from weekly FW records. Adherence was classified broadly as "good" (> 50 weekly supplements consumed), "medium" (25–50) or "poor" (< 25), taking into account length of trial participation. The target number of interviews was 15 per category, provided this allowed for data saturation and for inclusion of participants of varying age, marital status and education level. A FW initially contacted participants to arrange an interview with AC, who was known in the villages, having previously conducted focus groups to elicit community views on iron and anaemia [19]. AC explained that the interview was to explore what participants thought of the trial and what had influenced their adherence to supplements. Women generally agreed to be interviewed but if not, an alternative participant with similar characteristics and adherence level was approached. Individual written consent was obtained before each interview.

Most interviews were conducted in Mooré, the local language, in the village or at study headquarters in Nanoro. Individuals were asked to describe their circumstances and expectations of the study. The theoretical perspective was interpretive and derived from Symbolic Interactionism [20] and Identity Theory [21]. The premise was that individual choices (ie taking iron) reflected the several roles individuals fulfilled, albeit choice was constrained by societal and cultural norms and could change over the life course as individuals become tied to their role positions [22]. Interviews were recorded with permission, transcribed into French, which was checked (SG) and then sent to the external collaborator (LB). She advised on subsequent interviews and assessed when interviews yielded no new insights. LB and AC coded the transcripts separately by hand, forming the basis for a field visit, at which emerging themes were agreed. Interviews were analysed without knowledge of trial arm. Additional file S1 provides additional verbatim quotations to support the thematic analysis.

Results

Interviews were conducted with 39 young women, with one exclusion. Table 1 describes their socio-demographic characteristics and adherence categories. Factors affecting adherence were:

Dissatisfaction with taking tablets

Though few side effects were reported, body aches and fever attributed to supplements by ID 38 (poor adherence), which were more suggestive of malaria (for which she was treated) led to her dropping out of the trial. ID 19 (poor adherence) complained of itching, yet when pregnant, took antenatal daily iron with no apparent side effects. ID 17 (medium adherence) refused supplements at menses, saying it caused stomach cramps. Nausea was a problem for ID 15 (good adherence). With a few exceptions (Additional file 1, point a), the intrusiveness of weekly visits was tolerated although participants disliked delays when a FW made several visits in the same compound. Most dissatisfaction was expressed by ID 31 (medium adherence) who complained about the system for reimbursement of health care expenses, her follow-up when she married and moved village, discontinuation of weekly iron supplements when she became pregnant and switched to daily iron as part of routine antenatal care, and her husband's grievance that the FW did not greet him when she visited.

Mobility

Periodic absences disrupted adherence. The low level of education (Table 1) meant that respondents mainly attended to domestic chores and/or petty trading. Whereas young men frequently migrated to work in

Table 1 Socio-demographic characteristics and indicative level of adherence to supplements

N°	Current Age[a]	School Grade[b]	Occupation	Marital Status	Delivered Yes/No	Adhesion Level
1	18	4th Secondary	Student	Single	No	Good
2	18	4th Secondary	Student	Single	No	Medium
3	17	5th Secondary	None	Single	No	Medium
4	17	No Education	Petty Trade	Single	No	Good
5	17	No Education	Petty Trade	Single	No	Good
6	17	No Education	None	Single	No	Medium
7	21	6th Primary	None	Married	No	Medium
8	23	No Education	Petty Trade	Married	No	Medium
9	17	3rd Primary	Sewing	Single	No	Good
10	19	No Education	Sewing	Single	No	Good
11	20	No Education	None	Married	No	Poor
12	20	No Education	None	Married	No	Poor
13	16	No Education	None	Single	No	Poor
14	Excluded [c]					
15	23	6th Primary	None	Single	No	Good
16	20	2nd Primary	None	Single	No	Good
17	19	6th Primary	None	Single	No	Medium
18	21	3rd Secondary	Student	Single	No	Good
19	19	No Education	None	Married	Yes	Poor
20	21	2nd Secondary	Student	Single	No	Poor
21	17	No Education	None	Single	No	Poor
22	19	No Education	Petty Trade	Married	No	Good
23	16	No Education	None	Single	No	Medium
24	18	4th Secondary	Student	Single	No	Good
25	18	4th Secondary	Student	Single	No	Medium
26	16	No Education	None	Single	No	Good
27	19	No Education	None	Married	Yes	Poor
28	18	No Education	None	Single	No	Medium
29	18	No Education	None	Married	No	Good
30	16	No Education	None	Single	No	Poor
31	22	3rd Secondary	None	Married	Pregnant	Medium
32	18	No Education	None	Married	Yes	Medium
33	18	5th Secondary	Student	Single	No	Good
34	22	No Education	None	Single	No	Poor
35	17	3rd Secondary	None	Single	Yes	Poor
36	24	6th Secondary	Dressmaker	Single	Pregnant	Medium
37	18	No Education	None	Single	No	Poor
38	17	No Education	None	Single	No	Poor
39	16	5th Secondary	Student	Single	No	Good

[a]Reported age at time of interview, between 1 and 2 years after enrolment and commencement of supplementation
[b]Grade attained. French educational system: 6th grade denotes the first grade of Lower Secondary School. Entry into the 2nd (Upper Secondary) grade requires acquisition of Junior Secondary Education Certificate. Primary classes progress in ascending order
[c]Data from this participant was later rejected due to an RCT protocol violation

Côte d'Ivoire, girls were generally needed at home. ID 21 (poor adherence) was first sent to Côte d'Ivoire to care for her uncle's children but had returned to the village. Families living in Côte d'Ivoire tended to send daughters back to stay with the father's brother. ID 31 (medium adherence) herded cattle and looked after the younger children. Some were sent for domestic work elsewhere within Burkina Faso, and not always in accord with their own wishes. ID 28 (medium adherence) asked to visit her siblings in Côte d'Ivoire or Bobo-Dioulasso but instead was dispatched to the capital, Ouagadougou, to help her paternal uncle. She was recalled after two months to assist her grandmother. ID 34 (poor adherence) was in Bobo-Dioulasso for over a year, caring for her paternal grandfather. After returning from Ivory Coast and joining the study, ID 21 (poor adherence), still aged only 17 years, was sent to Ouagadougou for domestic work, returning home for the harvest season to work in the fields. ID 16 (good adherence), who was absent for two months while staying with her uncle in Ouagadougou, was also recalled, even though she wanted to stay in town where she had fewer chores and more young people for company.

Reliance on older daughters for domestic help probably accounted for the low level of schooling. ID 4 (good adherence) was living in a large household with her paternal uncle because her father was dead and her mother was absent. She has never been sent to school although younger girls in the compound attended. ID 3 (medium adherence) had been obliged to leave school, going to stay with her mother and aunt in Bobo-Dioulasso for five months to sell clothes on the market. She said she disliked housework, did not want to marry but if she did, would choose her own husband. ID 37 (poor adherence) was fearful of the uncle, became anxious when appearing to be idle, and did not attend the health centre when referred by the FW.

School attenders were apt to be mobile in school holidays, when they missed supplements. If they attended high schools in Nanoro and came back to study villages, they could be traced by FWs (eg ID 2 medium adherence), but not if they went elsewhere. Young women who had married into the study area periodically returned to their home villages (eg, ID 8 medium adherence) but generally did not stay for extended periods unless separating from a husband (eg, ID 11, poor adherence). Participants seemed unconcerned about missing doses and often did not inform the FW in advance of an intended move. When asked about her two months absence ID 28 (medium adherence) said,

No, I wasn't worried. When I returned I just continued taking it.

Individual and community interpretations of the purpose of iron supplementation

The purpose of giving iron supplements as described in briefings and information sheets was not recalled by most interviewees. There were some exceptions. ID 9 (good adherence) was literate, with a brother in University. She, together with her father and brother had read the information sheets and knew the supplements were iron and intended to improve the blood. ID 7 (medium adherence), ID 3 (medium adherence), ID 18 (good adherence), ID 25 (medium adherence) and ID 24 (good adherence) who were literate and/or current students (albeit older and struggling to get good grades) were also better informed. The community could not understand why men were not included or why female participants were nulliparous. It was stated by everyone that the trial was for "*young girls*" and excluded "*women.*"

Int: Tell me what women's illnesses you have already had.

P: I don't belong to the category of women.

Int: What's that?

P: I'm not a woman. I don't know.

Int: You don't belong with the women? You belong with the men?

P: No, I am a young girl. (ID 34 poor adherence).

The community initially believed that weekly supplements were contraceptives because iron tablets were strongly associated with pregnancy and antenatal care. This probably explains why, almost without exception, interviewees insisted they never discussed taking part in the trial with anyone – family or friends (Additional file 1, point b). Allowing "*young girls*" to join a trial providing contraception would be controversial so individuals did not readily admit to participation. Thus:

P: The young men say it is birth spacing medicine.

Int: And what do you say?

P: We are silent.

(ID 39 good adherence)

Given this interpretation, why did the community allow "*young girls*" to enrol in the trial?

– Free health care

Whether married or unmarried, young women needed male permission to enrol. Fathers/guardians knew the study provided a bed net and free treatment (Additional file 1, point c) and they sometimes overruled reluctant daughters. A husband's permission was required when young women married during the trial. Despite free treatment, new husbands wanted their wives to become pregnant and, hearing rumours about contraception, often demurred. ID11 (poor adherence) had married without telling her husband she was enrolled. She was lost to follow-up after marriage but, having left her husband, she requested to rejoin.

– Avoidance of unwanted pregnancy

Unmarried girls who became pregnant represented a community problem and were described as "spoilt." ID 35 (poor adherence), unmarried, became pregnant, was obliged to leave school and was working in her brother's shop to earn money. ID 27 (poor adherence) kept her pregnancy secret for as long as possible but eventually fled to the father's village (contrary to custom), delivered with a traditional attendant and planned to join her "husband" in Côte d'Ivoire.

– Infertility

Three married interviewees with infertility problems were motivated to take supplements associated with pregnancy. ID 29 (good adherence) had been married for three years with no child and her husband had taken a younger wife. He had not objected to her joining the trial, perhaps viewing the contraceptive issue as irrelevant in her case. She became pregnant and attributed her success to the supplement. ID 8 (medium adherence) and ID 7 (medium adherence) did not conceive and were disappointed.

Opinions on the value of supplementation
Whatever their expectations from the study, and the value accorded to free treatment, very few young women attributed any health benefit to the supplements (iron or folic acid) a themselves (Additional file 1, point d).

Discussion
Qualitative interviews showed that as "young girls" transitioned to adult women, changing roles and responsibilities often interrupted adherence to iron supplements. Had FWs not been assiduous in tracking participants and negotiating return to the trial, uptake would have been much lower. Adherence was boosted by free medical treatment, whereas the health promotion goal of building iron stores before pregnancy did not enthuse adolescents or communities.

This was the first large community iron supplementation trial of nulliparous young women living in a marginalised rural area. Adherence was closely monitored and qualitative interviews enabled us to interpret observed adherence patterns and explain periodic absences. In rural areas unmarried adolescent girls are an important source of domestic and agricultural labour, but it is difficult to establish whether such changes in residence constitute work or kin fostering [23]. Adolescents can be sent to relatives and strangers, move outside their villages, even between countries. Regionally, families migrate for work and tend to send adolescent girls home [24]. Relocation decisions are usually made by a father or a mother's brother, often following a critical event such as divorce, when a single parent or new wife, cannot or does not want to cope with a daughter from a previous marriage [25, 26]. Girls reported to us that such moves did not reflect their preferences, and conditions were variable, with the receiving household determining access to health or other benefits. Schooling, unplanned pregnancy and marriage put a brake on mobility. Most girls wanted to go to school yet, when the study was conducted, Burkina Faso had a female literacy rate for 15–24 year olds of 33.1% [27], with just 15.6% of girls in secondary education. Only in 2008 was the minimum age for admission into remunerated employment raised from 14 to16 years in support of obligatory education [28]. Domestic labour and education were catastrophically disrupted by an unplanned pregnancy [29] and, though we could not ascertain their number, many were suspected in cases lost to follow-up. Tradition dictated sending an unmarried pregnant girl away, ideally to a father's sister. Overtures for reconciliation started after the birth but paternal insistence on an alternative marriage alliance caused family breakdown. Parental control of a daughter's labour ceased at marriage and the mobility of married Burkinabè adolescents is highly restricted to prevent them running away [30]. Marriage often signalled a negative change in iron adherence.

The rationale for the safety trial was growing evidence that iron supplementation increases malaria infection risk so treatment had to be readily available for safety reasons. Access to health care was valued by adolescents but families may have pushed some girls to participate which could explain some negative attitudes towards the intervention [31]. The research team had not foreseen that supplements would be mistaken for contraceptives. Earlier focus groups indicated only that the function and elemental composition of iron were not well understood and anaemia was not regarded as an adolescent problem [19]. The community struggled with the rationale of giving iron to "young girls" in preparation for pregnancy as iron tablets were a recognised component of antenatal care. The concept of a health intervention to improve adolescent health in its own right has also to be established [32]. As in a school-based study in Dar-es-Salaam, iron supplements were assumed to be contraceptives [11]. In Tanzania this led to study withdrawals, yet enrolment was high in our trial, suggesting that some girls and families were not averse to contraception, even though it could not be discussed or admitted. AC possibly misread frequent silences, as interviewing adolescents, especially when illiterate and economically vulnerable, was challenging. Once aware, the research team did address this misconception and since many adolescents subsequently became pregnant, the notion was dispelled. This may have negatively affected adolescent interest in the supplements.

Conclusions

The 2030 Agenda for Sustainable Development cannot be met without investment in adolescent health and well-being [33]. Improving nutritional status is an important goal still to be achieved but, if iron supplementation of menstruating girls is perceived to be non-essential, it may be frustrated [34]. Recommended approaches to encourage uptake include strong communication components [11], counselling [35], social marketing with peer educators [36] and integrated adolescent health packages [37]. The evidence base for marginalized and non-school attending populations is lacking [7] as is the evidence for tailored and context-specific nutritional interventions [38]. Integrating prevention of iron deficiency and anaemia with other adolescent interventions may be preferable to stand-alone iron supplementation programmes. Our findings are encouraging in so far as they indicate that delivery of iron supplements as part of a pregnancy prevention strategy may not necessarily meet with parental opposition, if deemed to benefit the wider community. The iron regime (daily or intermittent, length, etc) will need to take account of the specific circumstances likely to interrupt adolescent adherence in each cultural setting, especially among girls who do not progress through secondary education. To ensure improved iron status, the regime must be delivered and adhered to, in line with the recommended guidelines.

Abbreviations

FW: Field Worker; INT: Interviewer; P: Participant; RCT: Randomised Controlled Trial

Acknowledgements

We gratefully acknowledge: the contribution and support of participating women, local communities, in the memory of his Majesty Naaba Tigré of Nanoro, study teams, including Blaise Kientaga, female field assistants, nurses, midwives, supervisors and doctors.

Funding

This work was supported by the National Institutes of Health (Grant Number U01HD061234-01A1; Supplementary -05S1 and -02S2), the National Institute of Child Health and Human Development, and the National Institutes of Health Office of Dietary Supplements. The funder played no role in the conduct or writing up of the study.

Authors' contributions

All authors (LB, AC, SG, TH, BB) contributed to the design of the study and writing of the manuscript. SG ran the trial in the field and AC conducted the qualitative interviews. LB and AC analysed the qualitative data; LB wrote the first draft. All authors assert ownership of, and responsibility for, the manuscript.

Ethics approval and consent to participate

The protocol was approved by the Liverpool School of Tropical Medicine, UK, Research Ethics Committee (LSTM/REC Research Protocol 10.55), the Institutional Review Board of the Institute of Tropical Medicine, Antwerp, Belgium (Reference IRB/AB/AC/016), the Antwerp University Hospital Ethics Committee (EC/UZA), the Institutional Ethics Committee of Centre Muraz (Comité d'Ethique Institutionnel du Centre Muraz, Reference 015–2010/CE-CM); the National Ethics Committee (Comité Ethique pour la Recherche en Santé, CERS) in Burkina Faso and the University of Manchester Ethics Committee. The study was performed in full compliance with the Declaration of Helsinki on human studies. The protocol summary (10PRT/6932) is available at http://www.thelancet.com

All subjects gave written informed consent in accordance with the Declaration of Helsinki. Individual and guardian written consents for minors were obtained from all non-pregnant women at recruitment with re-consent taken at entry to the pregnancy cohort.

Competing interests

The authors declare that they have no competing interest.

Author details

[1]Clinical Research Unit Nanoro, Institut de Recherche en Sciences de la, Santé, Direction Régionale du Centre-Ouest, Nanoro, Burkina Faso. [2]Department of Biomedical Sciences, Prince Leopold Institute of Tropical Medicine, Antwerp, Belgium. [3]Present address: Medical Mission Institute, Würzburg, Germany. [4]Liverpool School of Tropical Medicine and Institute of Infection and Global Health, University of Liverpool, Liverpool, United Kingdom; Global Child Health Group, Academic Medical Centre, University of Amsterdam, Amsterdam, The Netherlands. [5]Division of Cancer Sciences, Faculty of Biology, Medicine and Health, University of Manchester, Manchester, UK.

References

1. Thurnham DI. Nutrition of adolescent girls in low and middle income countries. Sight & Life. 2013;27:26–36.
2. World Health Organisation Worldwide Prevalence of Anaemia 1993-2005. In: de Benoist B, McLean E, Egli I, Cogswell M, editors. WHO Global Data Base on Anaemia. Geneva: World Health Orgnaisation; 2008.
3. Fernández-Gaxiola AC, De-Regil LM. Intermittent iron supplementation for reducing anaemia and its associated impairments in menstruating women. Cochrane Database Syst Rev. 2011;(Issue 12. Art. No: CD009218) https://doi.org/10.1002/14651858.CD009218.pub2.
4. Titaley CR, Dibley MJ. Factors associated with not using antenatal iron/folic acid supplements in Indonesia in the 2002/2003 and 2007 Indonesian demographic and health surveys. Asia Pac J Clin Nutr. 2015;24:162–76.
5. Galloway R, Dusch E, Elder L, Achadi E, Grajeda RHE, et al. Women's perceptions of iron deficiency and anemia prevention and control in eight developing countries. Soc Sci Med. 2002;55:529–44.

6. Nagata JM, Gatti LR, Barg FK. Social determinants of iron supplementation among women of reproductive age: a systematic review of qualitative data. Mat Child Nutr. 2012;8:1–18.

7. Denno DM, Hoopes AJ, Chandra-Mouli V. Effective strategies to provide adolescent sexual and reproductive health services and to increase demand and community support. J Adolesc Health. 2015;56:S22–41.

8. Zavaleta N, Respicio G, Garcia T. Efficacy and acceptability of two iron supplementation schedules in adolescent school girls in Lima. Peru J Nutr. 2000;130:462S–4S.

9. Shah BK, Gupta P. Weekly vs daily iron and folic acid supplementation in adolescent Nepalese girls. Arch Peds & Adolesc Med. 2002;156:131–5.

10. Agarwal KN, Gomber S, Bisht H, Som M. Anemia prophylaxis in adolescent school girls by weekly or daily iron-folate supplementation. Ind Pediatr. 2003;40:296–301.

11. Muro GS, Gross U, Gross R, Wahyuniar L. Increase in compliance with weekly iron supplementation of adolescent girls by an accompanying communication programme in secondary schools in Dar-es-salaam, Tanzania. Food Nutr Bull. 1999;20:435–44.

12. Salam RA, Hooda M, Das JK, Arshad A, Lassi ZS, Middleton P, et al. Interventions to improve adolescent nutrition: a systematic review and meta-analysis. J Adolsc Health. 2016;59:S29–39.

13. Low MSY, Speedy J, Styles CE, De-Regil LM, Pasricha SR. Daily iron supplementation for improving anaemia, iron status and health in menstruating women (review). Cochrane Database Systematic Reviews. 2016;(April 18, Issue 4. Art. No: CD00974736):608–24.

14. Brabin L, Roberts S, Gies S, Nelson A, Diallou S, Stewart CL, et al. Effects of long-term weekly iron and folic acid supplementation on lower genital tract infection – a double blind, randomized controlled trial in Burkina Faso. BMC Med. 2017;15(1):206. https://doi.org/10.1186/s12916-017-0967-5.

15. Lynch SR. The potential impact of iron supplementation during adolescence on iron status in pregnancy. J Nutr. 2000;30:448S–51S.

16. Brabin BJ, Gies S, Owens S, Claeys Y, D'Alessandro U, Tinto H, et al. Perspectives on the design and methodology of periconceptional nutrient supplementation trials. Trials. 2016;17:58.

17. Gal-Régniez A, Guiella G, Ouédraogo C, Woog V, Bassonon D, Singh S, et al. Protéger la prochaine génération au Burkina Faso: Nouvelle évidence sur les besoins de santé sexuelle et reproductive des adolescents. Report November. New York: Guttmacher Institute; 2007.

18. Derra K, Rouamba E, Kazienga A, Ouedraogo S, Tahita MC, Sorgho H, et al. Profile: Nanoro health and demographic surveillance system. Int J Epidemiol. 2012;41:1293–301.

19. Compaoré A, Gies S, Brabin BJ, Tinto H, Brabin L. "There is iron and iron…" Burkinabè women's perceptions of iron supplementation: a qualitative study. Matern Child Health J. 2014; Aug; DOI 10, 1007/s10995-014-1443-x

20. Mead GH. Mind, self, and society. Chicago: University of Chicago Press; 1934.

21. Stryker S, Statham A. "symbolic interaction and role theory." pp. 311–78 in handbook of social psychology, edited by G Lindzey and E Aronson. New York: Random House; 1985.

22. Stryker S, Burke PJ. The past, present and future of the identity theory. Soc Psychol Quart. 2000;63:284–97.

23. Thorsen D. Les enfants travailleurs domestiques : résultats d'une étude menée en Afrique de l'Ouest et centrale. UNICEF. 2012; https://www.unicef.org/wcaro/french/4494_7083.html.

24. Beauchemin C. Rural-urban migration in West Africa: towards a reversal? Migration trends and economic situation in Burkina Faso and Côte d'Ivoire. Popul Space Place. 2011;17:47–72.

25. Riisøen KH, Hatløy A, Bjerkan L. Travel to uncertainty. A study of child relocation in Burkina Faso, Ghana and Mali. FAFO Report 440. Oslo: Fafo Institute for Applied International Studies; 2004.

26. West CT. Domestic transitions, desiccation, agricultural intensification, and livelihood diversification among rural households on the central plateau. Burkina Faso Am Anthrop. 2009;111:275–88.

27. UNICEF. Statistics, Burkina Faso, provided at https://www.unicef.org/infobycountry/burkinafaso_statistics.html.

28. Ansell N. Children, youth and development. London and New York: Routledge; 2005.

29. Gorgen R, Maier B, Diesfeld HJ. Problems related to schoolgirl pregnancies in Burkina Faso. Stud fam. Planning. 1993;24:283–94.

30. Brady M, Saloucou L, Chong E. Girls' adolescence in Burkina Faso. A pivot point for social change: Pop Council, Ougadougou, Burkina Faso; 2007.

31. Paré Toe L, Ravinetto RM, Dierick S, Gryseels C, Tinto H, Rouamba N, et al. Could the decision of trial participation precede the informed consent process? Evidence from Burkina Faso. PLoS One. 2013;8(11) https://doi.org/10.1371/journal.pone.0080800.

32. Mason E, Chandra-Mouli V, Baltag V, Christiansen C, Lassi ZS, Bhutta ZA. Preconception care: advancing from "important to do and can be done" to "is being done and is making a difference". Rep Health. 2014;11(Suppl3):S8.

33. Global Accelerated Action for the Health of Adolescents (AA-HA!). Guidance to support country implementation. Summary. Geneva: World Health Organization; 2017. (WHO/FWC/MCA/17.05). Licence: CC BY-NC-SA 3.0 IGO

34. World Health Organisation. Guidelines. Daily iron supplementation of adult women and adolescent girls. 2016. ISBN 978 92 4 151019 6.

35. Vir SC, Singh N, Nigam AK, Jain R. Weekly iron and folic acid supplementation with counseling reduces anemia in adolescent girls: a large-scale effectiveness study in Uttar Pradesh, India. Food Nutr Bull. 2008; 29:186–94.

36. Berger J, Thanh HT, Cavalli-Sforza T, Smitasiri S, Khan NC, Milani S, et al. Community mobilization and social marketing to promote weekly iron-folic acid supplementation in women of reproductive age in Vietnam: impact on anemia and iron status. Nutr Rev. 2005;63:S95–S108.

37. Chandra-Mouli V, Williamson NE, Hainsworth G, McCarraher DR, Phillips SJ. Contraception for adolescents in low and middle income countries: needs, barriers, and access. Rep Health. 2014;11:1. http://www.reproductive-health-journal.com/content/11/S1/S1.

38. Johnson W, Moore SE. Adolescent pregnancy, nutrition, and health outcomes in low and middle income countries: what we know and what we don't know. BJOG. 2016;123:1589–92.

Comprehensive knowledge on cervical cancer, attitude towards its screening and associated factors among women aged 30–49 years

Alehegn Bishaw Geremew[1*], Abebaw Addis Gelagay[1] and Telake Azale[2]

Abstract

Background: Screening services for cervical pre-cancerous lesions is currently available for all women aged 30–49 years at public hospitals in Ethiopia. Though women's knowledge and their attitude are determinants for the uptake the screening service, there is limited information on these regards. Therefore, this study aimed to assess comprehensive knowledge on cervical cancer, attitudes towards the screening, and associated factors among women aged 30–49 years at Finote Selam town, northwest Ethiopia.

Methods: A community based cross-sectional study was conducted from March 30, to April 15, 2017. The sample size calculated for this study was 1224 and a cluster sampling technique was used to select the participants from three randomly selected kebeles. Epi-Info version 7 and Statistical Package for Social Sciences version 20 were used for data entry and analysis respectively. A binary logistic regression model was used. In multivariable logistic analysis, adjusted odds ratio with a 95% confidence interval was used to determine the presence and strength of associations between covariate and outcome variable.

Results: A total of 1137 women participated in this study. Nearly one third, 30.3% (95%CI: 27.7, 32.9) of the women had knowledge of cervical cancer, and 58.1% (95% CI: 55, 62.2) had a favorable attitude towards cervical cancer screening. In the multivariable analysis, having college and above education (AOR = 7.21, 95%CI: 3.41, 15.29), knowing someone with cervical cancer (AOR =5.38, 95%CI: 2.38, 12.15), and having a history of sexually transmitted diseases (AOR = 2.75, 95%CI: 1.24, 6.04) were significantly associated with knowledge on cervical cancer. Meanwhile, college and above educational status (AOR = 2.56, 95%CI: 1.14, 5.69), knowing someone with cervical cancer (AOR = 3.24, 95%CI: 1.14, 9.15), and having knowledge of cervical cancer (AOR = 3, 95%CI: 1.97, 4.29) were positively associated with favorable attitudes towards cervical cancer screening.

Conclusion: The proportion of women who had knowledge on cervical cancer was low where as relatively, a large proportion of the study participants in this study had favorable attitude towards cervical cancer screening. Educational status, knowing someone with cervical cancer, a history of sexually transmitted diseases was factors affecting both women's knowledge and their attitude. Having knowledge on cervical cancer was factor affecting attitude towards screening services. Provision of information, education, and counseling about the disease and screening service are mandatory to address their knowledge gap and to improve women's attitude towards screening service.

Keywords: Women aged 30–49 years, Knowledge, Attitude, Ethiopia

* Correspondence: alexbishaw@gmail.com
[1]Department of Reproductive Health, Institute of Public Health, College of Medicine and Health Science, University of Gondar, 196 Gondar, Ethiopia
Full list of author information is available at the end of the article

Plain English summary

Screening services for cervical pre-cancerous lesions are currently available for all women aged 30–49 years at public hospitals in Ethiopia. Though women's knowledge and their attitude are determinants for the uptake the screening service, there is limited information on these. Therefore, this study aimed to assess the comprehensive knowledge of cervical cancer, attitudes towards the screening, and associated factors among women aged 30–49 years at Finote Selam town, northwest Ethiopia.

A total of 1137 women participated in this study. Nearly one third, 30.3% of the women had comprehensive knowledge on cervical cancer, and 58.1% had a favorable attitude towards cervical cancer screening. Having college and above education, knowing someone with cervical cancer, and having a history of sexually transmitted diseases were significantly associated with comprehensive knowledge of cervical cancer. Meanwhile, college and above educational status, knowing someone with cervical cancer, and having comprehensive knowledge of cervical cancer were positively associated with favorable attitude towards cervical cancer screening. Therefore we recommended that provision of information, education, and counseling about the disease and screening service are mandatory to address the knowledge gap and to improve women's attitude towards screening services.

Background

Despite the fact that cervical cancer is preventable, it is reported that there were 485,000 cervical cancer cases and 236,000 deaths of women due to cervical cancer in 2013 worldwide [1]. Almost 87% of the deaths occurred in less developed regions, it was the second most commonly diagnosed cancer and the third leading cause of cancer death among females in less developed countries [2].

East Africa has the highest sub- regional incidence of cervical cancer in which the age standardised rate is 42.7 per 100,000 women, followed by Southern Africa with 31.5 per 100,000 women [3]. In Ethiopia, an estimated 7095 new cervical cancer cases were diagnosed, and 4732 die annually from it in 2012 [4]. New cases of cancer were diagnosed in the Black Lion specialized Hospital data set between 1997 and 2012, and the result revealed that 31.8% were cervical cancer patients [5].

The large geographic variations in cervical cancer rates reflect the presence of differences in the accessibility of screening service because the presence of screening service detects precancerous lesion and helps early initiation of treatment of the lesion before it progresses to cancer stage [6]. A population survey indicates the average cervical cancer screening in developing countries is 19%while it is 63% in developed countries and ranging from 1% to 73%respectively [7]. A meta-analysis noted that the risk of dying from cervical cancer was 35% lower among women invited to screening with cytology testing than among women who were not offered screening services [8].

Having knowledge on cervical cancer and it's screening is associated with the uptake of services [9], favourable attitudes towards cervical cancer screening is also associated with the uptake of screening services [10, 11]. Cervical cancer screening helps to detect pre-cancerous lesions before it advances to a cancerous stage which in turn reduces its related mortality rates. In Ethiopia, screening services for cervical pre-cancerous lesion is available for all women aged 30–49 years at public health institutions [12]. Women's knowledge on cervical cancer and their attitude for screening determine the uptake of service [13]. However, evidence on women's knowledge of cervical cancer and their attitude towards screening at the community level is very limited in Ethiopia. Therefore, a community based study was conducted to assess knowledge of cervical cancer, attitude towards its screening and associated factors among women aged 30–49 years at Finote Selam town, northwest Ethiopia.

Methods
Study design and setting

A community based cross-sectional study was conducted from March 30, to April 15, 2017 at Finote Selam town, northwest Ethiopia. Finote Selam town is located in West Gojam Administration Zone of the Amhara Regional State, northwest Ethiopia. According to the population projection of Ethiopia for all regions at woreda level 2017, the total population of the town is estimated to be 38,399. Out of these, 19,923 are male and 18,476 female [14]. At the moment, the town has five kebeles, the smallest administrative units. The total number of households was 5530.

Finote Selam town has one primary hospital, one public health centre, and four private clinics. Since April 2016, cervical cancer screening service and treatment for pre cervical lesion has been offered to women aged 30 to 49 years. For this study, all women aged 30–49 years living in Finote Selam town were the source population.

Sample size and sampling procedure

The sample size was determined using single population proportion formula ($n = (Z\acute{\alpha}/2)^2 p (1-p)/d^2$) with the following assumptions: 44.6% proportion of sufficient knowledge on cervical cancer, and 42.1% favourable attitude towards screening on the bases of a previous study done in Dessie, Ethiopia [11], A 95% level of confidence, 5 and 4% degree of precision for knowledge, and attitude respectively, two design effect, and 5% none response rate were used. The sample sizes calculated were 797 and 1224 for knowledge and attitude, respectively. Sample size was also calculated for factors using EPI info version

7 considering a 95% level of confidence, and 80% power. However, the sample size for factors were found less than the sample size calculated for the outcome variables (knowledge and attitude). So, we considered 1224 as sample size for this study.

Operational definitions

Having comprehensive knowledge on cervical cancer

Refers to women who answered mean value and above of the twenty knowledge questions [15].

Favourable attitude towards cervical cancer screening

refers to women who answered mean and above of the six attitude questions Six attitude questions were used with five likert scale measurement: strongly disagree, disagree, neither agree nor disagree, agree, and strongly agree. A woman who scored mean value and above was considered as having a favourable attitude.

Data collection instrument and process

The data collection tool (questionnaire) was developed by reviewing literature [11, 15–17]. The questionnaire was first prepared in English and translated to Amharic then back to English to ensure consistency. The questionnaire carried socio-demographic characteristics, risk of exposure to cervical cancer and reproductive health service utilization, knowledge and attitude assessing questions. The attitude questions were developed using a five level likert scale. Six female diploma and two BSc degree graduated midwives were recruited for data collection, and supervision, respectively. Face-to-face interviewer administered questionnaire was used.

To ensure data quality, a two day training was given to data collectors and supervisors. The questionnaire was pre-tested on 42 women who were living outside the selected kebeles to check the response, the clarity, and the appropriateness of the questions. The data collection and supervision were overseen by researchers to ensure completeness and consistency of data.

Data analysis

The data were checked for completeness, coded manually, and entered into EPI-info version 7 and transferred to SPSS version 20 for analysis. Descriptive statistics were expressed in numerical value, mean, standard deviation, and percentages. Both bivariate and multivariable logistic regression analyses were done to identify variables associated with knowledge on cervical cancer, and attitude towards screening.Variables with less than 0.2 P-value, in the bivariate analysis were entered into multivariable analysis to control potential confounders. Hosmer-Lemeshow goodness of fit test was used to check the model fitness. Adjusted odds ratio with 95% confidence interval was used to determine the presence, degree, and direction of association between covariates and the outcome variable.

Results

Socio demographic characteristics participants

A total of 1137 women participated in this study giving a response rate of 93.7%. Ten questionnaires were incomplete. The mean age of the participants was 37.4 years (SD $\pm$ 5.72 years). The majority (92.2%) of study participants were Orthodox Christians, two-thirds (66.4%) of the women were married, and nearly half 513(45.1%) had no formal education. Out of the total participants, 530(46.6%) reported that their main occupation was household activities. One quarter (24.5%) of the participants had less than 23 US$ family average monthly income, and 37.7% had more than 68 US $ (Table 1).

Women's risk of exposure and reproductive health services utilization

More than half of the women, 615 (54.1%), had the first sexual intercourse at the age of 16 or below. The mean age of the first sexual intercourse of the women was 16.4 years (SD $\pm$ 3.29 years). More than two-thirds of participants, 788(69.3%), had two or more sexual partners in their life time. One thousand sixteen (89.4%) women had history of at least one pregnancy and 1002 (88%) history of at least one child birth. Among women who had history of pregnancy, 579 (57%) had antenatal follow up during their last pregnancy. Out of the total participants 163(14.3%) had at least one history of abortion in their life time. Approximately three-fourths of the women, 830(73%) used modern contraceptive in their life time, and 14.6% had history of oral contraceptive use. During data collection, 590(51.9%) were using modern contraceptive. Only 49 (4.3%) of the women reported that they had history of sexually transmitted disease.(Table 2) Sixty-four (5.6%) participants reported that they knew persons with cervical cancer.

Knowledge about cervical cancer

The awareness of the women on cervical cancer was 34.3% (95%CI: 31.7, 36.9). The major source of information was the mass media for 163(41.7%), family, friends, and neighbors for 160(41%). The number of the participants who listed at least one symptom of cervical cancer was 240 (21.1%) (95%CI: 18, 24). The most commonly mentioned symptom for cervical cancer was intermenstrual bleeding 99 (8.7%). Most of the participants 897(78.9%) did not know any symptom of cervical cancer. Slightly less than a quarter, 264(23.2%) (95%CI: 19.6,26), of the participants identified at least one risk factor for the diseases. The most commonly mentioned, 138 (12.1%), risk factor for cervical cancer was multiple sexual partners.

Table 1 Socio-demographic characteristics of study participants in Finote Selam town, northwest Ethiopia, 2017

Characteristics	Frequency n = 1137(%)	Compressive knowledge		P-value	Attitude		P-value
		No	Yes		No	Yes	
Age							
30–34	372(32.7)	249	123	0.003	163	209	0.142
35–39	366(32.2)	241	125	0.001	130	236	0.001
40–44	200(17.6	145	55	0.137	83	117	0.80
45–49	199(17.5)	157	42		100	99	
Religion							
Orthodox	1048(92.2)	737	351		449	599	
Muslim	81(7.1)	51	30	0.16	25	56	0.037
Protestant	8(0.7)	4	4	0.22	2	6	0.322
Marital status							
Married	755(66.6)	29	28	0.001	13	44	0.001
Divorced	221(19.4)	523	232	0.73	301	454	0.50
Windowed	104(9.2)	159	62	0.257	110	111	0.970
Single	57(5)	81	23		52	52	
Educational status							
No formal education	513(45.1)	455	58		276	237	
Primary school	295(26)	220	75	.000	124	171	.001
Secondary school (9–12)	198(14)	81	117	.000	53	145	.000
College/university	131(11.5)	36	95	.000	23	108	.000
Occupation							
Household activities	530(46.)	434	96		270	260	
Self employed	254(22.3)	166	88	.000	87	167	0.000
Farmerand daily worker	169(15)	132	37	0.27	74	95	0.11
Government employed	98(8.6)	22	76	0.000	16	82	0.000
Private employee	73(6.4	31	42	0.000	27	46	0.027
Student	13(1.1)	7	6	0.017	2	11	0.024
Family average monthly income[a]							
< 22	278(24.5)	234	61		142	153	
22–45	344(30.3)	288	79	0.276	171	196	0.693
45–68	85(7.5)	47	24	.020	30	41	0.373
> 68	430(37.7)	223	181	.000	133	271	.000

[a]in USD

Out of participants, 259 (22.8%) (95%CI: 20, 27.3), mentioned at least one prevention methods of cervical cancer. Avoiding multiple sexual partners, 181 (15.9%), and early sexual intercourse, 60 (5.3%), were the most commonly mentioned ways of prevention. Nearly three-fourths participants, 866 (76.2%) reported that cervical cancer could not be treated even if diagnosed early stage. With regard to treatment of the diseases, surgery was the most frequently mentioned method by 175 (15.4%) followed by chemotherapy pointed out by 167 (14.7%) (Table 3). About 30.3% (95%CI: 27.7, 32.9) of the participants had comprehensive knowledge of cervical cancer (Fig. 1).

Women's attitude towards cervical cancer screening

The majority of the women, 1046 (92%), agreed on consulting a health care professional during inter-menstrual bleeding. About half of the participants, 586 (51.5%), agreed that any sexually active woman is at risk of acquiring cervical cancer, and 429(37.8%) participants agreed that cervical cancer could be transmitted sexually. Two-thirds 744 (65.4%) agreed that pre-cervical cancer lesion screening helped to prevent cervical cancer. Among respondents, 699 (61.5%) stated that pre cervical cancer screening was not harmful. Significant proportions of women (87%) agreed to screen for the future if screening was free of charge. The proportion of women who had

Table 2 Women's risk of exposure to cervical cancer and reproductive health services utilization in Finote Selam town, northwest Ethiopia

Characteristics		Frequency	Percent
Age at first sexual intercourse	<=16 years	615	54.1
	> 16 years	522	45.9
Life time number of sexual partners	One	349	30.7
	Two and more	788	69.3
History of pregnancy	Yes	1016	89.4
	No	121	10.6
History of child birth	Yes	1002	88
	No	135	12
ANC during the last pregnancy(N = 1016)	Yes	579	57
	No	437	43
Abortion experience during the life time	Yes	163	14.3
	No	974	85.7
PNC after the last child birth (N = 1002)	Yes	259	25.8
	No	743	74.2
Ever used modern contraceptive method in the life time	Yes	830	73
	No	307	27
Modern contraceptive use during data collection	Yes	590	51.9
	No	547	48.1
Self reported history of STI during life time	Yes	49	4.3
	No	1088	95.7
Knew person with cervical cancer	Yes	62	5.6
	No	1075	94.4

Abbreviation: *ANC* Ante Natal Care, *PNC* Post Natal Care, *STI* Sexually Transmitted Infections

favorable attitude towards cervical cancer screening was 58.1% (95% CI: 55, 62.2) (Fig. 1).

Factors associated with women's comprehensive knowledge on cervical cancer

The bivariate analysis showed that socio-demographic variables, such as age, marital status, education, occupation, average family monthly income, knowing anyone who had cervical cancer, and reproductive history including number of life-time sexual partner, gravidity, ANC service utilization, parity, PNC service utilization, ever use of modern contraceptives, currently using contraceptives and history of STD were significantly associated with the comprehensive knowledge score of cervical cancer at *P*-value of less than 0.2. In the multi variable analysis, educational status, knowing someone with cervical cancer, and history of STD remained significant.

Participants who attended primary school were nearly two times (AOR = 1.65, 95% CI: 1.05, 2.59) more likely to be knowledgeable on cervical cancer than those who did not attend formal education. Women who attend secondary school (grade 9–12) were more than five times (AOR = 5.59, 95% CI: 3.25, 9.63) more likely to be knowledgeable than those who did not have formal education. Study participants who attended college/university were seven times (AOR = 7.21,95%CI: 3.41,15.29) more likely to be knowledgeable than those who did not have formal education. Women who knew someone with

cervical cancer were five times (AOR = 5.38, 95% CI: 2.38, 12.15) more likely to be knowledgeable on cervical cancer compared to those who did not know cancer cases.

In the present study, women who had history of sexually transmitted diseases (STD) were nearly three times (AOR = 2.75, 95%CI: 1.24, 6.04) more likely to be knowledgeable than those who had no history of STD (Table 4).

Factors associated with a ttitude towards cervical cancer screening

According to the bivariate analysis, seven socio-demographic variables, age, religion, marital status, education, occupation, average family monthly income, knowing someone with cervical cancer, including nine other variables were significantly associated with attitude to cervical cancer screening at *P*-value of less than 0.2. In the multivariable analysis, three variables, such as educational status, knowing someone with cervical cancer and comprehensive knowledge about the diseases became significant with attitude towards cervical cancer screening at a P-value of less than 0.05.

Participants who attended college/university were 2.56 times (AOR = 2.56,95%CI:1.14,5.69) more likely to have a favorable attitude towards screening than those who did not attend formal education. Women who knew someone who had cervical cancer were three times (AOR = 3.24, 95% CI: 1.14, 9.15) more likely to have a favorable attitude towards cervical cancer screening.

Table 3 Knowledge of participants of cervical cancer by components among aged 30-49 years women in Finote Selam town, northwest Ethiopia, 2017

Variables	Frequency $n = 1137$	Percent
Symptom of cervical cancer		
Inter menstrual bleeding	99	8.7
Foul smelling vaginal discharge	95	8.4
Pain during sexual intercourse	69	6.1
Vaginal bleeding during and after sexual intercourse	20	1.8
Risk factors of cervical cancer		
Multiple sexual partners	138	12.1
Early sexual intercourse	67	5.9
HIV infection	43	3.8
HPV infection	40	3.5
Others	4	0.4
Prevention of cervical cancer		
Avoiding multiple sexual partners	181	15.9
Avoiding early sexual intercourse	60	5.3
Avoiding pregnancies	24	2.1
Screening for pre-cervical cancer lesions	22	1.9
Vaccination of HPV	4	0.4
Cervical cancer can be treated if diagnosed early stage	271	23.8
Treatment for cervical cancer		
Surgery	175	15.4
Chemotherapy	167	14.7
Radiotherapy	15	1.3

Abbreviation: *HPV* human papiloma virus
Note: Others = multiparty and oral contraceptive use

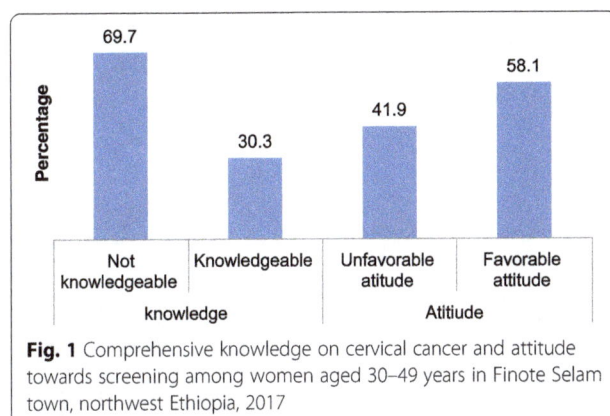

Fig. 1 Comprehensive knowledge on cervical cancer and attitude towards screening among women aged 30–49 years in Finote Selam town, northwest Ethiopia, 2017

Women who had comprehensive knowledge of cervical cancer were three times (AOR = 3.00, 95%CI: 1.97, 4.29) more likely to have a favorable attitude towards cervical cancer screening than their counterparts (Table 5).

Discussion

Knowledge of cervical cancer and attitude towards its screening are essential for the prevention of the disease. The current study was conducted to determine women's comprehensive knowledge on cervical cancer, attitude towards pre-cervical cancer screening and associated factors.

The study revealed that nearly one-third, 30.3% (95%CI: 27.2–32.9), of participants had comprehensive knowledge on cervical cancer. This finding is comparable with that of a community based study conducted in Gondar (31%), Ethiopia, among women aged 15 years and above [15]. This finding is higher than the finding 25% reported from Addis Ababa [18]. The possible reason for difference might be that the researchers used only 13 questions and 7/13 was used as the cutoff point to determine knowledge in the previous study. However, our result is lower than the finding reported by a community-based study in Uganda which noted 55% [19]. The possible reason for the difference from the study done in Uganda could be the variation in educational status between the two study populations. The majority of the participants in the Ugandan study completed primary school unlike ours in which nearly half of participants did not have formal education.

Ours study showed that 58.1% (95% CI: 55, 62.2) of the women had favourable attitude towards cervical cancer screening. This result was better than that of a study done in Dessie, Ethiopia which documented 42.1% [11]. The gap between our study and that of Dessie might be the high proportion of single (unmarried) participants in the Dessie study. There is evidence that single women have less favourable attitude towards screening [16]. However, the result is lower than the finding of a hospital-based study in India which reported 76% [16]. The difference between our and the study in India might be the study setting; hospitalized women might have high health seeking behaviour and better access to information. Our finding was also lower than that of a study conducted among market women in Nigeria noted 80.4% had favourable attitude towards screening [20]. The difference might be that in the Nigeria study the participants were shop owners/attendants aged 15 years and above, most of them with higher educational status.

In this study, educational status was positively associated with women's comprehensive knowledge on cervical cancer. Women who have primary, secondary and college/university education were more likely to have better knowledge on cervical cancer than those who did not have

Table 4 Bivariate and multivariable logistic regression analysis of factor associated with knowledge on cervical cancer among women aged 30–49 years Finote Selam town, northwest Ethiopia, 2017

Factors	Knowledge on cervical cancer		COR	95% CI	AOR	95%CI
	Not knowledgeable	Knowledgeable				
Age						
30–34	249 (66.9)	123 (33.1)	1.85	1.23–2.76**	1.27	0.72–2.43
35–39	241 (65.8)	125 (34.2)	1.94	1.29–2.90**	1.40	0.76–2.59
40–44	145 (72.5)	55(32.5)	1.42	0.89–2.24	1.33	0.68–2.59
45–49	157 (78.9)	42(21.1)	1		1	
Marital status						
Single	29(51)	28(49)	3.40	1.69–9.63*	0.92	0.32–2.62
Married	523 (69.3)	232(30.7)	1.56	0.95–2.54	0.81	0.38–1.72
Divorced	159 (72)	62(28)	1.37	0.79–2.37	0.94	0.42–2.12
Windowed	81 (77.8)	23(22.2)	1		1	
Educational status						
No formal education	455 (88.6)	58(11.4)	1		1	
Primary	220 (74.5)	75(25.5)	2.67	1.83–3.90***	1.65	1.04–2.59**
Secondary (9_12)	81 (40.9)	117(59.1)	11.33	7.64–16.79***	5.6	3.25–9.63***
College/university	36 (27.4)	95(72.6)	20.70	12.92–33.13***	7.21	3.41–15.28***
Occupation						
Home maker	434 (81.8)	96(18.2)	1		1	
Employed	53 (30.9)	118(69.1)	10.06	6.79–14.90***	1.66	0.89–3.08
Self employed	166 (65.3)	88(34.7)	2.40	1.70–3.36***	1.04	0.67–1.63
Farmer, daily labor	132 (78.1)	37(21.9)	1.26	0.87–1.94	1.37	0.81–2.33
Student	7 5 (53.8)	6(46.2)	13.87	1.27–11.78*	1.04	0.27–4.02
Family monthly income[a]						
< 22	234 (79.3)	61(20.7)	1		1	
22–45	288 (78.4)	79(21.6)	1.27	0.83–2.24	0.73	0.42–1.15
45–68	47 (66.1)	24(33.9)	1.96	1.11–3.45*	0.70	0.30–1.64
> 68	223 (55.1)	181(44.9)	3.11	2.20–4.38***	0.97	0.38–1.67
		Knowing anyone who had Cervical cancer				
No	775 (70.3)	298(29.7)	1		1	
Yes	17 (26.5)	47(73.5)	7.19	4.06–12.72***	5.38	2.38–12.2***
No of sexual partners						
One	218 (62.4)	131(37.6)	1		1	
More than one	574 (72.8)	214(27.2)	1.61	1.23–2.10**	1.38	0.95–2.06
Gravidity						
0	68 (56.1)	53(43.9)	1		1	

Table 4 Bivariate and multivariable logistic regression analysis of factor associated with knowledge on cervical cancer among women aged 30–49 years Finote Selam town, northwest Ethiopia, 2017 (*Continued*)

Factors	Knowledge on cervical cancer		COR	95% CI	AOR	95%CI
	Not knowledgeable	Knowledgeable				
1	73 (58.8)	51(41.2)	0.89	0.54-1.48	1.35	0.28-6.36
2-4	460 (60.6)	200(39.4)	0.56	0.37-0.82**	1.02	0.22-4.77
>=5	191 (82.3)	41(17.7)	0.28	0.16-0.45***	2.07	0.23-18.20
Parity						
Null-porous	79 (58.5)	56(41.5)	1		1	
1	88 (58.6)	62(41.4)	0.99	0.62-1.59	0.96	0.21-4.37
2-4	444 (70.1)	189(29.9)	0.60	0.41-0.88**	0.89	0.19-4.14
>=5	181 (82.6)	38 17.4	0.30	0.18-0.48**	0.53	0.06-1.78
ANC utilization for last pregnancy						
No	426 (76.80)	128(23.2)	1		1	
Yes	366 (62.7)	217(37.3)	1.97	1.52-2.55***	1.24	0.79-1.93
PNC utilization for last delivery						
No	642 (73.1)	236(26.9)	1		1	
Yes	150 (57.9)	109(42.1)	1.98	1.48-2.63***	1.19	0.80-1.78
Ever-use modern contraceptive						
No	263 (85.6)	44(14.4)	1		1	
Yes	529 (63.7)	301(36.3)	3.40	2.39-4.82***	6.54	0.54-87.64
Currently using contraceptive						
No	274 (68.6)	125(31.4)	1		1	
Yes	254 (58.9)	177(41.1)	1.57	1.14-2.03**	1.08	0.76-1.54
History of STD						
No	774 (71.1)	314(28.9)	1		1	
Yes	18 (36.7)	31(63.3)	4.5	2.34-7.70**	2.75	1.24-6.04**

[a]In USD, *COR* Crude odds ratio, *AOR* adjusted odds ratio, *CI* Confidence interval, *ANC* Ante-Natal care, *PNC* Post-Natal care, *USA* United States of America, 1: Reference category, *STD* Sexually transmitted disease, *:0.05 < p < 0.2, **:0.001 < p < 0.05, ***:p < 0.001

Table 5 Bivariate and multivariable analysis of factor associated with attitude towards cervical cancer screening among women aged 30–49 years Finote Selam town, northwest Ethiopia, 2017

Factors	Attitude towards screening		COR	95% CI	AOR	95%CI
	Unfavorable attitude	Favorable attitude				
Age						
30–34	163 (43.8)	209 (56.2)	1.29	0.91–1.82[*]	0.98	0.68–2.10
35–39	130 (35.5)	236 (64.5)	1.83	1.29–2.60[**]	0.73	0.42–1.27
40–44	83 (41.5)	117 (58.5)	1.42	0.95–2.11[*]	0.83	0.45–1.50
45–49	100 (50.2)	99 (49.8)	1		1	
Religion						
orthodox	449 (42.8)	599 (57.2)	1		1	
Muslim	25 (30.2)	56 (69.8)	1.80	1.03–2.73[*]	0.74	0.40–1.50
Protestant	2 (25)	6 (75)	0.74	0.14–3.96	0.36	0.05–2.22
Marital status						
Single	13 (22.8)	44 (77.2)	3.38	1.63–7.01[**]	2.08	0.74–5.87
Married	301(39.8)	454 (60.2)	1.50	1.00–2.27[*]	1.07	0.53–2.13
Divorced	110(49.7)	111 (52.3)	1.01	0.63–1.60	0.63	0.30–1.31
Windowed	52 (50)	52 (50)	1		1	
Education						
No formal education	276 (53.80)	237 (46.2)	1		1	
Primary	124 (42)	171 (58)	1.61	1.20–2.14[**]	1.32	0.90–1.95
Secondary (9_12)	53 (26.7)	145 (73.3)	3.16	2.22–4.56[***]	1.54	0.88–2.67
College/university	23 (17.5)	108 (82.5)	5.46	3.37–8.85[***]	2.56	1.14–5.69[**]
Occupation						
Home maker	270 (50.9)	260 (49.1)	1		1	
Employed	43 (25.1)	128 (74.9)	3.09	2.10–4.54[***]	0.74	0.38–1.44
Self employed	87(34.2)	167 (65.8)	2	1.46–2.71[***]	1.30	0.84–2.02
Farmer & daily labor	74 (43.7)	95 (56.3)	1.33	0.94–1.88[*]	1.67	0.94–2.67
Student	2 (15.3)	11 (84.7)	5.71	1.25–26.01[**]	1.7	0.32–9.00
Family average monthly income[a]						
< 22	142 (47.9)	153 (52.1)	1		1	
22–45	171 (46.5)	196 (53.5)	1.06	0.78–1.44	0.94	0.61–1.46
45–68	30 (42.2)	41 (57.8)	1.26	0.75–2.14	0.70	0.33–1.48
> 68	133 (32.9)	271 (67.1)	1.9	1.38–2.57[***]	1.14	0.69–1.89
Knowing anyone who had CCa						
No	464 (43.2)	609 (56.8)	1		1	
Yes	12 (18.7)	52 (81.3)	3.30	1.74–6.25[***]	3.24	1.14–9.15[**]
No of sexual partners						
One	127 (36.3)	222 (63.7)	1		1	

Table 5 Bivariate and multivariable analysis of factor associated with attitude towards cervical cancer screening among women aged 30–49 years Finote Selam town, northwest Ethiopia, 2017 (Continued)

Factors	Attitude towards screening		COR	95% CI	AOR	95%CI
	Unfavorable attitude	Favorable attitude				
More than one	349 (44.2)	439 (55.8)	0.72	0.55–0.93**	1.03	0.71–1.49
Gravida						
0	43 (35.5)	78 (64.5)	1		1	
1	51 (41.1)	73 (58.9)	0.78	0.47–1.32	1.10	0.26–4.61
2–4	264 (40)	396 (60)	0.82	0.53–1.23	1.29	0.29–5.74
>=5	118(50.8)	114 (49.2)	0.533	0.33–0.83**	1.70	0.19–14.63
ANC service utilization						
No	270 (48.7)	284 (51.3)	1		1	
Yes	206(35.3)	377 (64.7)	1.74	1.37–2.20***	1.07	0.72–1.57
Parity						
Nulparous	48 (35.5)	87 (64.5)	1		1	
1	62 (41.3)	88 (58.7)	1.93	1.24–3.00**	0.76	0.19–3.03
2–4	253 (39.9)	380 (60.1)	1.51	0.95–2.30*	0.78	0.18–3.38
>=5	113 (51.5)	106 (48.5)	1.60	1.17–2.18**	0.55	0.06–4.65
PNC service utilization for last delivery						
No	403 (48.5)	475 (52.5)	1		1	
Yes	73 (28.1)	186 (71.9)	2.16	1.59–2.92***	1.43	0.97–2.10
Ever use modern contraceptive						
No	172 (56)	135 (44)	1		1	
Yes	304 (36)	526 (64)	2.20	1.69–2.87***	2.00	0.44–9.07
Currently using contraceptive						
No	156 (39)	243 (61)	1		1	
Yes	149 (34.5)	282 (65.5)	1.52	1.14–2.03*	0.95	0.68–1.32
History of STD						
No	464 (42.6)	624 (37.4)	1		1	
yes	12 (24.4)	37 (75.6)	2.29	1.18–4.44**	1.27	0.55–2.93
Knowledge on Cervical cancer						
Not knowledgeable	407 (51)	385 (49)	1		1	
Knowledgeable	69 (20)	276 (80)	4.23	3.13–5.69***	3.00	1.97–4.29***

^{a}in USD, CCa Cervical cancer, COR Crude odds ratio, CI Confidence interval, AOR Adjusted Odds Ratio, ANC Ante-Natal care, PNC Post-Natal care, USA United States of America,1: Reference category, STD Sexually transmitted disease, *:0.05 < p < 0.2, **:0.001 < p < 0.05, ***:p < 0.001

formal education. Studies in the Democratic Republic of Congo [10], India [16], and Dessie, Ethiopia [11], reported similar findings. Similarly, in this study, it was found that educational status of women had a significant association with attitude towards cervical cancer screening. In the present study, women who had college and above educational status were more than two times more likely to have favorable attitude towards cervical cancer screening. Similar results were found by studies conducted in Eastern Uganda [19], and Addis Ababa [18].

The present study identified that the participants who knew someone with cervical cancer were five times more likely to be knowledgeable on cervical cancer than those who didn't know someone with cervical cancer. Studies conducted in Gondar [15], and Kenya [21] had similar findings. Our study revealed that women who knew someone who had cancer were 3.24 times more likely to have favorable attitude towards cervical cancer screening (AOR = 3.24, 95%CI: 1.14, 9.15).

Our finding showed that women who had history of STD were nearly three times more likely to be knowledgeable on cervical cancer than those who had not. A similar finding was reported by a study done on Asian Maldives [22]. This might be because of women who had STD might have contact with health professionals to get treatment for the disease during which they might be advised/counselled about the risks of unprotected sex, including the risk of viral infections, such as HIV, and the human papiloma virus plus their consequences and means of prevention. Thus, this communication might help them get information on cervical cancer. A study conducted in rural Kenya identified that family planning service utilization was positively associated with knowledge on cervical cancer [9]. In our study, no significant association was observed between knowledge on cervical cancer and obstetric service related variables such as ANC, family planning and post-natal service utilization. This may suggest that women who utilize maternal health services do not receive information on cervical cancer.

The finding in this study showed that women who had comprehensive knowledge of cervical cancer were three times more likely to have favorable attitude towards cervical cancer screening as compared to their counterparts. Previous studies done in Nepal [23], and a health facility-based study in Dessie Ethiopia [11], reported a similar finding. This shows that women who have adequate knowledge on cervical cancer might understand the nature disease (causes, symptoms, preventions, and treatments), and the benefits of screening which in turn make them have positive attitude towards screening. Since this study was conducted in urban setting that could not generalize for rural women. This might be the potential limitation of this study. Additionally, one of the independent variables

we considered was history of sexually transmitted diseases that might be exposed for social desirability bias. However, the authors tried to minimize this potential bias by providing adequate information for the study participants about the importance of telling the truth and confidentiality nature of the research.

Conclusion

In this study, it was identified that women's knowledge on cervical cancer was low, despite the high incidence of the disease in Ethiopia. Relatively, a large proportion of the study participants in this study had favorable attitude towards cervical cancer screening. Attending primary, secondary school and college, knowing someone who had cervical cancer and history of STD were factors associated to comprehensive knowledge on cervical cancer.

Attended college and above, knowing someone who had cervical cancer, and having comprehensive knowledge on cervical cancer were important factors for having favorable attitude towards cervical cancer screening. There is clear need for information sharing on cervical cancer, including its screening targeting women with less educated. Educational campaign on the disease and screening,involving the mass media in providing information to the women on cervical cancer, including screening service availability when the women visit health facilities for reproductive services are proposed.

Abbreviations
ANC: Ante Natal care; AOR: Adjusted Odds Ratio; CI: Confidence Interval; PNC: Post Natal care; SD: Standard Deviation; SPSS: Statistical Package for Social Sciences; STD: Sexually transmitted disease

Acknowledgements
We would like to extend our heart full gratitude to University of Gondar, Institute of public health for giving ethical clearance and the financial support for this study. Our heart full tank is extended to the study participants for their time and willingness to participate and to data collectors and supervisor for their commitment. Our appreciation also extended for Finote Selam town health office for their cooperativeness and provision of supportive letters.

Funding
University of Gondar sponsored this study. However, it has no role in manuscript preparation and publication.

Authors' contributions
ABG brought the idea. ABG, AAG, and TA equally contributed on proposal development, data collection process, data management and analysis, and write up. All authors have read and approved the manuscript.

Competing interests
All authors declared that they have no any competing interest.

Comprehensive knowledge on cervical cancer, attitude towards its screening and associated factors...

29

Author details

[1]Department of Reproductive Health, Institute of Public Health, College of Medicine and Health Science, University of Gondar, 196 Gondar, Ethiopia. [2]Department of Health Education and Behavioral Sciences, Institute of Public Health, College of Medicine and Health Sciences, University of Gondar, Gondar, Ethiopia.

References

1. Fitzmaurice C, Dicker D, Pain A, Hamavid H, Moradi-Lakeh M, MacIntyre MF, et al. The global burden of cancer 2013. JAMA Oncol. 2015;1:505–27.
2. Ferlay JSI, Dikshit R, Eser S, Mathers C, Rebelo M, et al. Cancer incidence and mortality worldwide: sources, methods and major patterns in GLOBOCAN 2012. Int J Cancer. 2015;136:E359–86.
3. UNFPA: Africa cervical cancer multi indicator incidence& mortality score card 2014.
4. Bruni L, Barrionuevo-Rosas L, Albero G, Serrano B, Mena M, Gómez D, Muñoz J, Bosch FX, de Sanjosé S. Human Papillomavirus and related diseases in Ethiopia. Summary report december 2016. ICO Information Centre on HPV and Cancer (HPV Information Centre). 2016. https://www.hpvcentre.net/statistics/reports/XWX.pdf.
5. Abate SM. Trends of cervical cancer in Ethiopia 2015. Cervical Cancer. 2015; 1:103.
6. Torre LA, Bray F, Siegel RL, Ferlay J, Lortet-Tieulent J, Jemal A. Global cancer statistics, 2012. CA Cancer J Clin. 2015;65:87–108.
7. Gakidou E, Nordhagen S, Obermeyer Z. Coverage of cervical cancer screening in 57 countries: low average levels and large inequalities. PLoS Med. 2008;5:e132.
8. Peirson L, Fitzpatrick-Lewis D, Ciliska D, Warren R. Screening for cervical cancer: a systematic review and meta-analysis. 2013;2:35. https://doi.org/10.1186/2046-4053-2-35.
9. Rosser JI, Njoroge B, Huchko MJ. Knowledge on cervical cancer screening and perception of risk among women attending outpatient clinics in rural Kenya. Int J Gynaecol Obstet. 2015;128:211–5.
10. Ali-Risasi C, Mulumba P, Verdonck K, Vanden Broeck D, Praet M. Knowledge, attitude and practice about cancer of the uterine cervix among women living in Kinshasa, the Democratic Republic of Congo. BMC Womens Health. 2014;14:30.
11. Andargie A, Reddy PS. Knowledge, attitude, practice and associated factors of cervical cancer screening among women in Dessie referral hospital and Dessie health center, Northeast Ethiopia. Glob J Res Anal. 2016;4
12. Federal Ministry Of Health Ethiopia: National Cancer Control Plan 2016–2020. October 2015.
13. Bayu H, Berhe Y, Mulat A, Alemu A. Cervical cancer screening service uptake and associated factors among age eligible women in Mekelle zone, northern Ethiopia, 2015 a community based study using health belief model. PLoS One. 2015;11:e0149908.
14. Population Projection of Ethiopia for All Regions at Wereda Level 2017 August 2013.
15. Getahun F, Mazengia F, Abuhay M, Birhanu Z. Comprehensive knowledge about cervical cancer is low among women in Northwest Ethiopia. BMC Cancer. 2013;13:2.
16. Bansal AB, Pakhare AP, Kapoor N, Mehrotra R, Kokane AM. Knowledge, attitude, and practices related to cervical cancer among adult women: a hospital-based cross-sectional study. J Nat Sci Biol Med. 2015;6:324.
17. Mitiku I, Tefera F. Knowledge on cervical cancer and associated factors among 15-49 year old women in Dessie town, Northeast Ethiopia. PLoS One. 2016;11:e0163136.
18. Belete N, Tsige Y, Mellie H. Willingness and acceptability of cervical cancer screening among women living with HIV/AIDS in Addis Ababa, Ethiopia: a cross sectional study. Gynecol Oncol Res Prac. 2015;2:6.
19. Mukama T, Ndejjo R, Musabyimana A, Halage AA, Musoke D. Women's knowledge and attitudes towards cervical cancer prevention: a cross sectional study in eastern Uganda. BMC Womens Health. 2017;17:9.
20. Ahmed SA, Sabitu K, Idris SH, Ahmed R. Knowledge, attitude and practice of cervical cancer screening among market women in Zaria, Nigeria. Niger Med J. 2013;54:316.
21. Sudenga SL, Rositch AF, Otieno WA, Smith JS. Knowledge, attitudes, practices, and perceived risk of cervical cancer among Kenyan women: brief report. Int J Gynecol Cancer. 2013;23:895–9.
22. Basu P, Hassan S, Fileeshia F, Mohamed S, Nahoodha A, Shiuna A, et al. Knowledge, attitude and practices of women in maldives related to the risk factors, prevention and early detection of cervical cancer. Asian Pac J Cancer Prev. 2014;15:6691–5.
23. Ranabhat S, Tiwari M, Dhungana G, Shrestha R. Association of knowledge, attitude and demographic variables with cervical pap smear practice in Nepal. Asian Pac J Cancer Prev. 2014;15:8905–10.

4

Temporal trends of preterm birth in Shenzhen, China: a retrospective study

Changchang Li[1,2,3], Zhijiang Liang[4], Michael S. Bloom[5], Qiong Wang[1,2], Xiaoting Shen[6], Huanhuan Zhang[1,2], Suhan Wang[1,2], Weiqing Chen[2], Yan Lin[7], Qingguo Zhao[4*] and Cunrui Huang[1,2*]

Abstract

Background: Preterm birth is the leading cause of child mortality under 5 years of age. Temporal trends in preterm birth rates are highly heterogeneous among countries and little information exists for China. To address this data gap, we investigated annual changes in preterm birth incidence rate and explored potential determinants of these changes in Shenzhen, China.

Methods: A total of 1.4 million live births, during 2003-2012, were included from the Shenzhen birth registry. Negative-binominal regression models were used to estimate the annual percent changes in incidence. To identify the potential determinants behind temporal trends, we estimated the contribution of each changing risk factor to changes in rate by calculating the difference in population-attributable risk fraction.

Results: Annual preterm birth incidence rates increased by 0.94% (95% CI 0.30%, 1.58%) overall, 3.60% (95% CI 2.73%, 4.48%) for medically induced, and 3.13% (95% CI 1.01%, 5.31%) for preterm premature rupture of membranes, but decreased by 2.34% (95% CI 1.62%, 3.06%) for spontaneous preterm labor. Higher maternal educational attainment (0.20 rate increase), lower proportion of inadequate prenatal care (0.15 rate reduction), more multipara (0.08 rate reduction), decreased proportion of preeclampsia or eclampsia (0.05 rate reduction), and larger proportion of young and older pregnant women (0.04 rate increase) were significant contributors to the overall change over time. Contributions of changing risk factors were different between preterm birth subtypes.

Conclusions: Preterm birth rate in Shenzhen, China increased overall during 2003-2012, although trends varied across three preterm birth subtypes. The rising rates were associated with changes in maternal education and age.

Keywords: Preterm birth, Incidence rate, Temporal trend, Medically induced preterm birth, Spontaneous preterm birth, China

Plain English summary

Complications from preterm birth (PTB) is the leading cause of neonatal and child mortality worldwide. Numerous studies have reported changes in PTB incidence over the past two decades. These finding showed that the temporal trends in PTB rates are highly heterogeneous among countries, but there is little information available for China.

China has the second greatest number of PTBs worldwide, with large disparities in PTB rates across different regions of the country. To better understand the temporal trends in PTB rates in mainland China, this study investigated changes in PTB rates by clinical subtype and explore potential determinants of the changes in Shenzhen, China.

Based on the data analysis, we found that preterm birth rate increased in Shenzhen between 2003 and 2012, yet with varied trends among three PTB clinical subtypes. In detail, incidence rates increased in late preterm and medically induced preterm birth, but decreased in preterm birth due to spontaneous preterm labor. Maternal education, parity and prenatal care visits played important roles in determining secular trends for PTB rates. In summary, the Shenzhen findings provided complementary evidence to confirm the increasing trends of PTB rates in mainland China. Moreover, this study also suggested that advanced and highly educated pregnant women should be the key

* Correspondence: zqgfrost@126.com; huangcr@mail.sysu.edu.cn
[4]Department of Public Health, Guangdong Women and Children Hospital, 521, 523 Xing Nan Street, Guangzhou 511442, China
[1]Department of Health Policy and Management, School of Public Health, Sun Yat-sen University, 74 Zhongshan Road #2, Guangzhou 510080, China
Full list of author information is available at the end of the article

target population groups for future clinical intervention and public health prevention strategies in developed area of China.

Background

Complications from preterm birth (PTB) is the leading cause of neonatal and child mortality worldwide [1]. Globally, it was estimated that 15 million babies yearly, were delivered preterm, which caused one million deaths in children under 5 years of age in 2013 [1, 2]. In addition to increased mortality, PTB infants are at higher risk for suffering chronic health conditions, and neurodevelopmental and learning impairment [3]. Preterm birth introduces enormous physical, psychological and economic costs. A study from Canada indicated that total national cost corresponding to PTB was at least $587.1 million in 2014. The cost per infant over the first 10 years of life was estimated to be $67,467 for early preterm births, $52,796 for moderate preterm births, and $10,010 for late preterm births [4]. Therefore, even a modest reduction in PTB would make for substantially reduced short and long-term costs.

The investigation of temporal trends in PTB rates is essential to inform policy and to design interventions for reducing the burden of PTB. Numerous prior studies have reported changes in PTB incidence over the past two decades. These findings showed that the temporal trends in PTB rates are highly heterogeneous among countries [2, 5]. A global study of 65 developed, Latin America, and Caribbean countries reported higher PTB rates for 2010 than for 1990, although PTB rates were stable for 14 countries, and 3 countries (Croatia, Ecuador, and Estonia) had a decline [2]. Findings from European countries suggested the PTB rate in Austria increased from 1996 to 2004, but then declined slightly between 2004 and 2008 [5]. Notably, variations in PTB clinical subtypes (spontaneous PTB and medically induced PTB) were also highly heterogeneous among different countries [5]. Factors possibly associated with changes in PTB rates include changes in obstetric population characteristics (e.g. older) and risk factors (e.g. multiple gestations), implementation of specific clinical practices (e.g. use of vaginal progesterone), and changes in public health policies and regulations (e.g. smoking bans in public places) [6, 7].

Existing studies of PTB rates have mainly focused on populations in Europe and North America, yet there is little information available for China [2, 5]. After India, China has the highest number of PTBs worldwide, with large disparities in PTB rates across different regions of the country [2, 8]. The incidence of preterm birth was higher in low-income regions than in high-income regions. The highest incidences were recorded in Southwest China and Northeast China. Only two previous studies investigated temporal trends in Chinese PTB rates during the past decades [9, 10], and the conclusions were inconsistent. PTB rates overall increased in mainland China's Hubei Province, but remained constant in Hong Kong. In an extended analysis, Hui and colleagues [10] suggested that the stable PTB rates in Hong Kong resulted from a pattern of decreasing preterm birth due to spontaneous preterm labor (S-PTB) coupled to increasing preterm birth following premature rupture of membranes (PROM-PTB). However, the trends in mainland China PTB subtypes remain unclear.

Identifying risk factors specific to PTB subtypes will assist clinicians and policymakers in designing interventions to prevent PTB. Hence, a good knowledge of temporal trends in the rates of PTB subtypes and the reasons behind changing rates may enhance PTB prevention [6, 11, 12]. To better understand the temporal trends in PTB rates in mainland China, this study aimed to investigate changes in PTB rates by clinical subtype and to explore potential determinants of the changes in Shenzhen, China.

Methods
Study design and setting

We conducted a retrospective cohort study of births in Shenzhen, which located in Guangdong Province in southern China. Shenzhen is the first Special Economic Zone in China, stemming from China's economic reform in 1980s. It is a megacity with a total population of about 11.9 million. During the past 30 years, the population of Shenzhen has experienced significant socioeconomic and health changes, reflecting the typical development of mainland China. Thus, Shenzhen provides an excellent opportunity to explore the drivers behind health changes in mainland China.

Data collection

We used the Shenzhen Birth Registry Database to capture data for all live births from January 1, 2003 to December 31, 2012 ($n = 1.42$ million). This birth registry database covers all midwifery clinics and hospitals, allowing for accurate PTB rate calculation. Furthermore, this system connects to a city-wide maternal and children health information system, what also allowed for capture of medical record data, including demographic and clinical information for both mother and newborn. The high validity and reliability of data from the Shenzhen Birth Registry Database was previously described [13].

To minimize variability in reporting over the study period, we excluded births: (1) Missing gestational (0.02%) or maternal (0.01%) ages; (2) With maternal age < 13 years or > 50 years (1.87%); or, (3) With gestational age < 22 weeks or > 46 weeks according to the distribution of gestational ages (0.36%) [14]. The flow of study population selection was shown in Additional file 1: Figure S1.

Measures

We collected all variables available from the electronic medical record, and selected the variables for inclusion as PTB risk factors based on the literature [3]. We extracted pregnancy and birth data for each live birth including date of birth, date of mother's last menstrual period (LMP), infant sex (male, female, hermaphrodite), delivery mode (vaginal, cesarean section), parity (0, ≥1), gestational hypertension (yes/ no), preeclampsia or eclampsia (yes/no), and number of prenatal care visits. The number of prenatal care visits was transformed into the adequacy of prenatal care utilization (APNCU) index [15], by calculating the ratio between the actual number of visits and the recommended number. According to the recommendation by the Institute for Clinical Systems Improvement (ICSI), a pregnant woman should be examined four times for the first 28 weeks of pregnancy, five times for 32 weeks, six times for 36 weeks, and 7-11 times for 37-41 weeks of pregnancy [16]. We classified the index into four groups: inadequate (< 50%), intermediate (50-79%), appropriate (80-109%) and appropriate plus (≥ 110%).

We also extracted maternal sociodemographic characteristics and chronic maternal conditions data. We categorized maternal education as no high school, high school and college, bachelor, and postgraduate degree. Chronic maternal conditions included clinically diagnosed hypertension, hepatopathy, nephropathy, and heart disease.

Classification of preterm birth subtypes

We defined PTB as live born infants at less than 37 completed weeks of gestation from the date of LMP, or corrected by first trimester ultrasound if discrepant by more than 7 days. We classified PTB into spontaneous preterm birth and medically induced preterm birth (MI-PTB) according to clinical presentation, and then categorized spontaneous preterm births as preterm premature rupture of membranes (PROM-PTB) and preterm labor (S-PTB). The classification criteria were as follows: (1) MI-PTB, defined as labor induction and/or elective cesarean section without PROM; (2) PROM-PTB, regardless of delivery mode or induction and status; and, (3) S-PTB, which included all non-PROM associated vaginal deliveries. Based on this classification scheme, remaining births that did not meet the criteria for PROM-PTB and MI-PTB were categorized as S-PTB [17].

Statistical analysis

We expressed incidence rate as the number of PTB infants per 100 live births [18]. We calculated annual PTB rates for the entire Shenzhen population and for specific groups defined by PTB subtypes, maternal age, and maternal education. We used negative-binomial regression models to estimate rate ratios (RR), with annual PTB rates operationalized as a count data. RRs were then transformed into the annual percent change (RR-1). We also analyzed changes in proportions of PTB subtypes across time. Risk factors associated with each PTB subtype were identified by using binominal logistic regression models. We included maternal age, and education, infant sex, pregnancy characteristics and chronic maternal conditions in the models. Adjusted odds ratios (AORs) and 95% confidence intervals (95%CI) were calculated to present the risk.

Finally, to analyze the contribution of changing risk factors to changes in PTB rate, we calculated the difference in population-attributable risk fraction (AF_p) for each changing risk factor. The Born Too Soon Preterm Prevention Analysis Group used this method to analyze drivers for increasing PTB rates in the U.S. [7]. The process for this approach follows:

i. Identify distributions of each risk factor for 2003-2007 and 2008-2012. We selected the year of 2007 as the cut-off year because Shenzhen PTB rates increased after 2007.

ii. Identify the PTB for every category of each risk factor during 2008-2012, using ORs generated from logistic regression models.

iii. Calculate AF_p for each PTB risk factor, and compute specific AF_p values for 2003-2007 and 2008-2012. We defined AF_{pi} and AF_p, where, AF_{pi} is the population attributed risk fraction for exposure category j of the ($j = 1....n$) ith risk factor, PF_j is the proportion of the total population in exposure category j for the ith risk factor, RR_j is the risk ratio for the exposure category j of the ith risk factor, approximated using ORs, and AF_p is the population attributable risk across all risk factors i [19]. The formulas were as follows:

$$AF_{Pi} = \frac{\sum_{j=1}^{n} PF_j(RR_j - 1)}{1 + \sum_{j=1}^{n} PF_j(RR_j - 1)} \quad (1)$$

$$AF_p = 1 - \prod_{i=1}^{n}(1 - AF_{Pi}) \quad (2)$$

Notably, the AF_{Pi} value of each risk factor for 2003-2007 was calculated by PF_j in 2003-2007 and RR_j in

2008-2012, whereas AF_{Pi} value for 2008-2012 was a result of PF_j and RR_j in 2008-2012.

iv. Multiply the AF_P by PTB rates in 2008-2012 and subtract the result for 2003-2007 from 2008 to 2012 (Formula 3). The difference was the projected increased in PTB rates between two study periods for each changing risk factor.

$$\text{Projected increase} = AF_{P2008-2012} \\ * rate_{2008-2012} - AF_{P2003-2007} \\ * rate_{2008-2012}$$

(3)

Sensitivity analysis

We performed a sensitivity analysis to ensure the robustness of our findings. Recognizing uncertainty in linear trends, we included year of delivery as a dummy variable into a negative-binominal regression model to examine changes in PTB rates by individual year.

All the analyses were conducted using R software (version 3.2.4; R Foundation for Statistical Computing, Vienna, Austria). An alpha level of 0.05 indicated statistical significance for a two-tailed test.

Results

Preterm birth rates in Shenzhen during the 10-year period 2003–2012

A total of 1.42 million births were recorded in the Shenzhen Birth Registry Database between 2003 and 2012. After excluding the 32,172 (2.25%) ineligible records and 2135 (0.15%) still births, we included 1.39 million (97.6%) live births in this study. There were 78,252 (5.7%) PTBs with PROM-PTB, S-PTB and MI-PTB accounting for 9.5%, 51.4% and 39.4% of overall PTBs, respectively. PTB rates among different maternal and infant groups are presented in Table 1. Subtype-specific PTB rates appeared to differ by maternal age and education. For example, S-PTB rates were higher in younger mothers and in less educated mothers, but MI-PTB rates were higher in older mothers and more highly educated mothers.

Time trends in preterm birth rate

Figure 1 shows that PTB rates increased from 5.6% in 2003 to 6.06% in 2012, corresponding to a 0.94% annual rise (95%CI 0.30%, 1.58%) (Additional file 1: Table S1). There were approximately 3.60% (95%CI 2.73%, 4.48%), and 3.13% (95%CI 1.01%, 5.31%) overall increases in MI-PTB and PROM-PTB, respectively, but S-PTB decreased by about 2.34% (95%CI 3.06%, 1.62%) per year during the study period. Time trends for PTB rates by infant

gestational age and maternal age and education are also presented in Fig. 1. Significant increasing trends were detected for moderate and late preterm (32- < 37 gestational weeks), older mothers (≥ 36 years) and mothers with higher educational attainment (vs. less than high school). As shown by the sensitivity analysis in Additional file 1: Table S1, the overall PTB rates were lower in 2005-2007 than in 2003, however the differences were not statistically significant as shown in Additional file 1: Table S2. In contrast, overall PTB rates in 2008, 2009, 2010, and 2012 were significantly higher than for 2003 (Additional file 1: Table S2).

Risk factors for preterm birth by subtype

As described by Table 2, statistically significant risk factors for PTBs included chronic maternal conditions, inadequate prenatal care and male infant sex. In contrast, multipara consistently decreased the risk. The effects of maternal age and education were less consistent across the three PTB subtypes. S-PTB was more likely to be associated with younger maternal age and lower education. We also detected associations between maternal chronic conditions and gestational complications with higher rates of PROM-PTB and MI-PTB, although with lower rates for S-PTB with gestational hypertension and pre-eclampsia or eclampsia.

Contributions of changing risk factors to changes in preterm birth rates

Table 3 describes the percentage of mothers for every category of each risk factor during 2003-2007 and 2008-2012. A notable increase in risk factor incidence occurred among older (≥ 36 years) mothers, mothers with higher educational attainment, multiparous women, and pregnant women with intermediate prenatal care. The changes in the incidence of chronic conditions, gestational hypertension, preeclampsia or eclampsia, and male infant were comparatively modest.

The contributions of risk factor changes to differences in PTB rates are shown in Fig. 2. Larger proportions of younger and older women and higher educational attainment were associated with rising PTB rates, but lower proportions of inadequate prenatal care visits, and mothers with preeclampsia or eclampsia contributed to declining PTB rates, as did more multipara. The magnitudes of projected rate increases differed across PTB subtypes as shown by Additional file 1 Table S3. However, chronic conditions and gestational hypertension had only modest effects on increases of PTB rates. The increasing overall PTB was unexplained by the combined effect of changes in sociodemographic and pregnancy characteristics (projected − 0.11% rate change). In more detail, 12.9% (0.08% /0.62%) of changes for MI-PTB were explained by the risk factors

Table 1 Descriptive Statistics of All Live Births and Preterm Births (PTB) in Shenzhen, China during 2003–2012

| | Live births | Term births | | Spontaneous preterm births [b] | | | | Medically induced preterm birth | |
| | | | | PROM-PTB | | S-PTB | | | |
		N	%	N	%	N	%	N	%
All live birth	1,385,882	1,307,570	94.35	7436	0.54	40,104	2.89	30,712	2.21
Maternal age (years)									
≤ 20	81,436	75,759	93.03	315	0.39	4375	5.37	987	1.21
21-35	1,230,521	1,164,107	94.60	6477	0.53	33,773	2.74	26,164	2.13
≥ 36	73,865	67,704	91.66	644	0.87	1956	2.65	3561	4.82
Maternal education									
Less than high school	599,640	565,404	94.29	2397	0.40	21,037	3.51	10,802	1.80
High school and college	498,618	469,616	94.18	2993	0.60	13,912	2.79	12,097	2.43
Bachelor	263,880	250,133	94.79	1884	0.71	4765	1.81	7098	2.69
Postgraduate	23,684	22,417	94.65	162	0.68	390	1.65	715	3.02
Parity									
0	857,543	808,052	94.23	5277	0.62	25,120	2.93	19,094	2.23
≥ 1	523,788	495,377	94.58	2139	0.41	14,778	2.82	11,494	2.19
Missing data	4491	–	–	–	–	–	–		
APNCU index [a]									
Inadequate	635,795	590,381	92.86	3711	0.58	27,182	4.28	14,521	2.28
Intermediate	388,153	366,230	94.35	2427	0.63	9716	2.50	9780	2.52
Appropriate	164,493	157,253	95.60	876	0.53	2458	1.49	3906	2.37
Appropriate plus	197,234	193,572	98.14	421	0.21	744	0.38	2497	1.27
Missing	147	–	–	–	–	–	–		
Maternal chronic conditions									
Yes	3152	2629	83.41	80	2.54	102	3.24	341	10.82
No	1,382,670	1,304,941	94.38	7356	0.53	40,002	2.89	30,371	2.20
Gestational hypertension									
Yes	5008	4496	89.78	72	1.44	101	2.02	339	6.77
No	1,380,814	1,303,074	94.37	7364	0.53	40,003	2.90	30,373	2.20
Preeclampsia or eclampsia									
Yes	16,208	12,644	78.01	102	0.63	309	1.91	3153	19.45
No	1,369,614	1,294,926	94.55	7334	0.54	39,795	2.91	27,559	2.01
Infant sex									
Male	752,163	707,283	94.03	4306	0.57	23,432	3.11	17,142	2.28
Female	633,466	600,123	94.74	3130	0.49	16,648	2.63	13,565	2.14
Hermaphrodite	193	164	84.97	0.00	0.00	24	12.44	5	2.59

[a]APNCU the adequacy of prenatal care utilization
[b]PROM-PTB preterm birth following premature rupture of membranesm, S-PTB preterm birth due to spontaneous preterm labor

considered, 25.0% (− 0. 10% /− 0. 40%) for S-PTB and 12.44% (0.02% /0.16%) for PROM-PTB, respectively.

Discussion

This study highlighted the time trends of preterm birth incidence rate by subtype, and investigated the reasons behinds the changing rates in China. Our results demonstrated that PTB rates increased from 5.59% to 6.06% in

Shenzhen, China, over the period 2003-2012, with high heterogeneity across three PTB subtypes. This increase predominantly took place in late preterm and MI-PTB, and the corresponding annual percent change (*APC*) were 1.34% and 4.19%, respectively. In stratified analyses according to maternal demographic characteristics, PTB rates rapidly increased in mothers with advanced age and high educational attainment, while these decreased

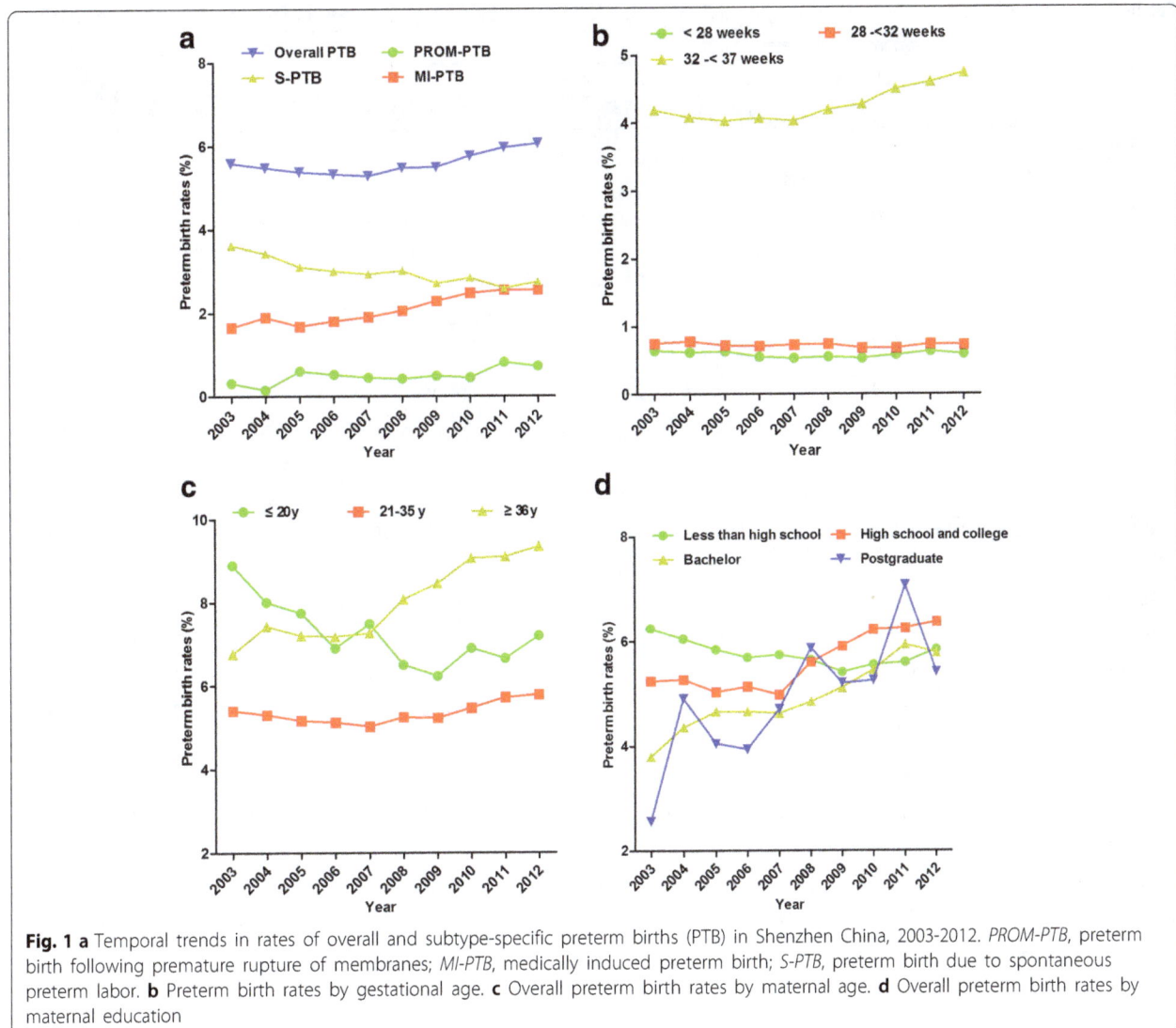

Fig. 1 a Temporal trends in rates of overall and subtype-specific preterm births (PTB) in Shenzhen China, 2003-2012. *PROM-PTB*, preterm birth following premature rupture of membranes; *MI-PTB*, medically induced preterm birth; *S-PTB*, preterm birth due to spontaneous preterm labor. **b** Preterm birth rates by gestational age. **c** Overall preterm birth rates by maternal age. **d** Overall preterm birth rates by maternal education

in younger and mothers with low education. In addition, we found that higher educational attainment, adjusted for maternal age, increased PTB rates (projected increase rate = 0.20%), especially in MI-PTB.

Increasing preterm birth rates and drivers behind the trends

The rising PTB incidence in Shenzhen was consistent with findings from Hubei, China, and also coincided with general trends worldwide [2, 9]. However, the Shenzhen increase (from 5.60% in 2003 to 6.06% in 2012) was slower than reported for Hubei (from 5.67% in 2001 to 10.5% in 2012) [9], but faster than for countries that successfully reduced PTB increase rates from 2001 to 2010, including Canada (from 7.4% in 2000 to 7.8% in 2010), New Zealand (from 7.4% in 2000 to 7.6% in 2010), and Lithuania (from 5.3% in 2000 to 5.4% in 2012) [7]. Different changes in PTB rates between geographic regions appear to be

associated in part with prenatal care access [3, 8]. For example, in high-income regions, pregnant women were more likely to obtain sufficient prenatal care, which may decrease the risk of obstetric complications, including PTBs [3, 8]. Our findings, suggesting a decrease in PTB in association with adequate prenatal care, further corroborate the importance of prenatal and maternal care resources in determining PTB rates, in particular moderate and late PTB.

In terms of reasons for increasing PTB rates over time in Shenzhen, we found that elevated MI-PTB and late preterm played important roles in driving PTB rates. However, the incidences of maternal conditions were stable or declined during the study interval. This apparent contradiction may be due part to changing standards of clinical practice in China, that encourage obstetric intervention (e.g. caesarean deliveries), as reported by Chang et al. [7]. The multivariable analysis showed that

Table 2 Multivariable Logistic Regression Analysis of Risk Factors for Preterm Birth (PTB) Subtypes in Shenzhen, China, 2003–2012

| | Spontaneous preterm birth [b] | | | | Medically induced preterm birth | |
| | PROM-PTB | | S-PTB | | | |
	β	AOR[c] (95% CI)	β	AOR[c] (95% CI)	β	AOR[c] (95% CI)
Maternal age (years)						
21-35	–	Reference	–	Reference	–	Reference
≤ 20	−0.400	0.670 (0.597, 0.753)	0.386	1.471 (1.422, 1.522)	−0.539	0.583 (0.546, 0.623)
≥ 36	0.706	2.026 (1.863, 2.203)	−0.026	0.974 (0.930, 1.021)	0.799	2.224 (2.141, 2.31)
Maternal education						
Bachelor	–	Reference	–	Reference	–	Reference
Less than high school	−0.791	0.454 (0.424, 0.485)	0.074	1.077 (1.040, 1.114)	−0.627	0.534 (0.516, 0.553)
High school and college	−0.334	0.716 (0.681, 0.771)	0.026	1.027 (0.992, 1.063)	−0.252	0.777 (0.753, 0.802)
Postgraduate	−0.071	0.931 (0.792, 1.096)	−0.153	0.858 (0.773, 0.953)	0.092	1.097 (1.013, 1.187)
Parity						
0	–	Reference	–	Reference	–	Reference
≥ 1	−0.528	0.590 (0.559, 0.623)	−0.236	0.790 (0.773, 0.807)	−0.114	0.892 (0.870, 0.916)
APNCU index [a]						
Appropriate	–	Reference	–	Reference	–	Reference
Inadequate	0.485	1.625 (1.504, 1.755)	1.075	2.929 (2.806, 3.057)	0.182	1.199 (1.155, 1.245)
Intermediate	0.399	1.490 (1.377, 1.611)	0.536	1.709 (1.634, 1.788)	0.206	1.228 (1.182, 1.276)
Appropriate plus	−1.068	0.344 (0.306, 0.386)	−1.405	0.245 (0.226, 0.266)	−0.735	0.479 (0.455, 0.504)
Maternal chronic conditions						
No	–	Reference	–	Reference	–	Reference
Yes	1.755	5.786 (4.617, 7.250)	0.571	1.770 (1.449, 2.162)	1.440	4.222 (3.730, 4.779)
Gestational hypertension						
No	–	Reference	–	Reference	–	Reference
Yes	1.008	2.740 (2.166, 3.467)	−0.319	0.727 (0.596, 0.886)	0.864	2.372 (2.109, 2.669)
Preeclampsia or eclampsia						
No	–	Reference	–	Reference	–	Reference
Yes	0.227	1.255 (1.029, 1.530)	−0.341	0.711 (0.634, 0.797)	2.378	10.782 (10.339, 11.244)
Infant sex						
Female	–	Reference	–	Reference	–	Reference
Male	0.168	1.183 (1.129, 1.239)	0.168	1.183 (1.159, 1.207)	0.082	1.085 (1.060, 1.111)
Hermaphroditism	−8.381	0.002 (0.000, 0.002)	1.459	4.301 (2.784, 6.644)	0.238	1.269 (0.515, 3.129)

[a]APNCU the adequacy of prenatal care utilization
[b]PROM-PTB preterm birth following premature rupture of membranes, S-PTB, preterm birth due to spontaneous preterm labor
[c]AOR adjusted odds ratio, CI confidence interval

changes in age and education among obstetric populations made important contributions to the increasing PTB rates. These findings suggest that cause of the rising PTB rates may be multifactorial, resulting from a higher number of high-risk pregnancies, coupled to more extensive implementation of reproductive interventions among older and more highly educated women, such as use of assisted reproductive technologies (ART) [20]. Unfortunately, data describing the use of ART services was not available for this analysis.

Except for the drivers for PTB rates, we found improving prenatal care was an important contributor to decreased PTB, especially in S-PTB. The strong contribution of prenatal care visits to PTB rate declines indicated that many women would have benefited from improved coverage of recommended basic antenatal care services [3]. In general, more opportunities for prenatal care exist with longer gestational age, potentially introducing reverse causation. To address this bias, we computed the APNCU index, which was standardized by gestational age to reflect the access to

Table 3 Distribution of Risk Factors for Preterm Birth (PTB) in Shenzhen, China, 2003- 2012

	Incidence rates (%)	
	2003-2007	2008-2012
Preterm birth [a]		
Overall-PTB	5.38	5.79
PROM-PTB	0.43	0.59
S-PTB	3.24	2.84
MI-PTB	1.81	2.43
Maternal age (years)		
21-35	90.71	87.78
≤ 20	4.62	6.54
≥ 36	4.66	5.68
Maternal education		
Less than high school	50.11	39.66
High school and college	32.79	37.66
Bachelor	16.26	20.51
Postgraduate	0.83	2.17
Parity		
0	66.57	59.40
≥ 1	33.43	40.10
Missing	0.00	0.50
APNCU index [b]		
Inadequate	54.81	40.93
Intermediate	14.84	30.14
Appropriate	15.61	14.4
Appropriate plus	14.73	15.3
Missing	0.00	0.02
Maternal chronic conditions		
No	99.81	99.76
Yes	0.19	0.24
Gestational hypertension		
No	99.79	99.56
Yes	0.21	0.44
Preeclampsia or eclampsia		
No	98.67	98.92
Yes	1.33	1.08
Infant sex		
Female	45.13	46.02
Male	54.85	53.97
Hermaphrodite	0.02	0.01

[a]*Overall-PTB* all preterm births, *PROM-PTB* preterm birth following premature rupture of membranes, *S-PTB* preterm birth due to spontaneous preterm labor, *MI-PTB* medically induced preterm birth
[b]*APNCU* the adequacy of prenatal care utilization

prenatal care. In China, a pregnant woman at least five prenatal care visits were recommended during pregnancy [21], while the international standard was 7-11 visits [16]. As a result, although proportions of inadequate prenatal care in China declined over time, 71.07% of mothers in our study received insufficient prenatal care. Hence, strengthening access to and delivery of prenatal care remains a critical strategy to help prevent PTB in China.

Future research directions
Still, as for PTB trends in China, several important research questions remain to be answered in the future. First, PTB incidence rates increased in both Shenzhen and Hubei, but whether there were differences in trends between these single centers and China as a whole remains unclear. Second, although we found that changes in maternal age and education drove PTB rates, the pathways for these effects are unclear. Third, the cause of temporal trends in PTB rates is likely to be multifactorial, a result of changing risk factor incidences, clinical practices, and public policies, while few studies have assessed the contribution of these potential drivers.

Strengths and limitations
Several previous studies, including a global estimation and two local investigations in China, have characterized recent trends in their rates of preterm birth overall [2, 9, 10]. Few studies, however, have documented the population-based temporal trends in PTB subtypes, and none has identified the determinants behind these trends. Rising PTB rates have been documented in Hubei, China, and the results of our study confirmed the increasing trends in a developed area of China. To our knowledge, this is the first study to characterize the time trends of PTB subtypes in mainland China, and to explore the reasons behind these trends.

The results of our study were limited by use of routinely collected registry data. This may have resulted in misclassified outcomes for some women. However, the high validity and reliability of the Shenzhen Birth Registry has been previously described [13], and an obstetrician reviewed each of the case records for accuracy, so we anticipate the impact was small. Next, we captured births only among women 13-50 years of age, and so may have missed PTB cases among higher risk ages. Yet, we defined the inclusion criterion according to the mean ages at menarche (12.76 years) and natural menopausal (50.76 years) in the Chinese population [22, 23], and so the impact is likely to have been modest. Third, in the analysis of determinants for PTBs, we also did not consider the association between cigarette smoking rates and PTB trends [24], as these data were unavailable in the birth registry. However, smoking prevalence has been stable in women according to the China National Health Services Survey [21]. A recent study showed that smoking prevalence was only 0.7% among

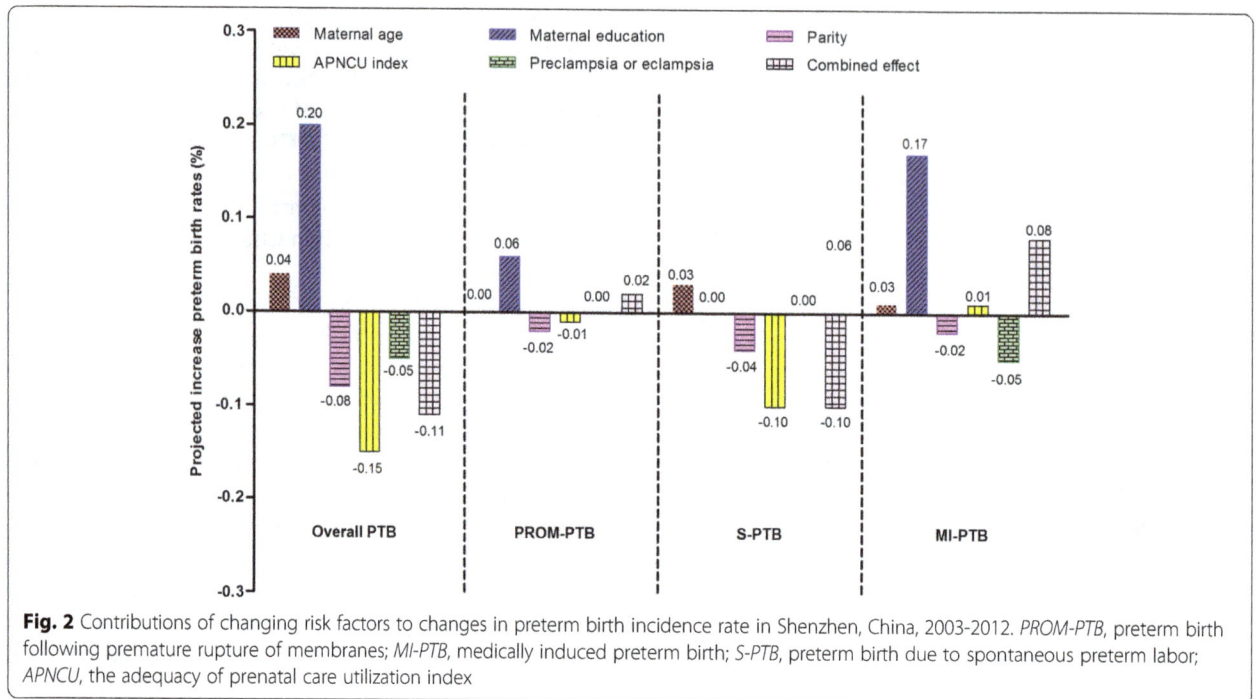

Fig. 2 Contributions of changing risk factors to changes in preterm birth incidence rate in Shenzhen, China, 2003-2012. *PROM-PTB*, preterm birth following premature rupture of membranes; *MI-PTB*, medically induced preterm birth; *S-PTB*, preterm birth due to spontaneous preterm labor; *APNCU*, the adequacy of prenatal care utilization index

women in Shenzhen [25], and so was unlikely to meaningfully bias our results.

Conclusions

In summary, the Shenzhen findings confirm the previous reports of an increasing trend for PTB rates in mainland China. Moreover, this study also suggested that older and more highly educated pregnant woman, should be key target population groups for clinical PTB interventions and public health PTB prevention strategies in developed areas of China. However, considering the wide variation of PTB rates among geographic areas, we suggest caution in generalizing the Shenzhen findings.

Preterm birth rate increased in Shenzhen between 2003 and 2012, yet with varied trends among three PTB subtypes. Maternal age, education, parity and prenatal care visits played important roles in determining secular trends for PTB rates. These findings represent potential targets for interventions or policies designed to reduce PTB. More knowledge on how these factors are associated with PTB in China is needed for shaping future prevention strategies. Our findings also highlight the importance of adequate prenatal care for reducing PTB in China.

Abbreviations

AF_P: Population-attributable risk fraction; *AORs*: Adjusted odds ratios; APC: Annual percent change; APNCU: The adequacy of prenatal care utilization; ART: Assisted reproductive technology; ICSI: Institute for Clinical Systems Improvement; LMP: Date of mother's last menstrual period; MI-PTB: Medically induced preterm birth; Overall-PTB: All preterm births; PROM: following premature rupture of membranes; PTB: Preterm birth; *RR*: Rate ratios; S-PTB: Preterm birth due to spontaneous preterm labor

Acknowledgements

Not applicable.

Funding

This work was supported by the Nature Science Foundation of Guangdong Province (2016A030313216), the Asia-Pacific Network for Global Change (CRRP2016-10MY-Huang).

Authors' contributions

CL and CH conceived of the study and supervised all aspects of its implementation. MB, QW, HZ and XS contributed to conceptualizing ideas and designing the study, QZ, ZL and YL provided input regarding analysis of the data, S.W and W.C interpreted findings, and reviewed drafts of the manuscript. All authors read and approved the final manuscript.

Competing interests

The authors declare that they have no competing interests.

Author details

[1]Department of Health Policy and Management, School of Public Health, Sun Yat-sen University, 74 Zhongshan Road #2, Guangzhou 510080, China. [2]Guangzhou Key Laboratory of Environmental Pollution and Health Risk Assessment, School of Public Health, Sun Yat-sen University, 74 Zhongshan Road #2, Guangzhou 510080, China. [3]Department of Biostatistics and Epidemiology, School of Public Health, Sun Yat-sen University, 74 Zhongshan Road #2, Guangzhou 510080, China. [4]Department of Public Health, Guangdong Women and Children Hospital, 521, 523 Xing Nan Street, Guangzhou 511442, China. [5]Departments of Environmental Health Sciences and Epidemiology and Biostatistics, University at Albany, State University of New York, Rensselaer, USA. [6]Center for Reproductive Medicine, The First Affiliated Hospital of Sun Yat-sen University, 74 Zhongshan Road #2, Guangzhou 510080, China. [7]Department of Children Health Care, Shenzhen Women and Children Hospital, Shenzhen, China.

References

1. Liu L, Oza S, Hogan D, Perin J, Rudan I, Lawn JE, et al. Global, regional, and national causes of child mortality in 2000–13, with projections to inform post-2015 priorities: an updated systematic analysis. Lancet. 2015;385:430–40.
2. Blencowe H, Cousens S, Oestergaard MZ, Chou D, Moller A-B, Narwal R, et al. National, regional, and worldwide estimates of preterm birth rates in the year 2010 with time trends since 1990 for selected countries: a systematic analysis and implications. Lancet. 2012;379:2162–72.
3. World Health Organization: Born too soon: the global action report on preterm birth. 2012.
4. Johnston KM, Gooch K, Korol E, Vo P, Eyawo O, Bradt P, et.al. The economic burden of prematurity in Canada. BMC Pediatr. 2014;14:93.
5. Zeitlin J, Szamotulska K, Drewniak N, Mohangoo A, Chalmers J, Sakkeus L, et al. Preterm birth time trends in Europe: a study of 19 countries. BJOG. 2013; 120:1356–65.
6. Schoen CN, Tabbah S, Iams JD, Caughey AB, Berghella V. Why the United States preterm birth rate is declining. Am J Obstet Gynecol. 2015;213:175–80.
7. Chang HH, Larson J, Blencowe H, Spong CY, Howson CP, Cairns-Smith S, et al. Preventing preterm births: analysis of trends and potential reductions with interventions in 39 countries with very high human development index. Lancet. 2013;381:223–34.
8. Zou L, Wang X, Ruan Y, Li G, Chen Y, Zhang W. Preterm birth and neonatal mortality in China in 2011. Int J Gynecol Obstet. 2014;127:243–7.
9. Xu H, Dai Q, Xu Y, Gong Z, Dai G, Ding M, et al. Time trends and risk factor associated with premature birth and infants deaths due to prematurity in Hubei Province, China from 2001 to 2012. BMC Pregnancy Childbirth. 2015;15:1.
10. Hui ASY, Lao TT, Leung TY, Schaaf JM, Sahota DS. Trends in preterm birth in singleton deliveries in a Hong Kong population. Int J Gynecol Obstet. 2014; 127:248–53.
11. Lackritz EM, Wilson CB, Guttmacher AE, Howse JL, Engmann CM, Rubens CE, et al. A solution pathway for preterm birth: accelerating a priority research agenda. Lancet Glob Health. 2013;1:e328–e30.
12. Morken N-H. Preterm birth: new data on a global health priority. Lancet. 2012;379:2128–30.
13. Liang Z, Lin Y, Ma Y, Zhang L, Zhang X, Li L, et al. The association between ambient temperature and preterm birth in Shenzhen, China: a distributed lag non-linear time series analysis. Environ Health. 2016;15:84.
14. Brown HK, Speechley KN, Macnab J, Natale R, Campbell MK. Neonatal morbidity associated with late preterm and early term birth: the roles of gestational age and biological determinants of preterm birth. Int J Epidemiol. 2014;43:802–14.
15. Partridge S, Balayla J, Holcroft CA, Abenhaim HA. Inadequate prenatal care utilization and risks of infant mortality and poor birth outcome: a retrospective analysis of 28,729,765 U.S. deliveries over 8 years. Amer J Perinatol. 2012;29:787–94.
16. Akkerman D, Cleland L, Croft G, Eskuchen K, Heim C, Levine A, et al. Routine prenatal care. Bloomington: Institute for Clinical Systems Improvement (ICSI); 2012.
17. Kamath-Rayne BD, DeFranco EA, Chung E, Chen A. Subtypes of preterm birth and the risk of Postneonatal death. J Pediatr. 2013;162:28–34. e2
18. Martin JA, Hamilton BE, Osterman MJ. Births in the United States, 2013. NCHS data brief. 2014;175:1–8.
19. Auger N, Le TUN, Park AL, Luo Z-C. Association between maternal comorbidity and preterm birth by severity and clinical subtype: retrospective cohort study. BMC Pregnancy Childbirth. 2011;11:67.
20. Xu XK, Wang YA, Li Z, Lui K, Sullivan EA. Risk factors associated with preterm birth among singletons following assisted reproductive technology in Australia 2007–2009–a population-based retrospective study. BMC Pregnancy Childbirth. 2014;14:1.
21. Center for Health Statistics and Information: An analysis report of National Health Services Survey in China, 2013.
22. Shao HF, Sun DM, Liu J, Tao MF. A survey for reproductive health of postmenopausal women in shanghai. J Reprod Med. 2014;23:703-8.
23. Song Y, Ma J, Hu P, Zhang B. Geographic distribution and secular trend of menarche in 9-18 year-old Chinese Han girls. Beijing Da Xue Xue Bao. 2011; 43:360–4.
24. Meijer WJ, Noortwijk AG, Bruinse HW, Wensing AM. Influenza virus infection in pregnancy: a review. Acta Obstet Gynecol Scand. 2015;94:797–819.
25. Mou J, Fellmeth G, Griffiths S, Dawes M, Cheng J. Tobacco smoking among migrant factory workers in Shenzhen, China. Nicotine Tob Res. 2013;15:69–76.

5

Improving usability and pregnancy rates of a fertility monitor by an additional mobile application

Martin C. Koch[1][*], Johannes Lermann[1], Niels van de Roemer[2], Simone K. Renner[1], Stefanie Burghaus[1], Janina Hackl[1], Ralf Dittrich[1], Sven Kehl[1], Patricia G. Oppelt[1], Thomas Hildebrandt[1], Caroline C. Hack[1], Uwe G. Pöhls[3], Stefan P. Renner[1] and Falk C. Thiel[4]

Abstract

Background: Daysy is a fertility monitor that uses the fertility awareness method by tracking and analyzing the individual menstrual cycle. In addition, Daysy can be connected to the application DaysyView to transfer stored personal data from Daysy to a smartphone or tablet (IOS, Android). This combination is interesting because as it is shown in various studies, the use of apps is increasing patients' focus on their disease or their health behavior. The aim of this study was to investigate if by the additional use of an App and thereby improved usability of the medical device, it is possible to enhance the typical-use related as well as the method-related pregnancy rates.

Result: In the resultant group of 125 women (2076 cycles in total), 2 women indicated that they had been unintentionally pregnant during the use of the device, giving a typical-use related Pearl-Index of 1.3. Counting only the pregnancies which occurred as a result of unprotected intercourse during the infertile (green) phase, we found 1 pregnancy, giving a method-related Pearl-Index of 0.6. Calculating the pregnancy rate resulting from continuous use and unprotected intercourse exclusively on green days, gives a perfect-use Pearl-Index of 0.8.

Conclusion: It seems that combining a specific biosensor-embedded device (Daysy), which gives the method a very high repeatable accuracy, and a mobile application (DaysyView) which leads to higher user engagement, results in higher overall usability of the method.

Keywords: Female contraception, Fertility monitor, Mobile application, Body basal temperature, Fertility awareness based method, FABM

Plain English summary

The menstrual cycle is one of the characteristic physiological processes of the female body and it is a central indicator of overall health in women of reproductive age. Continuous fluctuations of hormones result in commensurable physiological changes throughout the menstrual cycle. In the last decade, specific biosensor-embedded devices have been developed to assist women in monitoring, measuring and representing these aspects of their body. For such devices, the typical-use related pregnancy rate is still low but was significantly worse than the method-related pregnancy rate. This implies that usability and understanding of a method plays a major role in a fertility monitoring device and its safe effective use. It is reported, that trough the additional use of a mobile application the interest and motivation of a patient's health behavior increases significantly. The contraceptive effectiveness of the fertility monitor (Daysy) has already been demonstrated in an independent trial. The result of the **method related Pearl-Index** calculation obtained in the present study (0,6) differs only a little from what is reported by Freundl and colleges (0,7). However, if the

---
* Correspondence: martin.koch@uk-erlangen.de
[1]Universitätsklinikum Erlangen, Frauenklinik, Universitaetsstrasse 21-23, 91054 Erlangen, Germany
Full list of author information is available at the end of the article

focus is on the **typical-use related Pearl-Index**, it has significantly improved from 3,8 to 1,3. Independently, the **perfect-use efficacy (0,8)** of Daysy was calculated in this study.

We conclude, that it is possible through the present technology of Daysy and the additional, optional use of DaysyView to improve usability and enhance the typical- , method- and perfect -use pregnancy rates.

Background

The menstrual cycle is one of the characteristic physiological processes of the female body and it is a central indicator of overall health in women of reproductive age. Continuous fluctuations of hormones result in commensurable physiological changes throughout the menstrual cycle [1]. These include fluctuation in urine luteinizing hormone (LH), cervical mucus and body basal temperature (BBT). Women have been engaging in monitoring these physiological changes as signs of their fertility for many years. In the past, they have charted different signs of their menstrual cycle (temperature rise, cervical mucus changes) to determine the onset as well as the end of the fertile phase by pencil and paper (Symptothermal Method) [2]. In the last decade, specific biosensor-embedded devices have been developed to assist women in monitoring, measuring and representing these aspects of their body.

Most of these devices use a combination of BBT measurement and sophisticated statistical methods in addition to a comprehensive on-board database to identify the fertile and infertile phase of the menstrual cycle [3]. Other devices use the correlation between pulse rate and the menstrual phases to determine the individual fertile window [4]. The medical device Daysy (Valley Electronics AG, Zurich, Switzerland) is an electronic device that also exploits the described relationship between the menstrual cycle and fluctuations in body temperature by measuring and recording the BBT as an aid in ovulation prediction for planning and preventing pregnancy by identifying the fertile and infertile phase of the menstrual cycle. Since the advent of fertility monitors, the reliability and safety of such devices has been tested in different clinical trials [2, 3, 5, 6]. For example, in their retrospective clinical trial, Freundl, et al., concluded that the fertility monitors Babycomp and Ladycomp achieved a method-related Pearl-Index (PI) of 0.7 and a typical-use related PI of 3.8 over 12 months, placing in a similar safety range as the natural family planning method (NFP) [5].

Since Daysy is based on the fertility algorithm of Babycomp and Ladycomp from Valley Electronics GmbH, it was claimed that Daysy has a similar PI to these products that are ultimately bounded by the fertility awareness-based method (FABM) itself.

For some contraceptive methods, such as sterilization or copper intrauterine devices (IUD), the inherent efficacy is extremely high and proper that extreme low pregnancy rates are found in all studies (Table 1).

For the remaining methods, the typical-use related pregnancy rate is still low but was significantly worse than the perfect-use related pregnancy rate (Table 1). This implies that usability and understanding of a method plays a major role in a fertility monitoring device and its safe effective use. It is reported that through the additional use of a mobile application (app), the interest and motivation of a patient's health behavior increases significantly [7]. One reason is that people have the tendency to interact with, or check, their mobile devices regularly; this repeated reviewing is reinforced by immediate visible information [8].

Tracking of menstrual cycles via app has been announced to be a common form of self-monitoring to either avoid or achieve pregnancy. In the United States about 80% of 18–49 year olds own a smart phone and approximately 28% are using mobile healthcare apps. Of 90.088 healthcare apps in the Apple iTunes store, 7% (6300) are for women's health and pregnancy (Institute for Healthcare Informatics). Mobile fertility apps gain support, but the majority are lacking clinical evidence [9]. A current study reported by Setton and colleagues, concluded that apps used to predict the fertile window and dates of ovulation are generally inaccurate [10]. One reason is that there is a wide variation in each menstrual cycle. Even in women with a "perfect" 28-day cycle, the fertile window varies from cycle to cycle [11]. However, until the present time, no study has been reported considering the contraceptive effectiveness of a fertility monitor (Daysy) optionally connected with an App (DaysyView). This combination is interesting because as described above, it is shown in various studies that the use of apps is increasing patients´ focus on their disease or their health behavior. Mobile displays were effective in encouraging users to maintain activity level, and reminder notifications aimed at goal achievement were desirable features [12–16].

Table 1 % of woman experiencing an unintended pregnancy

Method	Typical-use related pregnancy rates % (Usage Safety)	Perfect-use pregnancy rates % (Method Safety)
Vasectomy [29]	0.15	0.10
IUD with Copper [29]	0.8	0.6
Oral Contraceptive/Pill [29]	9	0.3
Fertility App [25]	8.3	n/a
Natural Family Planning [2]	1.8	0.4
Male Condom [29]	18	2
Diaphragm [29]	12	6

In this study, we presented that through the additional use of an App and thereby improved usability of the medical device, it is possible to enhance the typical-use as well as the method-related pregnancy rates.

Methods

Digital fertility monitor

Daysy is developed and manufactured by Valley Electronics AG, and it is sold worldwide. The core technology for Daysy is based upon that of LadyComp and BabyComp and Pearly as developed by Valley Electronics GmbH. The function of the portable medical device is based on the thermal method, where BBT is measured orally in 30–60s at rest and immediately after waking up.

Daysy has an embedded temperature sensor that measures the temperature at a rate of 1/100 of a degree precision. In the first three cycles, Daysy "learns" to identify fertile days by an algorithm that had been created on the basis of validation group. The algorithm is created from a combination of two elements - tracking and learning new data (the daily basal body temperature, menstruation start and end date, accumulated historical cycle data) and statistical methods (eg. the temperature rise after ovulation), calculated from the database of real menstrual cycle data. A sustained increase of at least 0.2 °C at the expected time of ovulation is necessary to determine a temperature shift by the algorithm.

Further, this algorithm uses statistical methods based on the previous cycles to provide a prognosis of the ovulation data upon which the users can act. It then compares the predicted date to the calculated ovulation date at the end of a cycle to update its model. Therefore, these devices can provide relevant data to be used for improving the chances of successful conception. Daysy is a tool of the so-called fertility awareness-based method. These types of tools do not control contraception, but rather use quantitative data and statistical models based on this data to advise the users to be aware of the fertile days. During these days, one must use an alternative form of contraceptive such as a barrier method (condom, diaphragm, etc.) to avoid pregnancy or abstain from sexual intercourse, as practiced by the NFP method, to avoid pregnancy.

In Europe, Daysy is classified as a class I medical device according to the council directive 93/42/EEC of June 1993 according to Rule 5 of Annex IX. According to EN ISO 62304:2006, the software in Daysy is classified as class A: No injury or damage to health is possible. The user interface for Daysy is designed to be simple and easy to use. It consists of an embedded temperature sensor for taking measurements orally, a single button, a buzzer, a communication jack, and a series of colored LEDs. The fertility status and device state are displayed to the user through the LEDs. Daysy does not display the user's temperature.

Depending if the user wants to conceive or prevent a pregnancy, the color LED on Daysy can be acted upon different ways: a green LED indicates "infertile", a red LED indicates "fertile" and a yellow LED indicates "unsure."

The app DaysyView

DaysyView is a free mobile app that augments the Daysy fertility monitor.

With the app, users can choose to transfer their stored data from Daysy to a smartphone or tablet (IOS, Android). This information can then be viewed graphically by the user in a more convenient form.

DaysyView is a program for displaying data related to a woman's menstrual cycle to aid in ovulation prediction. It can be used stand-alone to log and display a graphical representation of this data, or in conjunction with Daysy to display the fertility status as well.

When paired with Daysy, DaysyView shows the previous, current and estimated fertility status of the user once the data has been synchronized. Further, DaysyView enables a detailed overview of a woman's individual menstrual cycle, temperature curves and numerous statistics. The app offers the opinion to share cycle information with medical or internal professionals to give the user individual advice or support.

Aim of the study

Methods of fertility awareness are often described as unsecure and scientifically not sufficiently evaluated. The aim of this study was to evaluate feasability, satisfaction and failure rate of the described FAB-method. By investigating the (unplanned) pregnancy rate and additional used contraceptive methods, the PI is calculated by standard approach concerning the safety of the method (perfect- and method-related pregnancy rates) and concerning the individual woman (typical-use related pregnancy rate). Anamnestic factors i.e. weight, height and cycle length/ regularity of patients are taken into account to detect possible weaknesses of this FAB-method.

Study design

All Daysy international purchasers which are already registered and having a DaysyView account, received an invitation via email. The invitation included a hyperlink to an online questionnaire (Additional file 1) as well as information about the content of the trial. A "reminder" to participate was sent out in the middle of the study period.

Study participants had to finish the questionnaire completely and in a true manner. The study was conducted between November 1st and December 31st 2016. In this period 6278 surveys were sent to eligible participants.

Every participant agreed to share her data anonymously for this research performed by the company and external researchers. The data was stored by the company under the serial number of Daysy. Only the principal scientists and medical professionals of the University Medicine Erlangen, University Medicine Mainz, and research staff of Valley Electronic AG had access to the stored personal data. The survey did not include any personal data except date of birth, height and weight. Among others, the survey included questions related to the individual cycle, means of contraception, occurrence of pregnancy and the additional use of the app.

The study protocol was reviewed and authorized by the regional ethics committee (FAU/ Erlangen/ 276_16B).

Statistical analysis
Pearl index
Evaluation of the fertility monitor effectiveness was based on the PI calculation.

It reflects the number of unintended pregnancies among all the cumulative years of exposure to unintended pregnancy [17]. The PI represents the number of failures per 100 woman-years exposure. According to literature, there are two methods to calculate the PI:

(i) The number of pregnancies is divided by the total number of months of exposure from the start of the method until the completion of the study. The quotient is multiplied by 1200 if the denominator is reported in months.

(ii) The number of pregnancies is divided by the total number of cycles of the users of a given method. The quotient is multiplied by 1300 if the denominator is reported in cycles.

In the present study, the second method, based on cycles, was used to calculate the PI due to the fact that the participants supplied information on the number of cycles.

The perfect-use as well as the method and typical-use related pregnancy rate (PI) was calculated separately.

Kaplan-Meier
One major problem of the PI is that it does not account for duration of exposure; the PI is reasonably reflective of contraception failure if duration of use is short (i.e. 6 to 12 months) and most users use the method for about the period of time [18]. In a life-table analysis or (in this case equivalently) the Kaplan-Meier approach, a separate failure rate is calculated for each month of use such that varying durations of use are not problematic. The result

at observation cycle 13 can roughly be compared to the PI. The Kaplan-Meier approach was used to calculate the overall effectiveness rates. Pregnancy due to both typical-usage safety as well as the method failure were included in the calculation [19, 20].

Pregnancy classification
As the basis for the calculation of the **perfect-use related PI** we used a modified model of Trussel and Grummer-Strawn for the calculation [21]. Thus, only women who have indicated that they were sexual active (> 13 cycles) but had no unprotected intercourse on a fertile "red" or "yellow" days shown by the fertility monitor were considered. Pregnancy rates during perfect use show how effective the fertility monitor can be, where perfect use is defined as following the direction of the fertility monitor. Due to the retrospective character of this study, it was not mandatory for participants to log whether and when they had protected/unprotected intercourse or the pregnancy intention before each cycle.

Unplanned pregnancies that are included to calculate the **typical-use related PI** have to be a result of a user error, namely having unprotected sexual intercourse on a "red" or "yellow" day, regardless of whether the user resorts to an additional contraceptive method. Pregnancy rates during typical-use shows how effective the fertility monitor is during actual use (including inconsistent or incorrect use).

Unplanned pregnancies that are included to calculate the **method-related PI** have to be a result of an absolute method error, or more exactly: An unplanned pregnancy has to be the result of unprotected intercourse on a "green day" shown by the fertility monitor (independent of inconsistent or incorrect use).

A general rule was: If a participant has indicated that she has become unintentionally pregnant, it was verified directly from the user's dataset. The definition of a pregnancy was an elevated temperature of longer than 18 days, or if the user stopped using the device within the luteal phase.

Results
Within the study 6278 contacted women, 1969 (31%) followed the invitation and 798 (13%) completed the survey. The total number of recorded cycles was 4738. The average age of participants was 29 years (Fig. 1a), whereby the fertility monitor was mainly used to avoid pregnancy (74.68% see Fig. 1b). Because the size and weight of the participants were queried, it was possible to determine the body mass index (BMI; kg/m [2]), which was 23.02 on average (Fig. 1c). Women over 25 years had a significantly elevated BMI compared to women between 20 and 25 years (Fig. 1c) in this study.

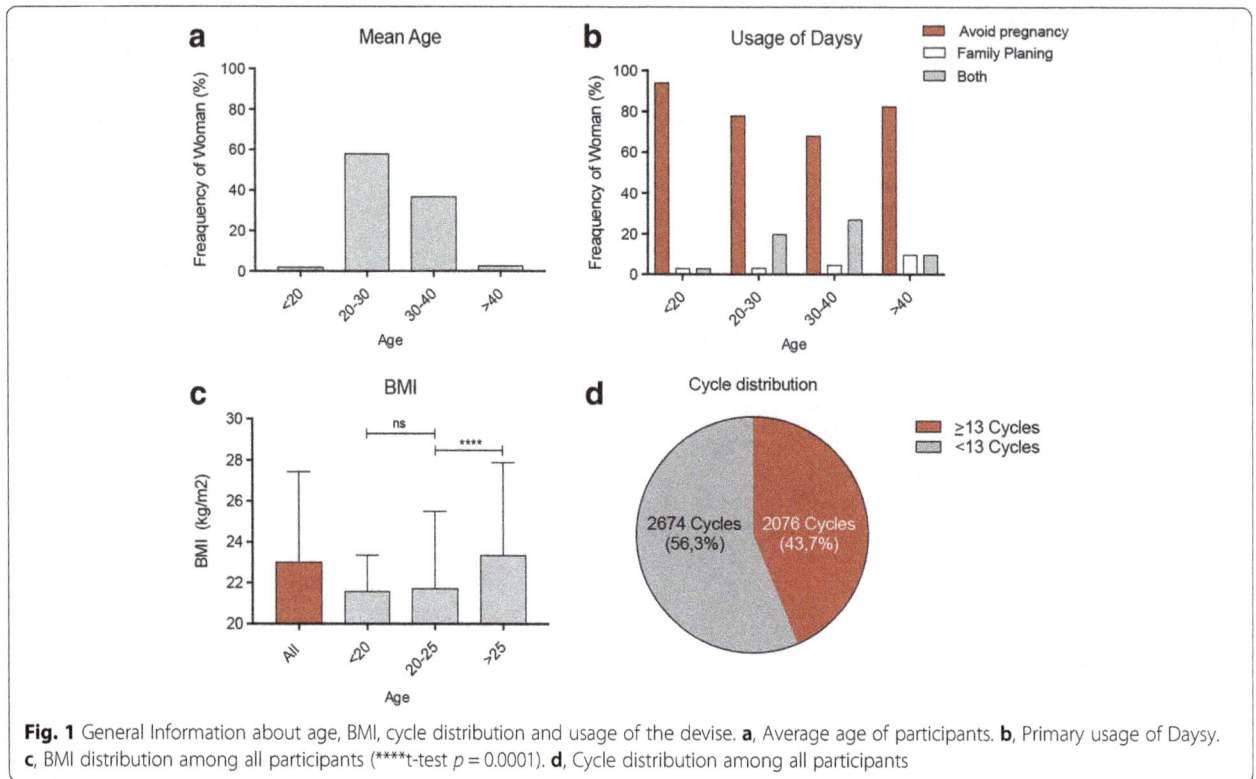

Fig. 1 General Information about age, BMI, cycle distribution and usage of the devise. **a**, Average age of participants. **b**, Primary usage of Daysy. **c**, BMI distribution among all participants (****t-test $p = 0.0001$). **d**, Cycle distribution among all participants

From 798 participating women, 524 (64%) indicated an additional contraceptive use (Fig. 2a). Out of the 493 respondents using additional precaution methods, 73% (358 out of 493) used the method during the fertile (red) phase, 22% (109 out of 493) used the method during the fertile and the infertile (green) phase of the menstrual cycle and 6% (27 out of 493) stated to use the additional method inconsistently (Fig. 2b). The analysis of the data showed that the male condom (93%) was the most

common additional contraceptive (Fig. 2c). Among the 493 women using an additional contraceptive method, 110 (22%) preferred several forms of contraception.

From a total number of 798 women using the fertility monitor for family planning, contraception or both, a total of 4750 cycles were identified. Through the internal database, all cycle data were double checked for their correctness. In five cases, the correctness (due to the lack of the serial number of the device) of the data could

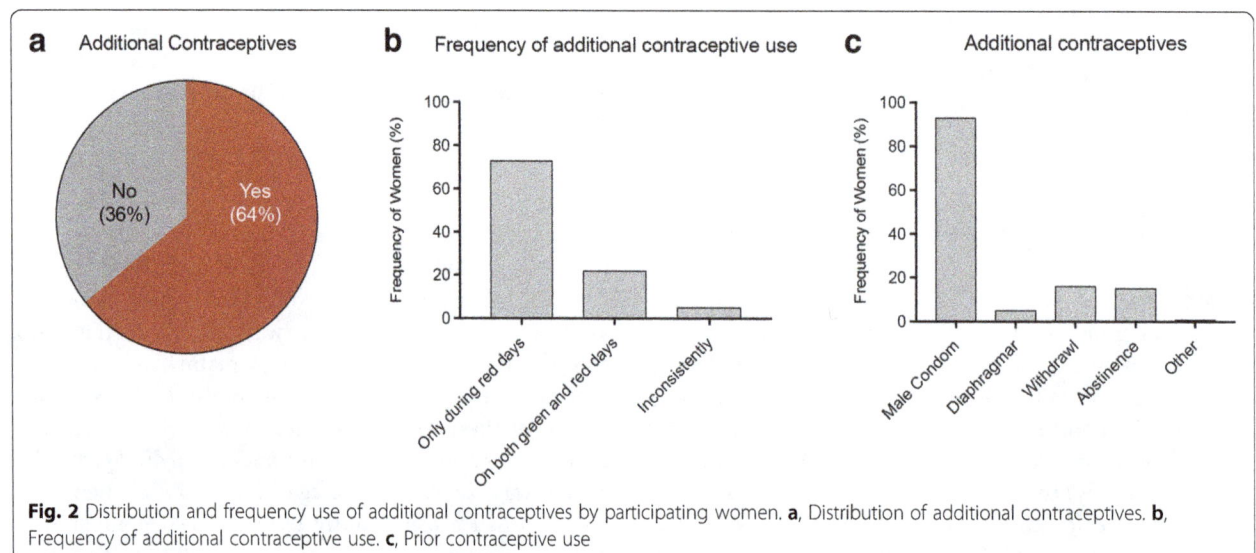

Fig. 2 Distribution and frequency use of additional contraceptives by participating women. **a**, Distribution of additional contraceptives. **b**, Frequency of additional contraceptive use. **c**, Prior contraceptive use

not be confirmed, these participants were excluded from the study.

668 respondents (2674 cycles in total) declared they had been using the fertility monitor for < 13 cycles (Fig. 1d). Their data was not taken into account when calculating the PI. Furthermore, 125 respondents (2076 cycles in total) reported they had been using the fertility monitor for > 13 cycles (Fig.1d). Among these 125 women, 2 women indicated that they had been unintentionally pregnant during the use of the device. Therefore, the total pregnancy- or typical-use related pregnancy rate is 2 × 1300 / 2076, which equals a PI of 1.252.

Counting only the pregnancies which occurred as a result of unprotected intercourse during the infertile (green) phase, we found 1 pregnancy, giving a method-related pregnancy rate of 0.626 according to the PI. To further calculate the perfect-use related pregnancy rate we calculate all cycles (1725 in total) in which the user was sexually active but stated to have had no unprotected intercourse on red (fertile) days for > 13 cycles. Therefore, the perfect-use pregnancy rate is 1 × 1300 / 1725, which equals a PI of 0.753.

The life-table shows for each month what the probability is that a woman becomes pregnant, as well as the typical-use related pregnancies by cycle (Table 2). The overall pregnancy-rates and its 95% confidence interval (CI) were calculated according to the Kaplan-Meier approach [19, 20]. The analysis shows that after 13 cycles of exposure, the typical-use related probability of an unintended pregnancy was 2.707% (Fig. 3 blue line). Focusing on women who claimed to have always had protected intercourse (independent of the fertility status), the probability of an unintended pregnancy decreases (n/s) to 1.92% after 13 cycles (Fig. 3 black line). The same value increases significantly to 10.82% probability if a woman is considered to have had unprotected intercourse on red (fertile) as well as on green (infertile) days (Fig. 3 imperfect use). If a woman had unprotected intercourse exclusively on green days (perfect-use related pregnancy rate), the probability of an unintended pregnancy was 2.19% (Fig. 3 perfect-use).

The average cycle length of all participants was 28.9 (± 3.52 SD) days. A closer analysis of the different age groups shows a significant difference in the cycle lengths (Fig. 4a). Thus, the length of the cycle decreases with increasing duration. The same trend is evident when women were asked for irregular cycles. When a fluctuation of 3–4 days is considered to be normal, 195 respondents (24.24%) reported to have irregular cycles. When women under 20 years are focused, the percentage of irregular cycles increases (41.18%). Because of the small number of participants under 20 ($n = 17$), the result is not significant (Fig. 4b). We found that when focusing all participants ($n = 798$) that 94.7% have a menstruation between 2 and 7 days. The result differs somewhat when only woman over 40 ($n = 22$) are considered. In this fraction of women, 10% (n = 2) have indicated that their menstruation lasts less than two days (Fig. 4c).

In the third section of the survey, women were asked if they used Daysy to get pregnant. Out of the whole cohort of 798 women, 69 (9.01%) answered the question with –yes-. Because according to the manufacturer, at least 3 cycles are required to precisely determine the fertile window, only woman with ≥ 3 (51 out of 69) cycles were considered for further evaluation. Among the 46 woman having sexual intercourse specifically on fertile (red) days, 18 (39.%) pregnancies were reported. In all cases, it took less than 1 year until the user conceived. For those who have not been pregnant while using Daysy, 6 (21.42%) already tried to conceive unsuccessfully before using the fertility monitor. A surprising observation was that of the women that wanted to become pregnant with the fertility monitor, 21.42% already had experience with NFP. Focusing all users, 40 out of 798 (5.01%) already had experience with NFP.

Regardless of for what the device was used, 90 out of 798 (11.2%) women reported to have experienced an abortion or miscarriage.

789 out of 798 (99%) of the questioned users would recommend the device to their friends. Surprisingly even the women who became unintentionally pregnant while

Table 2 Rate of unplanned pregnancies

Cycle #	Woman exposed	Cumulative Pregnancy	Cumulative pregnancy probability (%)	CI, lower Limit (%)	CI, upper Limit (%)
1	696	4	0.57	1.57	0.18
3	518	5	0.77	1.84	0.29
4	442	6	0.99	2.14	0.43
9	206	8	1.47	2.76	0.76
10	173	9	2.04	3.47	1.17
11	147	10	2,71	4.28	1.68
13	125	10	2,71	4.28	1.68

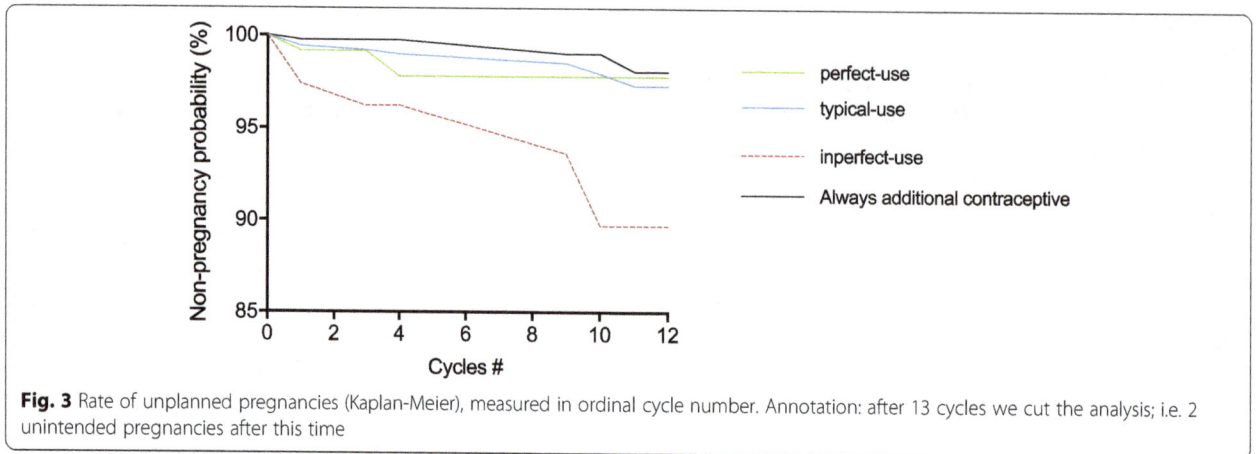

Fig. 3 Rate of unplanned pregnancies (Kaplan-Meier), measured in ordinal cycle number. Annotation: after 13 cycles we cut the analysis; i.e. 2 unintended pregnancies after this time

using the fertility monitor would recommend the device to a friend.

One of the main hypotheses of this study was that through the additional use of an App, and thereby improved usability of the medical device, it is possible to enhance the usage safety as well as the method safety rate. For this we asked the participating women about the frequency as well as the apprehension effect of the app. We found, that 516 out of 798 (64.66%) use the additional app DaysyView in a daily, 239 (29.24%) weekly and 44 (5.51%) monthly manner (Fig. 5). On closer inspection, it is noticeable that the usage decreases with the number of cycles. Thus, after 4 cycles, 74% of the women spent time daily by using the app, this frequency drops by 20% to 51% after 13 or more cycles. In return, the weekly and monthly usage increases (Fig. 5).

In addition, 84% of the participants indicated that they achieved a better understanding of themselves and their cycle through the additional use of the app DaysyView.

Because sharing data is a key opinion of apps, we also ask if DaysyView users use this option. Interestingly, 506 out of 798 (63.2%) woman stated that they shared personal cycle data with their partner, friends or healthcare professionals.

1 year after the study was started (November 1st, 2016) the status of 776 (98%) DaysyView accounts is "Ready", therefore DaysyView and the fertility monitor Daysy are still in use. 20 (2%) accounts and the corresponding serial numbers of the fertility monitor have been deleted from the server. Of the 778 remaining accounts, 618 (79%) were synchronized with the fertility monitor after June 1st 2017.

Discussion

The contraceptive effectiveness of fertility monitors has already been demonstrated in different trials [3]. Since the Daysy algorithm is identical to the fertility algorithm of Babycomp and Ladycomp from Valley Electronics GmbH it was claimed that Daysy has a similar method as well as typical-use related PI to these products (The perfect-use related PI was not part of the previous study). The result of the **method-related PI** calculation obtained in the present study (0.63) is comparable to that advertised by the manufacturer and differs only a little from what is reported by Freundl and colleges (0.7) [5]. However, if the focus is on the **typical-use related PI**, it has improved from 3.8 to 1.25. There are three

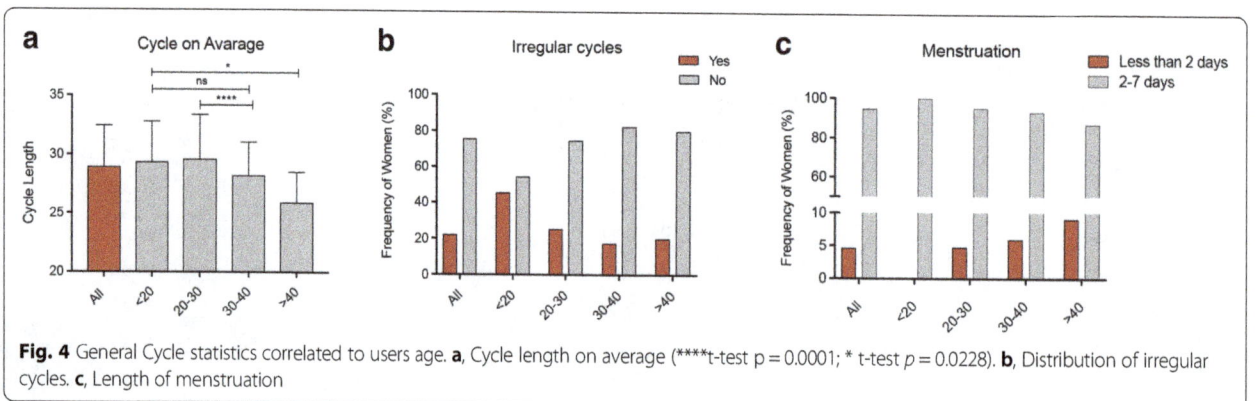

Fig. 4 General Cycle statistics correlated to users age. **a**, Cycle length on average (****t-test p = 0.0001; * t-test *p* = 0.0228). **b**, Distribution of irregular cycles. **c**, Length of menstruation

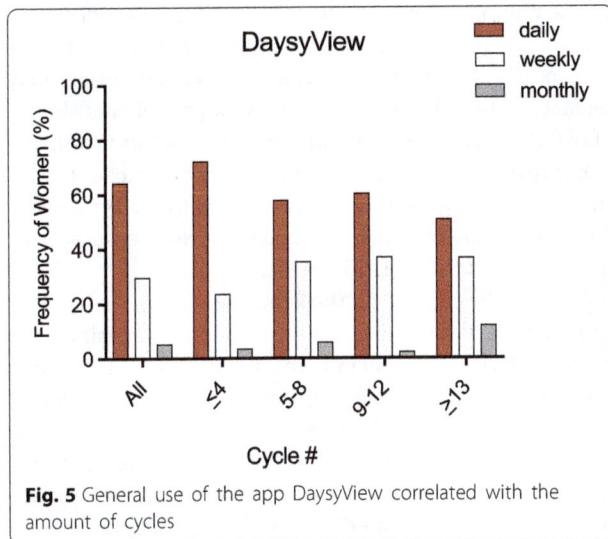

Fig. 5 General use of the app DaysyView correlated with the amount of cycles

reasons for the enhanced effectiveness of the fertility monitor Daysy. (1) It has been over 20 years since the research of Freundl et al. was published. The software, as well as the shape of the device, has improved and the amount of historical data has increased. (2) The sociodemographic characteristic of the users has changed. In 1997 Freundl reported, that 69% of the participants are between 19 and 29 years old. In the current study, this fraction decreases by 11% while the fraction of 30–39 years-old increases by 10% to 37%. As it is already shown across all methods, contraceptive failures were significantly higher among younger woman (those younger than 25) than among older peers [22] (3). The calculated value for the cycle computers Babycomp and Ladycomp means they are highly effective in recognizing the different phases of the menstrual cycle and their usage is connected with the risk similar to that of other known contraceptive methods.

The perfect-use related PI was 0.8. Considering the life-table analysis it was 2.19%. This results in the possibility to compare the effectiveness of the fertility monitor Daysy with current other study results focusing on fertility awareness-based methods. Compared to other methods based on FABM, the Daysy fertility monitor positions itself at the upper end [23, 24]. However, for the remaining methods, the typical-use related pregnancy rate is worse than the perfect-use related pregnancy rate. Looking at the fertility monitor examined here, one notices that the typical- and perfect-use related pregnancy rates are much closer together. Basically, there are two possible explanations for improved result. (1) Most of the fertility awareness based methods require that female users observe or measure their signs of fertility and transmit them accordingly for evaluation. This can lead to interpretation or rounding errors which are reflected in the typical-use of the method. With a perfect-use

related PI of 1 the algorithm used by an contraceptive mobile app has a very high safety [25]. If the typical-use related PI of 6.9 is considered, it becomes clear that the user in itself represents the greatest risk (which is our main hypothesis). The Fertility Monitor Daysy avoids this risk, women measure their basal temperature, which is stored on the device and automatically transmitted if necessary. This excludes rounding or interpretation errors. (2) The usability and understanding of a method plays a major role in a fertility monitoring device and its safe effective use. In the present study, users had the opportunity to use the additional app DaysyView as a display of their cycle data and thereby improve the usability of the medical device. Applications have the advantage of being available throughout the day, and they have the further ability to visualize complex cycle data in a simplified form. In the current study, the app DaysyView was used by 65% of the participants daily. Further, 84% of the participants indicated that they achieved a better understanding of themselves and their cycle through the additional use of the app DaysyView. The disadvantage of the app is that there is a kind of "wear-effect". Thus, after 13 cycles, the daily use drops down to 51%. One reason could be that users are better acquainted with the method and they do not need a daily observation of their cycle any longer. Another reason could be that female users have a greater confidence in the fertility monitor, so that a visual check of the fertility status is no longer considered necessary.

One year after the survey started, 98% of the participants' accounts were still active. If only the accounts that continue to be synchronized with the fertility monitor after 1st June 2017 are considered, it is still 79%. One way of explaining this discrepancy is, like already discussed above, that female users continue to use the fertility monitor, but no longer synchronize with the app. Another possibility is that, for pregnancy reasons, users do not use the fertility monitor during this time, and therefore do not synchronize further. Since participants only agreed during the period of the study (November 1st and December 31st 2016) that scientists had access to their data, this hypothesis could not be verified and will be part of further research.

The main reason for failure was unprotected (54%) as well as protected (46%) intercourse during the fertile phase (red days). As it is shown in Fig. 3 (inperfect-use) for the risk-taking women who had unprotected intercourse during the fertile time, the pregnancy probability increases significantly up to 10.82% after 13 cycles. This result is roughly comparable with the result that was found investigating the symptothermal method in 2007. It was reported that for this fraction who had unprotected intercourse during the fertile time, the pregnancy probability increases up to 7.5% per year [2].

In the current study, only 2 women indicated that they had unprotected intercourse during the infertile (green) phase and received an unintentional pregnancy. The probability of an unwanted pregnancy in this fraction is 2.2% which is slightly higher (n/s) than the incidence of women who have always used an additional contraceptive method (1.92%).

As already described: Through the digital analysis of temperature data, fertility monitors can reduce the risk of inaccurate or misinterpretation (as it is done by a computer) of fertility indicators and they can remind the user that a pregnancy risk exists on fertile (red) days but they cannot reduce the risk of the additional contraceptive methods or unprotected intercourse. It must be noted, that unwanted pregnancy is not a harm arising from the application of the device. It is a risk of FABM per se. Using fertility awareness-based methods means accepting this risk.

As discussed in the late 1970s, traditional BBT is not very effective in predicting the ovulation window to aid in conception [26]. This is because the method is only able to estimate the ovulation date after the fact. The software in Daysy uses statistical methods based on the previous cycles to provide a prognosis of the ovulation data upon which the users can act. It then compares the predicted date to the calculated ovulation date at the end of a cycle to update its model.

Daysy was used to achieve pregnancy in 9% of the participants. In 38% of cases there was a pregnancy within one year. Daysy was used on average for 8.5 months until the user conceived. Two studies showed that the fertility rates are perhaps higher than what we found in the current study. In the report published by Wang and colleagues, the authors found that – 50% became clinically pregnant in the first 2 cycles and > 90% in the first 6 cycles [27]. Another study analyzes the time to conception using FAB methods, and finds that for a fertile woman using FABM, the estimated cumulative probability of conception at 1, 3, 6, and 12 cycles was 38, 68, 81, and 92% [28].

The reason that our findings differ from the other results is that the largest share (70%) used Daysy for both, family planning as well as avoiding pregnancy (Fig. 1b). Thus, we don't exactly know when they "start" family planning.

Obviously, many women are convinced by this technology: 99% would recommend the device to their friends. Even all of the women who became unintentionally pregnant while using the fertility monitor would still recommend the device.

Limitations of the study

The retrospective design is a very time efficient and elegant way of answering new questions with existing data. The primary disadvantage of the retrospective study design is the limited control the researchers have over the data collection. The information provided by the participants may be inaccurate or biased by the fact that participants already know the device. To counter incorrect information, the data provided by the participants were double checked for their correctness from comparison with the internal database. With this measure, it could be further ensured that no doubts had taken part in the survey.

Another limitation of the study was that the fertility monitor Daysy is short time on the market, since the middle of 2014. By default, the majority of participants used the device less then 13 cycles (686 out of 798 or 2674 cycles in total). However, 125 respondents (2076 cycles in total) reported that they had been using the fertility monitor for more than 13 cycles. Thus, the typical-use and method-related PI could be calculated correctly. Due to the retrospective nature of the study, it was not possible to determine when and how often users had sexual intercourse on basis of each cycle. Thus, the calculation of the perfect-use pregnancy rate could only be calculated by analyzing all cycles in which the fertility monitor was correctly used. According to Trussel and Grummer-Strawn this could lead to a downwarded bias [21].

Conclusions

We conclude that it is possible through the present technology of Daysy and the additional, optional use of DaysyView, to improve usability and enhance the usage safety as well as the method safety rate. Therefore, it seems that combining a specific biosensor-embedded device, which gives the method a very high repeatable accuracy, and a mobile application which leads to higher user engagement results in higher overall usability of the method.

Abbreviations
App: Application; BBT: Basal Body Temperature; BMI: Body Mass Index; CI: Confidence Interval; etc.: et cetera; FABM: Fertility Awareness Based Methods; Fig.: Figure; iOS: i Operating System; IUD: Intrauterine Device; LED: ILight-emitting Diode; LH: Luteinizing Hormone; n/c: Not significant; NFP: Natural Family Planning; PI: Pearl-Index; SD: Standard Deviation; Tab.: Table

Acknowledgements
We thank Jessica Griger & Andrea De Groot for critical reading, advice and online support. JG is an employee at the Valley Electronics LLC, Maryland and has proofread the manuscript. ADG is a freelance customer service representative at the Valley Electronics AG and helped to design the questionnaire.
We also thank all women participating in this clinical trial.

Funding
This study was funded by the Valley Electronics AG, Zurich, Switzerland. NvdR is an internal scientist and employee of the company. NvdR analyzed the stored data. There are no other relationships or activities that could appear to have influenced the submitted work.

Capsule
With the fertility monitor Daysy and the additional use of a mobile application (DaysyView) improved usability as well as the pregnancy rates can be achieved.

Authors' contributions
SK, JL, SKR, SB, CCH and JH have substantially contributed to data acquisition and were revising it critically for important intellectual content. RD, PGO, TH, UGP and SKR substantially contributed to conception and design of the study and interpretation of data and were revising it critically for important intellectual content. MCK, FCT and NvdR substantially contributed to data acquisition, analysis and interpretation of the data, as well as conception of the study and drafting the article. All Authors gave the final approval for publication of the underlying version.

Competing interests
We have read and understood BMJ policy on declaration of interests and declare the following interests: This study was funded by the Valley Electronics AG, Zurich, Switzerland. NvdR is an internal scientist and employee of the company. NvdR analyzed the stored data. "All authors have completed the ICMJE uniform disclosure form at www.icmje.org/coi_disclosure.pdf and declare: no support from any organization for the submitted work, NvdR is employee at the Valley Electronics AG, Zurich; no other relationships or activities that could appear to have influenced the submitted work."

Author details
[1]Universitätsklinikum Erlangen, Frauenklinik, Universitaetsstrasse 21-23, 91054 Erlangen, Germany. [2]Valley Electronics AG, Marienstraße 16, 8003 Zurich, Switzerland. [3]Praxis, Kaiserstraße 26, 97070 Würzburg, Germany. [4]Klinik am Eichert, Frauenklinik, Eichertstraße 3, 73035 Göppingen, Germany.

References
1. Owen M. Physiological signs of ovulation and fertility readily observable by women. Linacre Q. 2013;80:17–23.
2. Frank-Herrmann P, et al. The effectiveness of a fertility awareness based method to avoid pregnancy in relation to a couple's sexual behaviour during the fertile time: a prospective longitudinal study. Hum Reprod. 2007;22:1310–9.
3. Freundl G, Frank-Herrmann P. G. C. Cycle monitors and devices in natural family planning. Endokrinol. 2010;7:90–6.
4. Shilaih M, de Clerck V, Falco L, Kübler F, Leeners B. Pulse rate measurement during sleep using wearable sensors, and its correlation with the menstrual cycle phases, a prospective observational study. Sci Rep. 2017;7:1294.
5. Freundl G, Frank-Herrmann P, Godehardt E, Klemm R, Bachhofer M. Retrospective clinical trial of contraceptive effectiveness of the electronic fertility indicator Ladycomp/Babycomp. Adv Contracept. 1998;14:97–108.
6. Binkiewicz P, Michaluk K, Demiańczyk A. Calculation of the Pearl Index of Lady-Comp, Baby-Comp and Pearly cycle computers used as a contraceptive method. Ginekol Pol. 2010;81:834–9.
7. Payne HE, Lister C, West JH, Bernhardt JM. Behavioral Functionality of Mobile Apps in Health Interventions: A Systematic Review of the Literature. https://doi.org/10.2196/mhealth.3335.
8. Oulasvirta, A., Rattenbury, T., Lingyi, @bullet, @bullet, M. & Raita, E. Habits make smartphone use more pervasive doi:https://doi.org/10.1007/s00779-011-0412-2.
9. Duane M, Contreras A, Jensen ET, White A. The performance of fertility awareness-based method apps marketed to avoid pregnancy. J Am Board Fam Med. 29:508–11.
10. Setton R, Tierney C, Tsai T. The accuracy of web sites and cellular phone applications in predicting the fertile window. Obstet Gynecol. 2016;128:58–63.
11. Wilcox AJ, Dunson D, Baird DD. The timing of the "fertile window" in the menstrual cycle: day specific estimates from a prospective study. BMJ. 2000;321:1259–62.
12. Miyamoto SW, Henderson S, Young HM, Pande A, Han JJ. Tracking health data is not enough: a qualitative exploration of the role of healthcare partnerships and mHealth technology to promote physical activity and to sustain behavior change. JMIR mHealth uHealth. 2016;4:e5.
13. Lubans DR, Smith JJ, Skinner G, Morgan PJ. Development and implementation of a smartphone application to promote physical activity and reduce screen-time in adolescent boys. Front public Heal. 2014;2:42.
14. Glynn LG, et al. Effectiveness of a smartphone application to promote physical activity in primary care: the SMART MOVE randomised controlled trial. Br J Gen Pract. 2014;64:e384–91.
15. Nollen NL, et al. Mobile technology for obesity prevention: a randomized pilot study in racial- and ethnic-minority girls. Am J Prev Med. 2014;46:404–8.
16. Carter MC, Burley VJ, Nykjaer C, Cade JE. Adherence to a smartphone application for weight loss compared to website and paper diary: pilot randomized controlled trial. J Med Internet Res. 2013;15:e32.
17. R, P. Factors in human fertility and their statistical evaluation. Lancet 607–11, (1933).
18. Trussell J, Portman D. The creeping pearl: why has the rate of contraceptive failure increased in clinical trials of combined hormonal contraceptive pills? Contraception. 2013;88:604–10.
19. Kaplan EL, Meier P. Nonparametric estimation from incomplete observations. J Am Stat Assoc. 1958;53:457.
20. Wilson EB. Probable inference, the law of succession, and statistical inference. J Am Stat Assoc. 1927;22:209–12.
21. Trussell J, Grummer-Strawn L. Contraceptive failure of the ovulation method of periodic abstinence. Fam Plan Perspect. 22:65–75.
22. Polis CB, et al. Typical-use contraceptive failure rates in 43 countries with demographic and health survey data: summary of a detailed report. Contraception. 2016;94:11–7.
23. AREVALO M, JENNINGS V, NIKULA M, SINAI I. Efficacy of the new TwoDay method of family planning. Fertil Steril. 2004;82:885–92.
24. Arévalo M, Jennings V, Sinai I. Efficacy of a new method of family planning: the standard days method. Contraception. 2002;65:333–8.
25. Scherwitzl, ☆ E Berglund et al. Perfect-use and typical-use pearl index of a contraceptive mobile app. Contraception. 2017; https://doi.org/10.1016/j.contraception.2017.08.014.
26. Lenton EA, Weston GA, Cooke ID. Problems in using basal body temperature recordings in an infertility clinic. Br Med J. 1977;1:803–5.
27. Wang X, et al. Conception, early pregnancy loss, and time to clinical pregnancy: a population-based prospective study. Fertil Steril. 2003;79:577–84.
28. Gnoth C, Godehardt D, Godehardt E, Frank-Herrmann P, Freundl G. Time to pregnancy: results of the German prospective study and impact on the management of infertility. Hum Reprod. 2003;18:1959–66.
29. Trussell J. Update on and correction to the cost-effectiveness of contraceptives in the United States. Contraception. 2012;85:611.

6

Knowledge and perspectives of female genital cutting among the local religious leaders in Erbil governorate, Iraqi Kurdistan region

Hamdia M. Ahmed[2], Mosleh S. Kareem[2], Nazar P. Shabila[1*] and Barzhang Q. Mzori[3]

Abstract

Background: Religious leaders are one of the key actors in the issue of female genital cutting (FGC) due to the influential position they have in the community and the frequent association of FGC with the religion. This study aimed to assess the knowledge and perspectives of the local religious leaders in Erbil governorate, Iraqi Kurdistan Region about different aspects of FGC.

Methods: In-depth interviews were conducted with a sample of 29 local religious leaders. A semi-structured questionnaire was used that included questions about their knowledge, understanding, and perspectives on different aspects of FGC such as the reasons for practicing it, their contact and communication with the community regarding the practice and perspectives about banning the practice by law.

Results: Participants believed that FGC is useful for reducing or regulating the sexual desire of women to prevent adultery and engagement in pre and extramarital sexual relations and to enhance hygiene of women. They indicated that there is no any risk in doing FGC if there is no excessive cut. Most participants indicated that FGC is attributed to the religion and some considered it a tradition mixed with the religion. People rarely ask the advice of the religious leaders regarding FGC, but they frequently complain about the effects of the practice. Participants did not support having a law to ban FGC either because they thought it would be against the religion's advice on FGC or it will not work.

Conclusions: The local religious leaders lack adequate knowledge about different aspects of FGC particularly the health consequences. There are different and disputing viewpoints about the reasons for practicing FGC, and there is poor support for having a law banning the practice. There is an essential need for enhancing the knowledge of the local religious leaders regarding FGC and its adverse effects on the women's health.

Keywords: Female genital cutting, Religious leaders, Women sexuality, Culture, Erbil governorate

Plain English summary

Female genital cutting (FGC) is the cutting or removal of part or all of the external female genitalia for non-medical reasons. FGC is commonly practiced in the Iraqi Kurdistan Region where the local religious leaders have an important role in the community. The aim of this study was to assess the knowledge and the viewpoints of local religious leaders in Erbil governorate, Iraqi Kurdistan Region of FGC.

In-depth interviews were conducted with 29 local religious leaders in Erbil governorate, Iraqi Kurdistan Region. Questions were asked about their knowledge, understanding, and viewpoints of different aspects of FGC. The local religious leaders believed that FGC is useful for reducing the sexual desire of women to prevent them from pre and extramarital sexual relations. They indicated that FGC would not cause any harm if the cutting is not excessive. Many of them thought that

* Correspondence: nazar.shabila@hmu.edu.iq
[1]Department of Community Medicine, Hawler Medical University, Erbil, Kurdistan Region, Iraq
Full list of author information is available at the end of the article

FGC is required by the religion and some considered it a tradition mixed with the religion. People rarely ask the advice of the local religious leaders regarding FGC, but they frequently come to them to complain about its complications. The local religious leaders did not support having a law to ban FGC because they thought it would be against the religion's advice on FGC.

The local religious leaders lack enough knowledge about FGC particularly the health complications. There is poor support for banning the practice by law. There is an important need for increasing the knowledge of the local religious leaders regarding FGC and its complications.

Background

Female genital cutting (FGC) is the cutting or removal of part or all of the external female genitalia for non-medical reasons. The World Health Organization classification describes four types of FGC: clitoridectomy, excision, infibulations, and other procedures [1].

It is widely recognized that FGC violates a series of human rights principles. It is also an important manifestation of gender inequality and discrimination [1, 2]. FGC has many serious implications for the health of girls and women. It often causes pain, bleeding, infection, and dysuria as immediate consequences of the procedure. It also causes chronic pain, chronic infections, poor quality of sexual life, birth complications, and psychological problems as long-term effects [1, 3, 4]. More than 125 million women have experienced some types of FGC in 29 countries across Africa and the Middle East while another 30 million girls are at risk of being cut in the next decade [5].

FGC is commonly practiced in the Iraqi Kurdistan region, which is particularly concentrated in Erbil and Sulaymaniyah governorates [5]. The prevalence of FGC in the Iraqi Kurdistan Region is around 40%. However, this prevalence varies by geographical locations from 4.6% in Duhok governorate to 62.9% in Erbil governorate and 55.8% in Sulaymaniyah governorate. The prevalence is close to 100% in some specific rural areas [6]. The most common type of FGC in the Iraqi Kurdistan Region is Type I (76–99%), which includes partial or total removal of the clitoris and/or the prepuce [7, 8].

The roots of FGC in the Iraqi Kurdistan Region are unclear. FGC is prevalent in Iraqi and Iranian Kurdish areas [9, 10] but rare in the rest of Iraq or the Turkish Kurdish area. FGC is deeply rooted in the cultural and social values and beliefs of the affected communities. Social and cultural traditions are considered important reasons for performing FGC in different countries, including the Iraqi Kurdistan Region (40.7% to 46.7%) [7, 8, 11]. Many people consider FGC a beneficial cultural practice and in the best interest of the child [12].

Many parents might subject their girls to FGC thinking that they are "protecting" them from being ostracized and socially excluded from the community [13]. FGC is believed to protect women's chastity through reducing libido. Therefore, it is usually associated with the cultural principles of modesty and femininity [12, 14].

In the Iraqi Kurdistan Region, the Domestic Violence Bill that was passed in June 2011 includes several provisions criminalizing female genital mutilation in Kurdistan. The bill listed female genital mutilation among 13 items of domestic violence. The bill sets penalties for encouraging and performing female genital mutilation practice with a fine, imprisonment and banning the health professionals from the practice [15]. The regional government also established the High Council of Women Affairs, a governmental agency directly linked to the Prime Minister's office and responsible for combatting all types of gender-based violence including FGM. Several civil society organizations are also actively involved in these efforts to reduce FGC practice [8].

Various reasons are given for practicing FGC in different communities. However, the practice has been linked to Islam in the predominantly Muslim communities, and there is a strong belief that every Muslim woman must be subjected to FGC [16]. Religious obligation or requirement is an important reason (38.8% to 50.3%) for practicing FGC in the Iraqi Kurdistan Region [7, 8]. In fact, FGC is not an Islamic problem and it is practiced in many non-Muslim communities. The practice predates Islam and there are many majority Muslim countries where the incidence of FGC is very limited [17]. The presence of religious scripts that explicitly prescribe or encourage FGC is usually denied in the literature. Some renowned Sunni and Shi'i Islamic scholars, including a scholar from the Iraqi Kurdistan region have dismissed any association between FGC and Islam and even issued fatwa[1] forbidding FGC [18–20]. However, many people still believe that FGC has religious support [21] and in some countries arguments inspired by Islamic law have been used to claim that FGC is an obligation in Islam (17). In the Iraqi Kurdistan Region, girls and women who are not cut might be considered to have haram[2] hands, and some people do not eat or drink from their hands [11]. These unexamined aspects of FGC might play a crucial role in the high prevalence of FGC in the Iraqi Kurdistan Region.

Understanding the views of different actors in the community about FGC is very important to uncover the motivations behind the practice and ensure the effectiveness of preventive programs. The limited research from the Iraqi Kurdistan Region has primarily assessed the prevalence of FGC and its associated factors. Research has rarely examined in an in-depth manner the knowledge and perspectives of the influential people in the community, such as the local religious leaders of this practice and their potential role in combating this harmful practice.

Stopping FGC needs to start at the grassroots level through the participation of all the key players in the community, such as religious leaders, advocates, and educators [22]. Religious leaders are one of the key actors in the issue of female genital cutting (FGC) due to the important position they have in the community and the frequent association of FGC with the religion. It has been suggested that religious leaders have a substantial influence on whether the practice persist or not [17]. Moreover, several programs show that rapid elimination of FGM can be achieved if communities, supported by religious leaders, decide to abandon the practice [23, 24]. Some reputed Islamic scholars in the Iraqi Kurdistan Region have publicly condemned the practice of FGC, while others preferred to stay silent or even encouraged the practice [20]. Therefore, this study aimed to assess the knowledge and perspectives of the local religious leaders in Erbil governorate, Iraqi Kurdistan Region about different aspects of FGC.

Methods

This interview-based qualitative study was conducted in Erbil governorate, Iraqi Kurdistan Region, from June 2016 to May 2017.

We selected a purposive sample of 40 local religious leaders to represent different geographical areas of Erbil governorate including both urban and rural areas, areas of the different socioeconomic conditions and areas with varying prevalence of FGC. The sample included both imams[3] and preachers (khateebs)[4] from the mosques and Islamic academic scholars from the College of Islamic Sciences and of different educational levels. We identified the participants by consulting two key contacts; an Imam and a scholar. One of the authors contacted the potential participants by phone and invited them to take part in the interviews.

A semi-structured questionnaire was developed and used to guide the in-depth interviews (Additional file 1). The questionnaire included questions about the demographic and professional characteristics of the participants. It also included questions about the knowledge, understanding, and perspectives of the local religious leaders of different aspects of FGC including the definition, types, performers, reasons for practicing it and the prevalence in the Kurdish community in addition to their contact and communication with the community and their perspectives about banning FGC by law. We purposely did not ask about their knowledge of the existing domestic violence law that also criminalizes FGC in the Iraqi Kurdistan Region not to influence their answers about their views on banning the practice by

law. The semi-structured questionnaire was pre-tested to determine the accuracy and the understanding of the questions. Two male surveyors interviewed the participants, and each interview lasted around one hour.

The study was approved by the Research Ethics Committee at Hawler Medical University. The participants were informed about the purpose, and the importance of the study and the informed consent was obtained before the interview. The anonymity of the participants was ensured throughout the different stages of the study.

Three researchers separately conducted the interviews (MSK; 12 interviews, BQM; 12 interviews and HMA; 5 interviews). All interviews were conducted in the Kurdish language. Most interviews were entirely audio recorded. For the few participants who did not agree to record their interviews, full notes were taken by the interviewer. The recordings were transcribed before being translated into the English language. The translation was verified by a native Kurdish speaker who was fluent in English. We used content analysis to analyze the translated transcripts qualitatively. This type of analysis aimed to approach the study topic without any preconceived ideas to allow new perceptions based on the collected data. The transcripts were reviewed by two authors independently. They compared their notes and reconciled any differences. The condensed meaning units were identified and summarized. Then, they were abstracted and labeled with codes. The emerging codes were used to obtain categories. The two authors further discussed these categories for identification and formulation of themes. A greater emphasis was placed on the themes repeated by more than one participant, themes of long discussions or strong feelings. The discordant views were included to underline differing knowledge or perceptions of the study participants.

The four criteria of transferability, credibility, dependability, and conformability were used to ensure the rigor of the study. This involved presenting sufficient quotations in the results section, using a semi-structured interview guide, checking some of the coded interviews by academic staff and conducting the preliminary analysis by two authors with the third author independently reviewing the process.

Results

Of the 40 local religious leaders, 29 agreed to participate in the study. The mean ± SD age of the participants was 48.9 ± 14.9 and ranged between 32 and 76 years. Twenty participants were Imams in mosques; 13 were from Erbil city center, and seven were from the towns and rural areas located within 60 km of Erbil city. The other 9 participants were Islamic academic scholars teaching at the College of Islamic Sciences in Erbil city. Four participants had a scientific certification to practice, eight had a diploma degree, seven had a bachelor degree, six had a master degree, and four had a Ph.D. degree. The 29 interviews provided a wide representation of views and sufficient saturation. The results have been categorized into the following seven categories: understanding of FGC, advantages and disadvantages of FGC, reasons for practicing FGC, contact with the community regarding FGC, the prevalence of FGC in the Iraqi Kurdistan Region, the geographical difference in the prevalence of FGC and banning FGC by law as shown in Table 1.

Understanding of FGC

The local name of circumcision (*khatana*), which is derived from the Arabic name, was primarily used by the participants during the interviews. However, some participants referred to other names used in religion such as "*khafedh*" which means to mitigate or reduce.

FGC was mostly defined as cutting off a part of the clitoris. Clitoris sometimes was called by its correct Kurdish name (*mitka*) or Arabic name (*bazr*), but most of the times a simulated name was used such as "the extra piece of meat at the upper part of the vulva," or it was simulated to "the chicken or rooster caruncle."

"As *sharia* says, this is from *the fiqh*[5] book, circumcision in women is cutting the furthest part of skin at the upper vulva." (Interview 23).

"Clitoris has its location in the upper part of the vulva of women. It becomes straight. Doctors should decide to cut or not and how much to cut. They do not cut more than the limit that damages it. So if it is required, they will only cut it and not anything below it or the side of it. The skin is like a caruncle of chicken or rooster that has a pile." (Interview 15).

"It is called reducing, which means dropping. It means reducing the heat of a woman's body, the heat of desire. When it is reduced a bit, the heat will not overcome the mind. Heat in *fiqh* means desire." (Interview 23).

Only one type of FGC was described by most participants, which was the cutting part of the clitoris. Sometimes reference was also made to the more extreme types that are not practiced in the Iraqi Kurdistan Region and in Islam, such as the Pharaonic circumcision that is practiced in Sudan and Egypt.

"There is only one type similar to men's circumcision. In men is the skin (foreskin) and in women is the clitoris." (Interview 15).

"There is light circumcision, let's say, and it is clear as it is cutting a part of the clitoris and is cut slightly. There is also a type that is done in Egypt and Sudan, which is called Pharaoh's circumcision. They exaggerate in cutting." (Interview 22).

There were different views about to whom FGC is usually performed in the Iraqi Kurdistan Region. Some participants indicated that FGC is needed for those having very large clitoris above the sides (labia) making the region ugly and it may be regarded as a congenital anomaly and very sensitive to sexual desire. They thought that if the clitoris is lower than the edges it does not need cutting. They stressed that medical professionals should decide this issue.

Some participants described the clitoris to be higher in some women, above the two edges of labia causing problems when erected such as annoyance to the husband during sex, and thus it requires cutting. They thought that the cut is according to the need and doctors knows to cut or not and how much to cut.

"Cutting is required when the clitoris is much higher than the sides and makes the area ugly and become very sensitive. I do not know about medical aspect, but it might become something annoying for the woman or is more enjoyable or not for the man; we do not know this. So if it is not large and is lower than the edges, it does not need cutting. *Fuqaha*[6] (Islamic jurists) and those who say FGC is *Sunnah*,[7] say if the clitoris is not higher it does not need cutting. If it is small, the cut might harm or take away the sexual pleasure." (Interview 19).

"Having this extra meat makes sex more enjoyable than not having it. This extra meat is different in some women as it is large and very high. This makes the organ of woman ugly. When the woman grows, the woman becomes annoyed by this organ during sex and many other things such as psychological problems. In some women, it is not very high and is not protruded outside, and it might not be seen at all." (Interview 19).

Another view was that FGC is practiced in areas of warm climate due to early maturity of girls and increased sexual desire.

"As *sharia* says and from reading the Fiqh books, the sexual desire of women is higher in the regions with the warmer climate, and always the sexual desire is stronger in the warmer areas. I think this is also

Table 1 The main categories and sub-categories of the results extracted from the interviews

Category	Sub-category	Participant's number with relevant quotation
Understanding FGC	Definition	15; 23
	Type	15; 22
	To whom	10; 17; 19; 23
	By whom	16
	Role of sharia[a]	5; 10; 19
Advantages and disadvantages	Reducing sexual desire	5; 23
	Better hygiene, reduced smell	5; 21
	No risk if well done	All
	Insufficient desire and pleasure	5; 16
Reasons for practicing FGC	The prophet said it	17
	In the sharia	27
	Culture NOT religion	20; 21; 28
	Regulating sexual activity	13; 15; 23
	Smell	5; 28
Contact of religious leader with the community regarding FGC	The families do not ask	14; 15; 16; 18; 24
	Complaints from men re sex	3; 5
	Hemorrhage post FGC	13
	Shame and right to complain	16; 17
	Unfaithful if no FGC	19
Prevalence of FGC in Iraqi Kurdistan	Decreasing	13; 21
	Unknown because secret for girls	23
Geographical differences inside and outside Iraqi Kurdistan	Shafi[b] vs. Hanafi[c] doctrine	5; 10; 16; 22
	Faith	5; 15
	Education	18; 21
	Weather/heat	5; 22
	Tradition	16
	Unclear	1
	Pressure groups	23

Table 1 The main categories and sub-categories of the results extracted from the interviews (Continued)

Category	Sub-category	Participant's number with relevant quotation
Banning FGC by law	Knowledge of the existing law	22
	Do not support	9; 12; 17; 29
	Call for expert opinion	13; 14

[a]Sharia is the religious law forming part of the Islamic tradition
[b]Shafi'i doctrine is one of the four schools of Islamic law in Sunni Islam. The Shafi school predominantly relies on the Holy Quran and the hadiths for sharia. Where passages of the Holy Quran and hadiths are ambiguous, the school first seeks religious law guidance from Ijma – the consensus of Sahabah (Prophet Muhammad's companions). If there was no consensus, the Shafi'i school relies on the individual opinion (Ijtihad) of the companions of Prophet Muhammad (peace be upon him), followed by analogy
[c]Hanafi doctrine is one of the four religious Sunni Islamic schools of jurisprudence. Hanafi doctrine derives Islamic law from the Holy Quran, and the hadiths containing the words, actions, and customs of the Prophet Muhammad (peace be upon him)

correct medically. These areas are different from the colder areas." (Interview 23).

Another view was that FGC is to be done only for women with high sexual desire and at risk of experiencing adultery.

"It is good to be done, but only for the women with high sexual desire. If you know she will indeed experience adultery, it is better to be done, but with her or her parents' permission." (Interview 10).

The last view was that FGC should be done for all girls and women.

"It needs to be done to every girl since one does not know who has a high sexual desire and who has not." (Interview 17).

Participants agreed that FGC is mainly practiced by traditional birth attendants in the Iraqi Kurdistan Region, but they stressed that it needs to be performed by female medical professionals or at least experienced traditional birth attendants to avoid complications.

"It was done by traditional birth attendants in the past. A woman was doing it. In my opinion, this is not good today in this situation. I do not like it. I prefer and if possible the people who are specialists in this field to do it. I prefer to be doctors and be a specialist in this area to do the work beautifully and not harming the woman." (Interview 16).

Participants who were the proponent of FGC argued that the sharia has already decided on it and it should be done to all girls. Other participants indicated that the parents need to decide on it and there is a need to have the father's consent, which is usually not done in the Iraqi Kurdistan Region. Others indicated that doctors should decide if it is required or not.

"*Sharia* decides, but there are different opinions on FGC among the different doctrines (madhabs)." (Interview 5).

"The decision is not by religion, but by a doctor and family." (Interview 10).

"In my opinion, parents should go to a doctor to examine the girl to see if it is the type that needs circumcision or not." (Interview 19).

Advantages and disadvantages of FGC

The participants mentioned different benefits of FGC and the primary focus was on reducing or regulating the excessive sexual desire that women have and the associated deviation, sin and community and social problems. Other advantages mentioned by the participants included enhancing the hygiene and cleanliness of the woman and avoiding the annoyance of the husband during sex.

"Women have a higher sexual desire than men. Cutting this piece of meat in women does not do anything harmful to women. We are a human being, and anything at its limit is a benefit. Cutting part of this piece of meat (clitoris) is for the benefit of the woman to curb this desire. Otherwise, it is possible that women's desire would be that high that she makes sin and exceed her limit." (Interview 23).

"It regulates or limits the sexuality and the desire of women." (Interview 5).

"FGC leads to cleanliness and hygiene of reproductive organ of the woman. It removes bad odor that many times happen due to some secretions that affect the woman. In the two small lips (labia minora) some secretions lead to bad odor in the woman organ and infection of the urinary tract." (Interview 5).

"From the medical aspect, we have many studies that say FGC has some benefits including taking away the odor, will not become a cause of annoyance for men during sex because in some women it is very long and reaches 3 cm." (Interview 21).

Most participants indicated that there is no any risk in doing FGC while some participants mentioned some disadvantages that only occur if there is excessive cut such as reduced or loss of sexual desire.

"It has harmful effects if it is done in a non-scientific way or if the organ (clitoris) is cut extensively that the woman loses all sexual feeling. This leads to a disaster of marital separation and results in many problems." (Interview 5).

"If a lot is cut, the first thing from the *sharia* aspect it, harms the body of the woman and harms the sex by losing sexual desire and pleasure. This woman will have less feeling, and when she gets married in the future, she might have problems." (Interview 16).

Reasons for practicing FGC

Most participants indicated that the practice of FGC is primarily attributed to the religion, while others considered it a tradition related to culture or a tradition mixed with the religion.

"FGC is related to the religion because the Prophet (peace be upon him) has said it. Even if it was practiced in the old times, it has come into the Islam *sharia* and became part of the *sharia*." (Interview 17).

"They say it is in *sharia* and it was done in the past. The tradition is mixed with religion." (Interview 27).

"It is primarily related to the culture, but people think it is related to the religion and apply it." (Interview 28).

"It is a tradition and cultural practice. In my belief, it has no relation with *sharia*. As I am aware, in the village where FGC was practiced, a preacher has mentioned in *khutba*[8] several times that FGC is risky and warned people of not disabling their children, but the people did not listen to him, and this is wrong." (Interview 20).

"In my opinion traditions and customs have their effect in the Iraqi Kurdistan Region. People do the work more due to being a tradition and custom. For example, they do not know religious scripts whether it is allowed or not, has sharia said that or not, but they depend on the daily behavior." (Interview 21).

Other reasons for practicing FGC that were frequently mentioned by the participants included reducing the sexual desire and regulating the sexuality of women as they considered women to have a high sexual desire by nature. Few participants said that FGC is practiced to enhance the hygiene of women as the women who are not cut might have a bad smell or stinking.

"The wisdom of doing FGC is to refine women's sexual feeling, which means to reduce the high sexual desire in women and decrease the mechanism leading to desire." (Interview 13).

"For women, mainly because they have an excessive desire and FGC reduces this desire a bit. It does not take away the desire, but will only reduce it." (Interview 15).

"It is called reducing, which means dropping. It means reducing the heat of a woman's body, the heat of desire. It does not mean weakening the desire. FGC will reduce the heat a bit, so it will not overcome the mind." (Interview 23).

"In the two small lips (labia minora), some secretions lead to bad odor in the woman's organ and infection in the urinary tract. This FGC takes away this type of allergy in the woman's reproductive organ. FGC leads to cleanliness and hygiene of the reproductive organ of the woman and removes the bad odor that many times happen due to a group of secretions that affect the woman." (Interview 5).

"I do not support this (FGC) to be done if it is related to sexual desire. However, if it is related to other things such as leading to annoyance or harm during sex or if there is odor or related to a disease, it can be done. If a woman is chaste and has strong faith, she can control her desire." (Interview 28).

Contact with the community regarding FGC

Most participants indicated that nobody has come to ask them for advice on FGC. Some stated that few people have come to ask and these included both men and women, poor and rich, and educated and uneducated. In past times when some of the participants were working in the rural areas, people used to come to ask for their advice on FGC.

"Until now, few people have come to ask questions about FGC; whether to do it or not, is it a *Sunnah* or not. They say that some people tell them to do it and some others say do not do it and they do not have a clear answer about it." (Interview 14).

"In this area, till now 2-3 women have contacted me asking whether to do it or not. I think it is something that has become less common." (Interview 18).

"Nowadays, very few people come to ask me. In the past when I was working in a village, many people used to come to ask me "should we circumcise this girl or not?" I was saying circumcise her. There was a woman in our village knowing to perform the practice like a doctor." (Interview 15).

A participant indicated that people are now asking more about the topic as the media started to talk about banning it.

"The rate of asking in this situation is more than the past. In the past, it was less; now people ask more about this topic because this issue is now raised more frequently in the community and even in media." (Interview 16).

A participant indicated that these sensitive things are usually not discussed among men because of shame.

"Actually, these things are less discussed among men, as it is considered a shame. Sometimes there were complaints and have been mentioned to me." (Interview 24).

Most participants indicated that they had received people complaining of FGC particularly husbands complaining of loss of sexual desire of their wives and even asking if they can remarry because of that. Few examples of other complications such as bleeding were also mentioned. Some participants said that some people might not complain directly from the effect of FGC, but when they are asked about the causes of other problems such as divorce, they exclusively refer to the lack of sexual desire in women that is resulted from FGC.

"People complain a lot that their wives are circumcised, and their sexuality is zero. The circumcised woman always feels shortage in front of man regarding sex." (Interview 3).

"Yes, Muslims complain from the FGC, and the reason is mainly related to performing this practice by unskilled people. The complaint basically leads to marital separation, cheating, and many family problems." (Interview 5).

"Yes, a woman was talking about her young daughter who had excessive cut and bleeding for many days. The performer has either cut a lot or did not know how to cut it." (Interview 13).

Participants indicated that many people do not come to talk to them due to the sensitivity of the topic of FGC and feeling ashamed to talk about it.

"Yes, many people have come to ask. They are ashamed to ask or ask very shamefully because it is a sensitive topic. From the *sharia* aspect, nothing should be ashamed of and be asked about, but there is some shame on this issue." (Interview 16).

There were some extreme views that nobody should complain about this issue because it is the *sharia* issue.

"Nobody has complained, but they have no rights to complain because this is a right of Muslim and Muslims should be committed with *sharia. Sharia* says it is an obligation (*wajib*)[9] for some and *Sunnah* for some. Those who do it, it is a reserve to avoid sin and those who do not do it and consider it a *Sunnah*. God's willing, they will not be sinners. Nobody has a right on another because the Muslim should be committed to the *sharia*." (Interview 17).

One participant talked about complaints of not having done FGC and leading to extramarital sex.

"A woman called me asking for advice. She had a number of daughters, and all were circumcised except one of them. All the daughters were grown up based on religion and shame, and all got married. She said that the non-circumcised daughter was cheating on her husband (extramarital sexual relationship). So I immediately related this cheating to the lack of circumcision." (Interview 19).

Prevalence of FGC in the Iraqi Kurdistan region

There was some general agreement among the participants that FGC was common in the region in the past, particularly in rural areas and it is much reduced nowadays. It was affected by the role of particular Imams in the community in the past, and it is decreased as education and awareness of people is improved.

"In my opinion, FGC is decreasing gradually in the Iraqi Kurdistan Region, and this is attributed to the people' education (awareness). It was mainly done in nomads and tribes because these communities lacked an adequate number of scholars. A person is an enemy of what he does not know." (Interview 13).

"It is not done in the area where I live in Erbil. However, it was practiced in my father's and my in-law's families who are from Rawanduz district. It was done for the children, but after the situation has changed and the education level is increased, they also stopped doing it." (Interview 21).

Some participants argued that it is hard to know how common the practice is since it is mainly done in secret for girls, not like boys.

"It is possible, but it is not clear because usually, FGC is practiced in secret. It is different for boys because this is the tradition and culture of Kurds. In the past, even in the Islamic *sharia*, boy's circumcision was associated with celebration, but for the girl, it is usually hidden. This was done in the villages in the past." (Interview 23).

Geographical difference in the prevalence of FGC

Participants did not have adequate knowledge about the observed difference in the prevalence of FGC in the different governorates and areas of the Iraqi Kurdistan Region or by countries. When they were told about that and asked about the reasons for such difference, they provided different reasons for that. Some attributed that to the difference in the religious doctrines as they thought that Erbil and Sulaymaniyah people follow Shafi'i doctrine that considers FGC an obligation while those in Duhok follow the Hanafi doctrine that considers FGC a *Sunnah*. They also attributed the difference in the prevalence among the countries largely to the difference in doctrine. Others attributed it to the difference in people's commitment to the Shafi'i doctrine and the faith.

"The reason for the high prevalence of FGC in the Iraqi Kurdistan Region and Egypt is related to being on Shafi'i doctrine. In the Shafi'i doctrine, FGC is an obligation for both men and women." (Interview 5).

"Because Imam Shafi'i considered it an obligation and the people in these places (Erbil and Sulaymaniyah) follow Shafi'i doctrine, but Duhok people follow another doctrine." (Interview 10).

"Doctrines have a great role, particularly in these places that we mentioned like the Iraqi Kurdistan Region because Imam Shafi'i had a particular opinion, which was different from that of other scholars such as Imam Abu Hanifa, Imam Ahmadi, and Imam Maliki. For Imam Shafi'i, it is an obligation for women and men both." (Interview 16).

"The difference is due to not taking the order as decisive, not like the Holly Quran script that is decisive. Those who have complete satisfaction with Shafi'i, take it as cutting off and consider FGC an obligation." (Interview 22).

"From religion aspect, the people in Erbil and Sulaymaniyah are more religious and have more commitment to doctrines than Duhok people." (Interview 5).

"Not practicing FGC is related to the weak faith. People in some regions or countries have weak faith. I have lived with some of them, and they do not fast or pray until becoming old age. So if the people do not fast or pray, how do they practice FGC?" (Interview 15).

Other participants attributed this difference to the level of the education and awareness of the people in the different regions, particularly with the effect of the awareness campaigns against FGC. They generally thought that FGC is less prevalent in the people having a higher education and awareness level.

"There is a group of things, including the violence against women program, improved education, and increased awareness about family relations problems and sexual weakness of women in the future. The people are not ready to do this harm to their girls any longer." (Interview 21).

"It is related to the educational aspect of the region. For example, the people of Sulaymaniyah city read more and see more, but some people in the rural area and other places in the Iraqi Kurdistan Region are less educated. The people have heard that this is a Sunnah and many people have done it." (Interview 18).

Some participants explained the difference by the difference in the weather in the different regions.

"The weather has a significant role in this procedure. Duhok is colder than the other areas." (Interview 5).

"In the areas where FGC is practiced, it mainly goes back to customs. In Sudan and Egypt, the area is warm, and FGC is practiced there. It is even practiced in the German area (south of Sulaymaniyah and east of Kirkuk) which I think is warm." (Interview 22).

Some other participants attributed this difference to the tradition or could not find a reason for that.

"FGC has remained in these places as a tradition." (Interview 16).

"The answer is very difficult, as not everybody talks about it, and there is no special medical facility that people can visit to have accurate statistics. Therefore, I cannot decide on it. This difference is not clear to me." (Interview 1).

Other participants argued that the human and women's rights groups have done a bad thing by raising this issue of FGC.

"It depends on the explanation by scholars and religious Imams and preachers. We actually must follow the *sharia*. In the past, we did not have any dispute on this. Now the women's rights say clearly that it is a *haram* thing done to women. What they say I think is not *sharia* and not from the women's rights aspect because who have created a woman and made a plan for her knows better than you and me. How the God will violate the rights of a woman from the desire aspect." (Interview 23).

Banning FGC by law

The participants were not asked about their knowledge of the presence of the already existing domestic violence bill that criminalizes FGC in the Iraqi Kurdistan Region. However, only one participant stated that he is aware of the existence of such a law when the participants were asked about their opinion of banning FGC by law.

"FGC is banned by the domestic violence law. When I was writing my Ph.D. thesis, I referred to that project that was submitted to the parliament for discussion at that time." (Interview 22).

Most participants did not support having a law to ban FGC because they thought that it would be against the *sharia* and religious advice on FGC or it will not work. Some participants argued that having a law banning FGC will become something suspicious and people will oppose it.

"I do not support banning FGC by law." (Interview 9).

"I do not agree with banning FGC by the law because a law cannot ban it." (Interview 12).

"It is not good to ban FGC by law. It is better to have it optional and everybody to do what they like." (Interview 17).

"The families who frequently practice FGC, for example, those in Garmian area, even if there are a hundred laws, if they are not convinced of it, they do not follow it. But if they have religious Imams and preachers with them, it will for sure have an effect." (Interview 29).

Other participants argued that there is a need to have a law to regulate the practice based on advice from religious and medical experts either to practice it or not. Some participants even suggested establishing a committee including the local religious leaders to prepare effective legislation about FGC that could be acceptable by the people.

"There should be a law issued and the general *fatwa* committee in the Iraqi Kurdistan Region with experts in this field to sit together in addition to women's organizations and report it in the media. The media should have a role. If it is a good thing, all people let do it. If it is not good, people will know about it. Now there is some knowledge about it, and it is generally less commonly practiced." (Interview 13).

"I support to be regulated by law and not prohibited; to be regulated by the law so not everybody can perform this procedure. But to be regulated by the law, from the medical and psychological aspects to consider the person who performs it and the one who is performed for." (Interview 14).

Discussion

The participants had a good understanding of the definition of FGC. However, their definition and description were mainly focused on type I FGC. This might be related to the fact that type I FGC is the most common type practiced in the Iraqi Kurdistan Region [7, 8] and today's position of some Islamic scholars urges Muslims practicing FGC to adopt the most moderate form of FGC [25].

There was a consistent emphasis among the participants on the necessity of FGC for the girls and women in areas of the warmer climate. The participants even related the high prevalence of FGC in warmer climate areas of the Iraqi Kurdistan Region such as Garmian area to that. It is often believed that women become sexually mature earlier in the warmer climate and their sexual desire/arousal is higher than those in the colder climate. This belief is sometimes related to the Islamic religion since early Islam started in the warm climate area of Saudi Arabia and child marriage was common in the pre-Islam time in that region. However, there is no clear evidence to prove this association of early sexual maturity to the warmer climate [26], and we believe that there is no any association between the women's sexuality and the climatic condition.

The participants believed that the women with larger clitoris need FGC due to having a higher sexual desire. However, there is no clear proof that women with larger clitoris will have a higher sexual desire. Even a study revealed that sexual function was improved in women with a smaller-sized clitoris [27].

The traditional birth attendants are primarily responsible for performing FGC in the Iraqi Kurdistan Region [7, 8] and the participants were aware of this fact. Although they emphasized the need for the medicalization of FGC, we believe that this will not reduce the long-term complications of FGC, has no any benefits and violates the code of medical ethics. It can even result in a setback in the efforts to ban this harmful practice [28].

The participants mentioned different benefits of FGC and the primary focus was on the claimed reducing or regulating the excessive sexual desire to prevent adultery and engagement in pre and extramarital sexual relations. However, FGC clearly violates the rights of women since women have the right to have sexual health and to feel sexual pleasure for the full psychophysical well-being of the person [29]. Moreover, it has been shown that women with FGC do not significantly differ from those without FGC in the mean sexual desire score. Other advantages of FGC mentioned by the participants included enhancing hygiene and cleanliness. FGC is seen as ensuring the hygiene of the female genitalia, which in their natural form are wrongly classified as unclean. It is believed that the girl who is not circumcised has a bad odor because she is not clean and even some people consider the food she prepares *haram* [11, 25]. In fact, FGC has no any proved benefits, and the serious health and psychosocial consequences surpass any claimed benefits.

Most participants indicated that there is no any risk in doing FGC while some participants mentioned some disadvantages that only occur if there is excessive cut such as reduced or loss of sexual desire. However, there is clear evidence that all forms of FGC, including type I, can cause a high rate of complications [30]. The other common complications of FGC include excessive bleeding, delay in or incomplete healing, and tenderness in addition to reduced libido and psychological problems in long terms [3, 7, 8]. The high prevalence rate of FGC and the proportion of medical complications show that FGC is a matter of public health concern. Girls who undergo FGC before ten years of age, which is the case in the Iraqi Kurdistan Region, seem to be more vulnerable to serious complications than those who are older at the time of FGC [3].

Most participants indicated that the practice of FGC is attributed to the religion and some considered it a tradition mixed with the religion. In many settings, an important contribution to the practice of FGC is a religious obligation [31, 32]. Dictate of religion is an important reason (38.8% to 50.3%) for practicing FGC in the Iraqi Kurdistan Region [7, 8]. The presence of religious scripts that explicitly prescribe or encourage FGC is usually denied in the literature [20]. However, FGC and circumcision, in general, have been mentioned in some *hadiths* and some scholars argue that it is at least permissible in Islam as the Prophet (peace be upon him) has not prohibited it. Many people still believe that FGC has religious support, particularly in Islam [21]. Concerning Islam's view about FGC, some readings of the *hadith* suggest that Islam requires FGC and in some countries arguments inspired by Islamic law have been used to suggest that prohibiting FGC could be un-Islamic [17]. However, this interpretation is questioned by some religious scholars who disagree about whether Islam requires, encourages, permits, or discourages the practice [21]. We strongly believe that there is no any association between Islam religion and FGC. In fact, there is not a single verse in the Holy Quran that can be used as a basis for FGC. However, it includes many verses that condemn any practice that harms the human being. Moreover, the tradition from the *Sunnah* of the Prophet Muhammad (peace be upon him) in support of FGC is not authentic [16]. FGC is practiced in many non-Muslim communities, and the practice predates Islam. Besides, there are many countries of Muslim majority, including those following the Shafi'i school where FGC is not practiced at all [17]. Some renowned Islamic figures have denied any association between FGC and Islam. For example, Sheikh Ali Gomaa, formerly the Grand Mufti of Egypt and then Sheikh Al-Azhar, issued a fatwa forbidding and criminalizing FGC since there is a medical consensus on the harm caused by the

procedure [18]. A similar fatwa was also issued by Mohammad Hussein Fadlallah, the Shia Grand Ayatullah of Lebanon [19]. Professor Mustafa Zalmi, a renowned Islamic academic scholar from the Iraqi Kurdistan Region, denied any association between FGC and Islamic religion and that the Holy Quran clearly forbids any harmful action or action that its harm is more than its benefits such as FGC [20]. The High Committee for Issuing Fatwas in Iraqi Kurdistan Region issued a fatwa about FGC in 2010, which indicated that the practice is not prescribed in Islam, but predates it. The fatwa does not absolutely prohibit FGC as it says parents may opt to circumcise their daughters, but it is better to avoid the practice because of the negative health consequences [33, 34].

Although almost all Muslims in the Iraqi Kurdistan Region follow the Shafi'i school, which considers FGC an obligation, not all of them practice FGC. While FGC has roots in the Islamic religion as indicated by many religious leaders, the survival and the continuation of the practice in some areas of the Iraqi Kurdistan Region and near complete lack of the practice in other areas indicate that FGC has primarily become a cultural tradition. Many Muslims of the Shafi'i doctrine in the Iraqi Kurdistan Region do not practice FGC at all, and many have not even heard about it. Although people might be aware of the disadvantages of FGC, they cannot abandon the practice due to cultural beliefs and social pressure. Therefore, the culture plays an important role in practicing FGC in the Iraqi Kurdistan context. Social and cultural traditions are considered important reasons for performing FGC in different countries, including the Iraqi Kurdistan Region (40.7% to 46.7%) [7, 8, 11]. Many people consider FGC a beneficial cultural practice. Parents might subject their girls to FGC thinking that they are "protecting" them from being ostracized and socially excluded from the community [13]. By a careful examination of all aspects of the problem, it is clear that FGC is not an Islamic problem and the practice can only be regarded as a cultural practice rather than a religious one.

Having nobody or few people asking the advice of Imams and preachers about FGC might indicate that their role in the practice might not be so important. Some participants indicated that people approached them more when they were working in rural areas. This fact, in addition to the high prevalence of FGC in the rural areas where poverty and lack of education are common, makes the religious leaders having a major say in banning the practice. Asking the advice of religious leaders of FGC is common in other settings such as Somalia [35].

Most participants indicated that they had received people complaining of FGC particularly husbands complaining of loss of sexual desire of their wives. Imams and preachers are not like health professionals to be in direct contact with the victims of FGC, but they come into indirect contact with some social problems resulting from FGC particularly through their role in marriage, divorce or when mediating over social problems. This highlights the important role they have in the community as they become indirectly exposed to the problems in the society. Mentioning such experience in this field also highlights the long-term social and psychological problems that result from FGC that lead to damaging the woman's life.

The participants did not support having a law to ban FGC either because it will be against the *sharia* and religious advice on FGC or because they thought it would not work. While there is a need for strong laws and their enforcement to prevent people subjecting their daughters to the practice [36], lack of knowledge and awareness about these laws has remained a major concern [37, 38]. Many people think that raising the awareness of the people and actively involving religious leaders in combating FGC is more important than issuing or enforcing legislation. It is very important to have and enforce a law for combating FGM and prosecuting FGM practitioners and people who subject their daughters to the practice. However, legislation alone cannot end a harmful practice that is falsely linked to the religion and is embedded in the culture and traditions. There is a need for adopting proper mechanisms for enforcing such laws and raising the awareness of the people about their existence. In religious societies, it is important to have any law supported by the religion so that people accept and follow it.

Limitations

This study is limited to Erbil governorate. However, some participants were originally from different areas of the Iraqi Kurdistan Region or had working experience outside Erbil governorate, and they comprehensively talked about their experience in these areas. Therefore, the results can partly provide an idea about the FGC problem in the Iraqi Kurdistan Region in general.

Conclusions

The local religious leaders lack adequate knowledge about different aspects of FGC particularly the health consequences. There are different and disputing viewpoints about the reasons for practicing FGC, and there is poor support for having a law banning the practice. The different sectors of the government and the society, including the local religious leaders, need to take a strong stance against this unacceptable practice of FGC that is considered a severe violation of human rights. They also need to initiate vigorous action to stop this practice and protect young girls and women from its severe physical, psychosocial and reproductive consequences. There is an essential need for enhancing the knowledge of the local

religious leaders regarding FGC and its adverse effects on the women's health to motivate them to take a leading role in advising the people about this harmful practice. The local religious scholars and the Ministry of Endowments and Religious Affairs need to provide a clear message with clear evidence to the local religious leaders about FGC and the view of the Islamic religion on this practice. Topics on FGC could be integrated into the curriculum of the religious schools. Thus,

Endnotes

[1]A *fatwa* in the Islamic faith is a non-binding but authoritative legal opinion or learned interpretation that a qualified jurist could give on issues about the Islamic law

[2]*Haram* is any act that is forbidden by Allah (God).

[3]Imam is an Islamic leadership position, and it is most commonly used as the title of a worship leader or prayer leader of a mosque and the Muslim community.

[4]*Khateeb* is a person who delivers the sermon (*khutbah*) during the Friday prayer and Eid prayers. The *khateeb* is usually the imam, but the two roles can be played by different people.

[5]*Fiqh* is Islamic jurisprudence, is the human understanding of the *sharia*.

[6]*Fuqaha* (singular Faqih) is an Islamic jurist, an expert in *fiqh*, or Islamic jurisprudence and Islamic Law Contents.

[7]*Sunnah* includes the specific words, habits, practices, and silent permissions (or disapprovals) of the Prophet Muhammad (peace be upon him).

[8]*Khutba* serves as the primary formal occasion for public preaching in the Islamic tradition. Such sermons occur regularly at the noon congregation prayer on Friday.

[9]*Wajib* or its synonym *fard* is one of the five types of rules into which *fiqh* categorizes acts of every Muslim. It denotes a religious duty commanded by Allah. The Hanafi doctrine, however, makes a distinction between *wajib* and *fard*, the latter being obligatory and the former merely necessary.

Abbreviation

FGC: Female genital cutting

Acknowledgements

This publication was made possible through the support of the John Templeton Foundation, via The Enhancing Life Project. Such support did not include involvement in the design of the study, the collection, analysis, and interpretation of data, or the writing of the manuscript.

Funding
Not applicable.

Authors' contributions
NPS contributed to the inception, design, analysis, interpretation, drafting the research manuscript and final approval of the revised manuscript for publication. HMA contributed to the inception, design, data collection, interpretation, editing, revision and final approval of the manuscript for publication. MSK contributed to the data collection, interpretation and editing, revision and final approval of the manuscript for publication. BQM contributed to the inception, design, data collection and editing and final approval of the manuscript for publication.

Competing interests
The authors declare that they have no competing interests.

Author details
¹Department of Community Medicine, Hawler Medical University, Erbil, Kurdistan Region, Iraq. ²College of Nursing, Hawler Medical University, Erbil, Kurdistan Region, Iraq. ³Directorate of Health, Erbil, Kurdistan Region, Iraq.

References
1. World Health Organization. Eliminating female genital mutilation: an interagency statement. Geneva, Switzerland: WHO; 2008.
2. Fisaha KG. Female genital mutilation: a violation of human rights. J Pol Sci Pub Aff. 2016;4:198.
3. Bjälkander O, Bangura L, Leigh B, Berggren V, Bergström S, Almroth L. Health complications of female genital mutilation in Sierra Leone. Int J Womens Health. 2012;4:321–31.
4. Mgbako C, Cave A, Farjad N, Shin H. Penetrating the silence in Sierra Leone: a blueprint for the eradication of female genital mutilation. Harv Hum Rights J. 2010;23:111–40.
5. UNICEF. Female genital mutilation/cutting: a statistical overview and exploration of the dynamics of change. New York: UNICEF; 2010.
6. Central Statistics Organization (CSO) and Kurdistan Regional Statistics Office (KRSO). Iraq multiple indicator cluster survey 2011, final report. Baghdad: CSO and KRSO; 2012.
7. Saleem RA, Othman N, Fattah FH, Hazim L, Adnan B. Female genital mutilation in Iraqi Kurdistan: description and associated factors. Women & Health. 2013;53:537–51.
8. Yasin BA, Al-Tawil NG, Shabila NP, Al-Hadithi TS. Female genital mutilation among Iraqi Kurdish women: a cross-sectional study from Erbil City. BMC Public Health. 2013;13:809.
9. Pashaei T, Rahimi A, Ardalan A, Felah A, Majlessi F. Related factors of female genital mutilation (FGM) in Ravansar (Iran). J Women's Health Care. 2012;1:108.
10. von der Osten-Sacken T, Uwer T. Is female genital mutilation an Islamic problem? Middle East Quarterly. 2007;14:29–36.
11. Shabila NP, Saleh AM, Jawad RK. Women's perspectives of female genital cutting: Q-methodology. BMC Womens Health. 2014;14:11.
12. Costello S. Female genital mutilation/cutting: risk management and strategies for social workers and health care professionals. Risk Manag Healthc Policy. 2015;8:225–33.
13. UNICEF. Legislative reform to support the abandonment of female genital mutilation/cutting. New York: UNICEF; 2010.
14. UNICEF. Changing a harmful social convention: female genital mutilation/cutting. New York: UNICEF; 2005.
15. Iraqi Kurdistan Parliament. [Law number 8: Combating family violence in Iraqi Kurdistan Region]. Waqaehi Kurdistan 2011;122:6–9. Arabic.
16. Asmani IL, Abdi MS. De-linking Female Genital Mutilation/Cutting from Islam. Population Council; 2008.
17. Wodon Q. Islamic law, Women's rights, and state law: the cases of female genital cutting and child marriage. The Review of Faith & International Affairs. 2015;13(3):81–91.
18. Islamopedia. Grand Mufti of Egypt Ali Gomaa denounces female circumcision and calls the practice a punishable offense following an international Islamic conference of scholars. http://www.islamopediaonline.org/fatwa/grand-mufti-egypt-ali-gomaa-denounces-emale-circumcision-and-calls-practice-punishable-offense. Accessed 5 Jan 2018.
19. Islamopedia. Grand Ayatollah Fadlallah responds to the question: "Is it true that Islam intends to inhibit and control lust in women with circumcision?" http://www.islamopediaonline.org/fatwa/grand-ayatollah-fadlallah-responds-question-it-true-islam-intends-inhibit-and-control-lust-wom. Accessed 5 Jan 2018.
20. Al-Zalmi MI. female genital mutilation: side effects and its banning in Quran. Erbil: Shahab press; 2011. Arabica
21. Hayford SR, Trinitapoli J. Religious differences in female genital cutting: a case study from Burkina Faso. J Sci Study Relig. 2011;50(2):252–71.
22. Yirga WS, Kassa NA, Gebremichael MW, Aro AR. Female genital mutilation: prevalence, perceptions and effect on women's health in Kersa district of Ethiopia. Int J Women's Health. 2012;4:45–54.
23. UNFPA, UNICEF. Annual report of the UNFPA-UNICEF joint programme on female genital mutilation/cutting: accelerating change. 2012. https://www.unfpa.org/sites/default/files/pub-pdf/UNICEF-UNFPA%20Joint%20Programme%20AR_final_v14.pdf. Accessed 5 Jan 2018.
24. Tomkins A, Duff J, Fitzgibbon A, Karam A, Mills EJ, Munnings K, Smith S, Seshadri SR, Steinberg A, Vitillo R, Yugi P. Controversies in faith and health care. Lancet. 2015;386:1776–85.
25. Berg RC, Dedison EA. Tradition in transition: factors perpetuating and hindering the continuance of female genital mutilation/cutting (FGM/C) summarized in a systematic review. Health Care Women Int. 2013;34:837–59.
26. Parent AS, Teilmann G, Juul A, Skakkebaek NE, Toppari J, Bourguignon JP. The timing of normal puberty and the age limits of sexual precocity: variations around the world, secular trends, and changes after migration. Endocr Rev. 2003;24(5):668–93.
27. Vaccaro CM, Fellner AN, Pauls RN. Female sexual function and the clitoral complex using pelvic MRI assessment. Eur J Obstet Gynecol Reprod Biol. 2014;180:180–5.
28. Serour GI. Medicalization of female genital mutilation/cutting. Afr J Urol. 2013;19(3):145–9.
29. Catania L, Abdulcadir O, Puppo V, Verde JB, Abdulcadir J, Abdulcadir D. Pleasure and orgasm in women with female genital mutilation/cutting (FGM/C). J Sex Med. 2007;4(6):1666–78.
30. Kaplan A, Hechavarría S, Martín M, Bonhoure I. Health consequences of female genital mutilation/cutting in the Gambia, evidence into action. Reprod Health. 2011;8:26.
31. Ali AAA. Knowledge and attitudes of female genital mutilation among midwives in eastern Sudan. Reprod Health. 2012;9:23.
32. Ashimi A, Aliyu L, Shittu M, Amole T. A multicentre study on knowledge and attitude of nurses in northern Nigeria concerning female genital mutilation. Eur J Contracept Reprod Health Care. 2014;19:134–40.
33. Kurdistan Islamic Scholars Union. Female circumcision: an explanation by the high Committee of Fatwa. 2010. http://www.zanayan.org/t_detail.php?section=2&id=26376. Accessed 10 Jan 2018.
34. Human Rights Watch: Iraqi Kurdistan: FGM Fatwa positive, but not definitive. 2010. https://www.hrw.org/news/2010/07/17/iraqi-kurdistan-fgm-fatwa-positive-not-definitive. Accessed 10 Jan 2018.
35. Fried S, Warsame AM, Berggren V, Isman E, Johansson A. Outpatients' perspectives on problems and needs related to female genital mutilation/cutting: a qualitative study from Somaliland. Obstet Gynecol Int. 2013;2013:165893.
36. Center for Reproductive Rights. Female genital mutilation (FGM): legal prohibitions worldwide. New York: Center for Reproductive Rights; 2008.
37. Dorkenoo E, Morison L, Macfarlane A. A statistical study to estimate the prevalence of female genital mutilation in England and Wales. UK: Foundation for Women's Health, Research and Development (FORWARD); 2007.
38. Malik IA, Shabila NP, Al-Hadithi TS. Women's knowledge of the domestic violence legislation in Erbil, Iraq and their response to spousal violence. J Fam Viol. 2017;32(1):47–53.

7

Gender role attitudes, awareness and experiences of non-consensual sex

Xiayun Zuo[1], Chaohua Lou[1*], Ersheng Gao[1], Qiguo Lian[1] and Iqbal H. Shah[2]

Abstract

Background: Non-consensual sex (NCS) among young people, an important subject with public health and human rights implications, was less studied in China. This study is to investigate the NCS awareness and victimization of university students in Shanghai, China and whether they were associated with adolescent gender-role attitudes.

Methods: Gender-role attitudes, awareness and victimization of different forms of NCS were examined among 1099 undergraduates (430 males and 669 females) in four universities in Shanghai using computer-assisted self-interview approach.

Results: University students held relatively egalitarian attitude to gender roles. Gender difference existed that girls desired to be more equal in social status and resource sharing while more endorsed the submissiveness for women in sexual interaction than boys. They held low vigilance on the risk of various forms of NCS, with the mean score on perception of NCS among boys (5.67) lower than that among girls (6.37). Boys who adhered to traditional gender norms were less likely to aware the nature of NCS ($\beta = -0.6107$, $p = 0.0389$). Compared with boys, higher proportion of girls had been the victims of verbal harassment, unwanted touch, fondling, and penetrative sexual intercourse. Multivariable analysis revealed that girls who held more traditional gender-role attitudes were more vulnerable to physical NCS (OR = 1.41, $p = 0.0558$).

Conclusions: The weakening but still existing traditional gender norms had contributions in explaining the gender difference on the low vigilance of NCS and higher prevalence of victimization among university students in Shanghai, China. Interventions should be taken to challenge the traditional gender norms in individual and structural level, and promote the society to understand the nature of NCS better as well as enhance negotiation skills of adolescents and young people that prevent them from potentially risky situations or relationships.

Keywords: Perception, Non-consensual sex, Victimization, Gender roles, University students, China

Plain English summary

With the aim to understand the gender-role attitudes, the awareness and victimization of non-consensual sex (NCS) among Chinese university students and the relationship between gender-role attitudes and NCS awareness and victimization, this study conducted quantitative analyses using data from a computer-assisted self-interview survey among university students. A total number of 1099 undergraduates aged between 18 and 24 from four universities in Shanghai were included in the analyses. Results showed that undergraduates held egalitarian attitudes to gender roles, and girls desired to be more equal in societal status and resource sharing whole more endorsed the submissiveness of women in sexual interaction than boys. They held low awareness on the risk of NCS and such awareness among boys was even lower. Compared with boys, higher proportion of girls had been the victims of verbal harassment, unwanted touch, fondling, and penetrative sexual intercourse. The relationship between gender-role attitudes and NCS awareness and victimization varied between gender: boys who adhered to traditional gender norms were less likely to aware the nature of NCS, while

* Correspondence: louchaohua60@163.com
[1]Key Laboratory of Reproduction Regulation of NPFPC, SIPPR, IRD, Fudan University, 779 Laohumin Road, Shanghai 200237, China
Full list of author information is available at the end of the article

girls who held more traditional gender-role attitudes were more vulnerable to physical NCS. Such findings suggested gender-sensitive interventions should be developed to question the traditional gender norms in the individual and structural level, and promote adolescents to understand the nature of NCS better as well as keep away from potentially risky situations or relationships.

Background

Non-consensual sex (NCS), interchangeably used as sexual abuse, sexual violence and sexual coercion, in general was operationalized to encompass a range of behaviors including unwanted penetrative sex, attempted rape, unwanted touch, as well as non-contact forms of abuse such as, verbal harassment or forced viewing of pornography. These acts may include any coercive situations that the victims lack of realistic choices available to prevent or redress the situation, for example physical violence, threats, intimidation, emotional manipulation and deception [1]. The issue of NCS among adolescent and young people is an important subject with not only public health implications, but also a violation of human rights with legal concerns as well. Significant numbers of young people, particularly girls and young women but also boys and young men, are exposed to NCS around the world places [2, 3]. Meanwhile, young people may be less equipped than adults to avoid incidents of NCS and may have fewer choices available to them to cope with such incidents. A growing number of studies show that experience of NCS during childhood and adolescence often adversely affects their subsequent psychological, behavioral, and reproductive outcomes [4–8].

A large body of research on adolescent NCS, with unspecified definitions and varying in research population and research methods have produced varied findings. For example, a wide range of prevalence from less than five to over 50 % is noted among adolescents from multiple countries [1, 9, 10]. Most surveys that report on this subject ask a fairly general question, usually on the line of "Have you even been forced to engage in sex?". Diversity of evidence obtained from such measurement might be partially attributed to the dynamic nature of young people's interpretations of NCS. For instance, young people who submit to the pressure of a partner's demands for sex as an expression of commitment may not respond affirmatively to a general question on "forced" sex. Marston found that young unmarried girls in Mexico identified sexual experience as non-consensual only if the perpetrator was someone with whom they didn't have a romantic relationship [11]. Young people's interpretation of NCS could be influenced by the sociocultural context and legal framework that young people live in. In some settings, early marriage is encouraged and young women are socialized to believe it is their duty to accept the sex from their

husband even if they are not willing to do so [12]. It is, therefore, quite important to provide precise and detailed interpretation of NCS and obtain youth's interpretation on them when conducting research on NCS among young people in particular sociocultural context.

NCS is influenced by multiple risk factors existing at different levels, from the individual to the community and societal level. Scholarly efforts have highlighted the role of gender norms. Gender norms, as defined by The World Health Organization, refer to beliefs about women and men, boys and girls that are passed from generation to generation through the process of socialization. They change over time and differ in different cultures and populations. Gender norms lead to inequality if they reinforce mistreatment of one group or sex over the other, or differences in power and opportunities [13]. UNAIDS reported at the macro level that sexual violence against women appears to be more common in settings where gender roles are rigidly enforced and where masculinity is associated with toughness and dominance while femininity with submissiveness [14]. Some empirical research in developed countries suggested the effects of individual attitudes to gender norms: young women who explicitly endorsed traditional gender beliefs were particularly disempowered during sexual interactions and at higher risk for NCS [15, 16]; male adolescents who supported traditional gender norms and beliefs in the inferiority of women and girls were more likely to report sexual violence and perpetration of intimate partner violence [17, 18]. Nevertheless some studies have failed to find significant association between NCS victimization and individual gender-role attitudes [14, 19, 20]. However, to our knowledge, no such studies on gender-role attitudes and victimization or perpetration of NCS have been conducted in China with specific cultural context on gender norms. Such findings would be extremely relevant to informing future NCS research and practice efforts.

China, with a traditional Confucian culture influenced deeply for thousands of years, has initiated many adolescent sexual and reproductive health research and programs. Most of these assume that young people's sexual experience, except rape, is voluntary. Few studies have considered the issue of NCS, however, in fairly general and ambiguous way, asking questions like "Have you ever been forced to engage in sex?" [21, 22]. There is no particular research to examine views on and prevalence of different kinds of NCS among young people, while anecdotal accounts suggest such incidents are not rare. The dearth of such evidence can probably compromise the beneficial effects of adolescent sexual and reproductive health promotion programs that remain largely uninformed of the evidence of appropriate strategies and interventions.

The traditional Confucian culture in China has strict doctrines linking unequal gender stratification and distribution of power and resources by its core of "Three obedience" (*san cong*) particularly for women, namely women subordinate to men in every stage of life: daughters to their fathers, wives to their husbands, and in widowhood, to their sons. Female were not allowed to go "out" to school but were expected to stay home learning skills of housework to raise family after getting married [23]. A woman should always be modest and submissive in manner, otherwise it could damage the reputation of her family, and the man was expected to be responsible and gentlemanlike. Chastity was particularly required of women that they should not only remain virginal until marriage but also maintain absolute fidelity toward their husbands, whether he was alive or dead. Women should be kept passive and sexually innocent in relationship with men. This was not the case for men. With the "open" policy in effect since the late 1970s, considerable changes in economy and globalization of social culture have taken place, and the traditional Confucian ideals of gender roles have been weakening gradually [24]. There is rapid rise in percentage of women getting high level of schooling and entering the labor market. More men and women are working in less traditional careers and sharing family and household responsibilities. Increasing number of adolescents and youth are now engaged in premarital sex [25]. However, the current attitudes to gender roles among adolescents were not known when they are witnessing these changes.

Thus, to better informing the programs and policies in China, the current study objectives include examining the awareness and victimization of NCS among a sample of university students, examining their attitudes to gender roles, and demonstrating evidence of associations between attitudes to gender roles and NCS awareness and victimization.

Methods
Sample and procedures
Four universities in Shanghai were selected purposively in 2009 to represent different academic rankings. From four types of disciplines, i.e. engineering, science, liberal arts and arts (including music, painting, movie etc.) in each selected university, one department, and then third-year students were randomly selected to achieve the sample size of male and female students. Only the third-year students were chosen due to two considerations – anticipation of more sexually active (consensual or non-consensual) adolescents among higher grade students and the fact fourth-year students are usually out of school preparing for graduation field work and, therefore, difficult to reach. The unequal sample size among male and female students was determined by the prevalence of non-physical and physical childhood sexual abuse with gender difference among adolescents suggested by a study conducted in China [26]. Totally 1099 students (430 males and 669

females) aged 18–24 years (mean age: 21.5 years) were recruited and voluntarily participated in the study with informed consent (accounting for 69.1~ 88.8% of students in each selected department). Four male and 3 female students refused to participate in the study. Nearly all of the students (99.8%) were unmarried and majority of them (88.1%) lived in the dormitory. One-third of them had lived in rural areas before entering the university. About 43% and 38.9% of respondents respectively reported their parent's educational level as high/vocational/technical school and college or above. Most of them (88.4%) had relatively good feeling about their family life and about one in two regarded their campus life as good. About 29.5% and 16.6% of male and female subjects reported they had experienced sexual intercourse, including consensual and non-consensual.

After obtaining their informed consent, university students were organized to fill the questionnaire in computer classrooms during the lunch break. With the computer-assisted self-completion interview (CASI), each participant read and answered questions on a computer without interposition of interviewers, who were trained to assist respondents, when necessary, in understanding questions and in handling any emergency during the survey. Information about respondents' views on and experience of NCS, relevant feelings, reactions and consequences, their attitudes to gender roles, among other topics was collected anonymously. In addition to providing anonymity, CASI allows for programmed consistency checks and skip patterns that reduce errors, and it eliminates the need for an additional data entry step after the assessment is completed. All study procedures were approved by the institutional review board of Shanghai Institute of Planned Parenthood Research (SIPPR) and WHO Research Ethics Review Committee.

Measures
Attitudes to gender roles
Six typical questions were asked to ascertain respondents' views about the gender division of roles in family, in social resource allocations and in sexual relations: (1) "household should be led by men", (2) "in general, boys should get more schooling than girls", (3) "when jobs are scarce, men should have more right to job than women", (4) "women should have same opportunities as men in leadership", (5) "it is acceptable for a husband to beat his wife in some situations", (6) "a woman should not be the first to show a man that she likes him". For each question, the response was measured on 3-point ordinal scale from disagreed (0), uncertain (1), and agreed (2). We reversed the fourth question, and then summed students' responses to get an index with the maximum of 12. The higher the score, the traditional the students' values and

the less egalitarian gender-roles they held. The median of the composite index was 2.

Awareness on NCS

We adopted the definition of NCS provided by Jejeebhoy, et al. [1]. Accordingly, nine episodes on different kinds of NCS were listed, containing verbal harassment via communication technologies (short message, telephone and on the Internet, etc.), forced viewing of pornographic material or video, forced exposure to exhibitionism, watched secretly while changing clothes or in similar situations, secret pictures or flashing disseminated on the Internet without permission, sexually suggestive talking, unwanted touch, foundling, as well as forced penetrative sex through threats, intimidation, emotional manipulation, deception, material and non-material incentives. Respondents were asked whether each mentioned episode was NCS and responses were scored "1" if they answered in affirmative and "0" if they answered negatively or "didn't know". These scores were summed up for the composite index (maximum score was 9) to reflect the respondent's overall perception of NCS.

Experience of NCS

Likewise, to avoid ambiguity, different forms of NCS aforementioned were separately listed to measure whether respondents had experienced such incidents. A typical question on one form of NCS was "have you ever encountered someone touching the private parts of your body or someone touching you with his/her private parts of body that made you feel uncomfortable or embarrassed?". We tried to get the prevalence of each form of NCS to make our results comparable to those from other studies.

Control variables

The demographic variables – gender, age, discipline, residence, feeling about family atmosphere and current campus life, and parent's educational level were included in the multiple regression analysis as control variables. All these variables, including parent's educational level were self-reported by university students. Parent's educational level was determined by the higher level of his/her father and mother to partially reflect the socioeconomic status of respondent's family.

Analysis

The original data collected via the electronic questionnaire were managed by Microsoft Access, which can be transferred into SAS dataset. The transformed data then were checked and analyzed using SAS statistical package 9. As gender was an important factor in understanding sexual issues, all analyses were stratified by gender (male, female).

Preliminary analysis used chi-square, t-test and ANOVA to examine the gender difference of attitudes to gender roles, and perception and experience of NCS. Then, multiple-regression (general linear model) and logistic regression were used to determine the influence of gender-role attitudes on experience of NCS among university students, adjusting for the effects of demographic covariates.

Results

Attitudes to gender roles

The responses supporting traditional gender roles ranged from 1% to 47% (Table 1). More than 20% of students endorsed the unequal position in family and social resource allocation between males and females. Only 2.9% of students accepted the physical violence against woman by her husband. Compared with girls, higher percentage of boys favored the resource sharing and power dominance of males. However, in sexual relations,

Table 1 Distribution of respondents' attitudes to gender roles, by sex of the respondent (%)

Items of traditional gender roles	Total ($n = 1099$)	Male ($n = 430$)	Female ($n = 669$)
Household should be led by men.			
Disagree	46.95	26.98	59.79
Uncertain	21.93	25.81	19.43
Agree	31.12	47.21	20.78
In general, boys should get more schooling than girls.			
Disagree	62.24	55.81	66.37
Uncertain	16.56	20.93	13.75
Agree	21.20	23.26	19.88
When jobs are scarce, men should have more right to a job than women.			
Disagree	64.15	43.95	77.13
Uncertain	15.20	24.19	9.42
Agree	20.66	31.86	13.45
Women should have same opportunities as men to leadership positions.			
Disagree	6.01	10.00	3.44
Uncertain	9.83	18.60	4.19
Agree	84.17	71.40	92.38
It is acceptable for a husband to beat his wife in some situations.			
Disagree	91.08	81.86	97.01
Uncertain	6.01	12.79	1.64
Agree	2.91	5.35	1.35
A woman should not be the first to show a man she likes him.			
Disagree	71.43	81.16	65.17
Uncertain	22.11	16.05	26.01
Agree	6.46	2.79	8.82

All were significant at $p < 0.001$ compared between male and female respondents higher proportion of girls accepted the traditional dogma of submission for females than did boys. The mean score of gender-role attitudes was higher for boys than for girls (3.59 vs 2.10), which meant boys held more gender-unequal attitudes. Even within groups of similar characteristics, such gender difference was found consistently.

Perception of NCS

For ease of description, the median splits were performed on the score of gender-role attitudes to categorize respondents as relatively traditional (score > 2) or egalitarian (score < =2) in their gender ideology. The analysis revealed students' low awareness of non-consensual sex in terms of the general perception score, with 5.67 as the mean score of recognition among boys, a little lower than among girls (6.37). Males who held more egalitarian attitudes had higher composite score of the recognition than those who held more unequal attitudes (6.02 vs. 5.45, $p = 0.048$). While among girls, the score of general recognition were of no significant difference between those favoring egalitarian or unequal attitudes (6.44 vs. 6.24, $p = 0.378$).

The proportion of male and female students who were aware of coercion on typical scenarios varied between 48.1~ 93.4%, with higher recognition of the kinds of physical sexual coercion including unwanted touch, fondling and penetrative sex (Table 2). Compared with girls, lower proportion of boys viewed events like forced watching of pornographic materials, disseminating private pictures without permission, unwanted fondling, and forced penetrative sex as NCS. Among boys, higher proportion of those who held egalitarian gender-role attitudes viewed unwanted touch, fondling and penetrative sex as non-consensual than those holding unequal

attitudes, while the two groups of boys held no different views on the non-physical coercion. Among girls, however, no associations between gender-role attitudes and views on all forms of NCS were found.

Experience of NCS

Most frequently mentioned experience of NCS was unwanted touch, reported by 27.2% and 63.3% respectively among boys and girls. About 50% of all boys and girls reported experiencing verbal harassment via short message, telephone and on the Internet. Also, about 20% of boys and 33.9% of girls had encountered sexually suggestive comments. Lower rate, about 7.7% of boys and 13.9% girls reported experiencing unwanted fondling, and less than 2% of boys and about 8% of girls reported attempted forced penetrative sex. About 1.9% and 5.2% of boys and girls respectively had encountered forced sexual intercourse, which accounted for 6.3% and 31.5% of sexually active boys and girls respectively (Table 3). We also found association of gender-role attitude and different forms of NCS experience. Among boys, lower percentage of those who held egalitarian attitudes to gender roles reported having experienced sexually suggestive comments and unwanted fondling. Lower percentage of girls holding egalitarian attitudes reported being victims of unwanted touch and forced penetrative sex.

Association between gender role attitudes and NCS awareness and victimization

Table 4 presents the results from General Linear Model (GLM) of students' awareness of NCS, with the score of awareness as the dependent variable. The independent variables included gender-role attitudes, and the

Table 2 Proportion of students who perceived the risk of NCS, grouped by sex of the respondent and gender-role attitudes (%)

Items on NCS	Male			Female		
	Total	Gender-role attitudes Score		Total	Gender-role attitudes Score	
		<=2 (n = 164)	> 2 (n = 266)		<=2 (n = 438)	> 2 (n = 231)
Score (mean)	5.67	6.02	5.45*	6.37#	6.44	6.24
Verbal harassment via communication technology	48.14	50.61	46.62	51.87	52.28	51.08
Forced watching porn	57.44	62.20	54.51	65.32#	66.44	63.20
Forced exposure to exhibitionism	60.70	64.63	58.27	76.38#	78.08	73.16
Watched secretly while changing clothes or in similar situations	54.42	56.10	53.38	60.09	60.50	59.31
Disseminating secret pictures/flash without permission	53.26	53.05	53.38	61.73#	62.10	61.04
Sexually suggestive comments	48.37	52.44	45.86	53.96	54.11	53.68
Unwanted touch/frottage	75.81	82.32	71.80 *	84.45	85.16	83.12
Unwanted fondling	80.00	87.20	75.56 *	89.54#	90.41	87.88
Unwanted penetrative sex	88.60	93.29	85.71*	93.42#	94.52	91.34

#significant at $p < 0.01$ compared between gender
*significant at $p < 0.05$ compared between two groups holding different gender-role attitudes within boys or girls

Table 3 Percentage distribution of students experiencing different forms of NCS, grouped by sex of the respondent and gender-role attitudes (%)

Forms of NCS	Male			Female		
	Total	Gender-role attitudes Score		Total	Gender-role attitudes Score	
		<=2 (n = 164)	> 2 (n = 266)		<=2 (n = 438)	> 2 (n = 231)
Verbal harassment via communication technology	47.67	48.17	47.37	49.48	50.46	47.62
Sexually suggestive comments	20.00	15.24	22.93*	33.93[#]	32.42	36.80
Unwanted touch/frottage	27.21	26.22	27.82	63.23[#]	60.50	68.40*
Unwanted fondling (n)	7.67 (33)	4.27 (7)	9.77* (26)	13.90[#] (93)	13.01 (57)	15.58 (36)
Attempted rape (n)	1.40 (6)	0.61 (1)	1.88 (5)	8.07[#] (54)	6.62 (29)	10.82 (25)
Completed forced sex (n)	1.86 (8)	1.22 (2)	2.26 (6)	5.23[#] (35)	3.42 (15)	8.66[*] (20)

[#]significant at $p < 0.01$ compared between gender
*significant at $p < 0.05$ compared between two groups holding different gender-role attitudes within boys or girls

demographic variables as covariates. Gender-role attitudes were negatively associated with the perception of NCS among boys ($\beta = -0.6107$, $p = 0.0389$), which meant boys who had more traditional attitudes of gender roles were less likely to recognize the coercion of specific events. However, gender-role attitudes were not significantly associated with perceptions of NCS among girls, controlling for the background characteristics included in the analysis.

Table 5 shows results of students' experience of physical sexual coercion using logistic regression, controlling for demographic covariates. Here, for efficiency of analysis and ease in interpretation, we merged together all those who reported having had experienced either unwanted touch, fondling, attempted or actual penetrative sex as one category of having experienced physical NCS. The positive association between traditional gender-role attitudes and experience of physical NCS was not found among boys, but marginally significant (OR = 1.41, $p =$ 0.0558) among girls. It seemed that girls who held more traditional gender-role attitudes were more likely to be the

victims of physical NCS. We also analyzed the association between gender-role attitudes and experience of verbal NCS (face-to-face and via technology together or respectively) and no associations were found (data not shown).

Discussion

To promote the awareness of the problem of NCS, adolescent health and rights advocates are calling for more research and an increased emphasis on its prevention. It is essential to better understand adolescents' perceptions of NCS to effectively address it, as self-disclosure is critical in identifying such events. This study, involving a range of NCS, was the first study of its kind in China that examined university students' perception of NCS. It found most unwanted physical contacts were viewed as abusive by majority of university students, while non-physical sexual violence was viewed as such by half of them. Their perception of NCS was, therefore, affected by the intrusiveness of the sexual act, and physical contact seemed to be the recognized threshold. This finding is consistent with those from US and Korean studies [27, 28]. In China, any act of

Table 4 Results of multiple regression (generalized linear model) assessing the influencing factors of perception of NCS, by sex of the respondent

Variables	Male		Female	
	Coefficient (β)	p-value	Coefficient (β)	p-value
Gender-role attitudes	−0.6107	0.0389	−0.1269	0.5642
Discipline [a]				
Literal arts	−0.0398	0.9312	0.7158	0.0104
Science	0.4269	0.3902	0.5256	0.1665
Engineering	0.2781	0.5099	1.0271	0.0004
Residence before entering university [b]	−0.0851	0.8005	−0.3830	0.1131
Parent' s highest education	0.4002	0.0652	0.1732	0.2665
Feeling about family atmosphere	0.1329	0.7185	0.3592	0.1509
Feeling about campus life	−0.0370	0.8663	−0.1521	0.4021

[a]arts as the reference
[b]rural area as the reference

Table 5 Results of logistic regression assessing the influencing factors of physical NCS experience, by sex of the respondent

Variables	Male		Female	
	Coefficient (β)	OR (95%CI)	Coefficient (β)	OR (95%CI)
Gender-role attitudes	0.0870	1.09 (0.70–1.69)	0.3440	1.41 (0.99–2.01)
Discipline [a]				
Literal arts	−0.0132	0.75 (0.38–1.47)	0.0487	0.99 (0.63–1.54)
Science	−0.4091	0.51 (0.24–1.08)	0.0701	1.01 (0.55–1.84)
Engineering	0.1505	0.88 (0.48–1.62)	−0.1790	0.79 (0.50–1.24)
Residence before entering university [b]	−0.1619	0.85 (0.52–1.39)	0.4938	1.64 (1.13–2.37)
Parent's highest education	−0.0814	0.92 (0.67–1.27)	−0.0043	0.99 (0.78–1.27)
Feeling about family atmosphere	0.3581	1.43 (0.86–2.39)	0.6343	1.89 (1.18–3.01)
Feeling about campus life	−0.0779	0.92 (0.67–1.28)	−0.0968	0.91 (0.68–1.21)

[a]arts as the reference
[b]rural area as the reference

rape against women or girls has been included in the law with relatively clear definition and accountability of perpetrators. However, sending pornographic message, indecent behavior and intentionally exposing one's body to others, and sexual harassment against women were ambiguously included in different laws and regulations since 2005 without clear penalty regulations. Such legalization status might limit the attention of the whole society to non-physical sexual violence and restrict the provision of education and further services for victims or survivors. This could partly explain the lower awareness on non-physical sexual violence among university students.

As found in other studies, females were much more likely to experience NCS than males. However, NCS rates were non-trivial rates for male university students. This pointed out the necessity that prevention programs reach out to men as potential victims. The most frequently reported form of NCS among university students was unwanted touch. However, unwanted touch is often overlooked by the public mainly owing to its seemingly less intrusiveness. The extent of negative effects in the aftermath of unwanted touch as compared to more intrusive NCS needs to be further studied. The forced penetrative sex was found to be higher (31.5%) among sexually active female students, compared to what has been reported in other studies conducted in Chinese universities [29]. The differences in the phrasing of questions and the types of NCS used in different studies may in part explain the divergence in findings. The emergence of sexual harassment through short message, telephone or the Internet relevant to today's adolescents is serious because of the growing number of adolescents using these technologies, which was also indicated by other studies [30, 31]. The wide application of information technology and the Internet endow sexual harassment with more versatile and hidden forms, requiring an urgent attention by policy makers and sexual education or service practitioners.

The study documents the transition from traditional gender norms to support for the egalitarian gender roles among university students in Shanghai. Over half of the students supported equal gender roles, while some were undecided. Gender difference was found in the adherence of the egalitarian gender roles. Girls expressed to be more equal in social status and resource sharing, while persistently showing the traditional gender role of female submissiveness in sexual interactions. This study found female university students who held traditional gender-role attitudes were more likely to be victims of NCS. Valuing deference and subordination could affect women's behaviors generally as well as during sexual encounters. Wigderson and Katz found college women invested in feminine deference were less assertive in refusing unwanted advances, and being less assertive in turn appeared to increase the risk of sexual assault [32]. In addition, as the still entrenching traditional gender norms expected women to be virgin and uninformed about sexual matters before marriage, young girls were less likely to have enough sexual knowledge and negotiation skills, and hence were unable to express their consent to sex or to resist sexual advances. This study also found the gender differences in the interpretation of NCS and the negative influence of traditional gender roles on perception of NCS among male university students. Men who held dominant masculine norms were more inclined to justify the sexual violence, especially when the violence toward women and girls. Extensive research has documented that men with more traditional gender role ideologies are significantly more likely to report sexual coercion and relationship violence [17, 18, 33, 34], and there has been emphasis on challenging traditional masculine ideologies in the programs involving boys and men in other countries [35–37]. This study also pointed a critical need to challenge the traditional masculine norms in China.

Gender-role attitudes had no impact on NCS experience among male students. As most of male students (50–58%) encountered male-to-male sexual coercion while majority of female students (80–98%) encountered heterosexual coercion, traditional gender norms do not adequately explain the experience of male-to-male sexual coercion. Further research should therefore explore the impact of traditional gender norms on young men's role as perpetrators and the underlying factors influencing the homosexual sexual violence among college males. Besides, no association was found between gender-role attitudes and overall perception on NCS among female students. It is possible that gender norms have several dimensions and the scale used in this study didn't capture meticulously the ideologies as perceived by today's university students that affect their awareness on NCS. Therefore, further research should investigate the potential dimension of gender role perceptions among young university students in terms of how these perceptions might be related to vigilance of NCS risks.

The results of the current study point out the need to not only improve the policy and legislation on kinds of NCS, but also educate the public on the variety of situation which constitute NCS. Such actions could significantly boost the identification and support services for the victims and survivors. Specifically, relevant policies and legislation should provide explicit definition on each kind of NCS and provide operable and detailed punishment regulations. Education programs should serve to increase the adolescents' vigilance of "danger" signs, especially when the case of sexual coercion does not fit the stereotype. Meanwhile, education programs should increase the NCS awareness of relevant professionals, emphasize that appropriate actions are taken when professionals recognize such cases, and thus increase the probability that adolescent and youth would receive potential mental, health, and legal support. The possibility that males could be potential victims of NCS should not be overlooked in the prevention and support services and programs. The findings also offer a strong justification to question the weakening but still entrenched traditional gender norms, both passive femininities and dominant masculinities, that favor coercion against women and have devastating impact on women's ability to assert themselves in sexual encounters and relationships. Young men need to better understand women's rights and learn skills to resolve conflicts. Young women should be empowered with negotiation and self-protection skills that would build their self-esteem and prevent them from potentially risky situations or relationships. Challenging harmful gender norms and unequal power between males and females requires going beyond individual level efforts to challenging gender inequalities at the structural level [38]. Support from the whole society, including family, school, media, government institutions and law enforcement, should be mobilized to eliminate the harmful gender norms and discriminatory practices.

Several limitations of the study are noteworthy. First, only six items were included in our exploratory study to reflect Confucian-based gender norms. Our conclusion for the effect of gender norms are considered tentative and appropriate scale to capture gender-role ideologies perceived by today's adolescents should be developed in future research. Second, this study didn't collect information regarding respondents as perpetrators for the reason that respondents would have feared punishment or stigma and were less likely to report it. Therefore, the effects of traditional gender-role attitudes on acts of perpetrators couldn't be explored. Third, data were based on self-reporting. Although computer-assisted self-interviewing method has proved to reveal higher prevalence rates for sensitive and stigmatized behaviors [39], recall bias cannot be ruled out. Fourth, the participants were recruited from four universities in Shanghai. The social norms and environment in these universities may have influenced the knowledge and information available to students as well as their assessment of harassment. Therefore, the results from this study cannot be considered to be representative of Chinese youth. Finally, given that the study was cross-sectional, causal interpretation of relationship cannot be drawn. For these limitations, results from this study should be considered exploratory in nature though they provide important insights on gender-role attitudes, perceptions and experience of NCS among university students in Shanghai.

Conclusion

This study found university students in Shanghai, China held relatively egalitarian attitude to gender roles and low awareness on NCS, but faced relatively high risk of being the victim of NCS. The weakening but still existing traditional gender norms had negative effects on the vigilance of NCS among male students and victimization among female students. The present study suggested the need of challenging the harmful gender norms both in individual and structure level while promoting policy and legislation as well as education and support programs on NCS, in order to help adolescents and young people to understand the nature of NCS better and enhance sexual self-efficacy and negotiation skills that prevent them from potentially risky situations or relationships.

Abbreviations
95%CI: 95% confidence interval; NCS: Non-consensual sex; OR: Odds ratio

Acknowledgements
We would like to acknowledge all the participants and the university faculties for participating in this study.

Funding

This study was supported by World Health Organization (No. A65308) and Innovation-oriented Science and Technology Grant from NPFPC Key Laboratory of Reproduction Regulation (CX2017-05).

Authors' contributions

XZ and QL conducted the data analyses and manuscript writing; CL, EG and IS designed the study and the outline of the manuscript. XZ designed the questionnaire and collected the data. All authors read and approved the final manuscript.

Competing interests

The authors declare that they have no competing interests.

Author details

[1]Key Laboratory of Reproduction Regulation of NPFPC, SIPPR, IRD, Fudan University, 779 Laohumin Road, Shanghai 200237, China. [2]Department of Reproductive Health and Research, World Health Organization, Geneva, Switzerland.

References

1. Jejeebhoy SJ, Bott S. Non-consensual sexual experiences of young people in developing countries: an overview. In: Shireen J, editor. Sex without consent: young people in developing countries; 2005.
2. Barth J, Bermetz L, Heim E, et al. The current prevalence of child sexual abuse worldwide: a systematic review and meta-analysis. Int J Public Health. 2013;58(3):469–83.
3. World Health Organization. Responding to children and adolescents WHO have been sexually abused. WHO clinical guidelines. Geneva: World Health Organization [WHO]; 2017.
4. Behnken MP, Le YCL, Temple JR, et al. Forced sexual intercourse, suicidality, and binge drinking among adolescent girls. Addict Behav. 2010;35(5):507.
5. Biglan A, Noell J, Ochs L, et al. Does sexual coercion play a role in the high-risk sexual behavior of adolescent and young adult women? J Behav Med. 1995;18(6):549–68.
6. Noell J, Rohde P, Seeley J, et al. Childhood sexual abuse, adolescent sexual coercion and sexually transmitted infection acquisition among homeless female adolescents. Child Abuse Negl. 2001;25(1):137.
7. Roode TV, Dickson N, Herbison P, et al. Child sexual abuse and persistence of risky sexual behaviors and negative sexual outcomes over adulthood: findings from a birth cohort. Child Abuse Negl. 2009;33(3):161.
8. Miller E, Decker MR, McCauley HL, et al. Pregnancy coercion, intimate partner violence and unintended pregnancy. Contraception. 2010;81(4):316–22.
9. Cáceres CF, Vanoss MB, Sid HE. Sexual coercion among youth and young adults in Lima, Peru. J Adolesc Health. 2000;27(5):361–7.
10. Sumner SA, Mercy AA, Saul J, et al. Prevalence of sexual violence against children and use of social services - seven countries, 2007-2013. MMWR Morb Mortal Wkly Rep. 2015;64(21):565–9.
11. Marston C. Chapter 19: pitfalls in the study of sexual coercion: what are we measuring and why?. Sex without consent young people in developing countries, 2005.
12. Amado LE. Sexual and bodily rights as human rights in the Middle East and North Africa. Reprod Health Matters. 2004;12(23):125–8.
13. World Health Organization. Gender mainstreaming for health managers: a practical approach. 2011.
14. Joint United Nations Programme on HIV/AIDS. Sex and youth: contextual factors affecting risk for HIV / AIDS. Geneva: UNAIDS; 2016.
15. Nicola C, Ward LM, Ann M, et al. Femininity ideology and sexual health in young women: a focus on sexual knowledge, embodiment, and agency. Int J Sex Health. 2011;23(1):48–62.
16. Katz J, Tirone V. Women's sexual compliance with male dating partners: associations with Investment in Ideal Womanhood and Romantic Well-Being. Sex Roles. 2009;60(5–6):347–56.
17. Reed E, Silverman JG, Raj A, et al. Male perpetration of teen dating violence: associations with neighborhood violence involvement, gender attitudes, and perceived peer and neighborhood norms. J Urban Health. 2011;88(2):226–39.
18. Nydegger LA, Difranceisco W, Quinn K, et al. Gender norms and age-disparate sexual relationships as predictors of intimate partner violence, sexual violence, and risky sex among adolescent gang members. J Urban Health. 2016;94(2):1–13.
19. Franklin CA. Physically forced, alcohol-induced, and verbally coerced sexual victimization: assessing risk factors among university women. J Crim Just. 2010;38(2):149–59.
20. Koss MP. The hidden rape victim: personality, attitudinal, and situational characteristics. Psychol Women Q. 1985;9(2):193–212.
21. Cheng Y, Kang B, Wang T, et al. Case-controlled study on relevant factors of adolescent sexual coercion in China. Contraception. 2001;64(2):77–80.
22. Wu J, Wang L, Zhao G, et al. Sexual abuse and reproductive health among unmarried young women seeking abortion in China. Int J Gynaecol Obstet. 2006;92(2):186–91.
23. Zuo X, Lou C, Gao E, et al. Gender differences in adolescent premarital sexual permissiveness in three Asian cities: effects of gender-role attitudes. J Adolesc Health. 2012;50(3):18–25.
24. Zhang N. Gender role egalitarian attitudes among Chinese college students. Sex Roles. 2006;55(7–8):545–53.
25. Zheng XY, Chen G, Han YL. Survey of youth access to reproductive health in China. Population & development, 2010.
26. Chen J, Dunne MP, Han P. Child sexual abuse in China: a study of adolescents in four provinces. Child Abuse Negl. 2004;28(11):1171–86.
27. Ko CM, Koh CK. The influence of abuse situation and respondent background characteristics on Korean nurses' perceptions of child sexual abuse: a fractional factorial design. Int J Nurs Stud. 2007;44(7):1165.
28. O'Toole AW, O'Toole R, Webster S, et al. Nurses' responses to child abuse. J Interpers Violence. 1994;9(2):194–206.
29. Feng ZQ, Wang HM, Yong-Zhong LI. Survey of behaviors detrimental to health in adolescents in urban area of Hainan Province. China Trop Med. 2007;7(2):283-5.
30. Bonomi AE, Anderson ML, Nemeth J, et al. Dating violence victimization across the teen years: abuse frequency, number of abusive partners, and age at first occurrence. BMC Public Health. 2012;12(1):637.
31. Arafa AE, Elbahrawe RS, Saber NM, et al. Cyber sexual harassment: a cross-sectional survey over female university students in upper Egypt. Int J Community Med Public Health. 2018;5(1):61-5.
32. Wigderson S, Katz J. Feminine ideology and sexual assault: are more traditional college women at greater risk? Violence Against Women. 2015;21(5):616.
33. Santana MC, Raj A, Decker MR, et al. Masculine gender roles associated with increased sexual risk and intimate partner violence perpetration among young adult men. J Urban Health. 2006;83(4):575–85.
34. Reyes MN, Foshee VA, Niolon PH, et al. Gender role attitudes and male adolescent dating violence perpetration: normative beliefs as moderators. J Youth Adolesc. 2016;45(2):350–60.
35. Das M, Ghosh S, Miller E, et al. Engaging coaches and athletes in fostering gender equity: findings from the Parivartan program in Mumbai, India. Summary report. New Delhi: International Center for Research on Women [ICRW]; 2012. 181(6): 775-786
36. Singh AK, Verma R, Greene M, et al. Promoting gender equity as a strategy to reduce HIV risk and gender-based violence among young men in India. 2010.
37. Ricardo C, Eads M, Barker G. INTERNATIONAL: engaging boys and young men in the prevention of sexual violence: a systematic and global review of evaluated interventions. Promundo; 2011. http://www.svri.org/sites/default/files/attachments/2016-04-13/menandboys.pdf. Accessed 13 Mar 2018.
38. Amin A, Chandramouli V. Empowering adolescent girls: developing egalitarian gender norms and relations to end violence. Reprod Health. 2014;11(1):1–3.
39. Le LC, Blum RW, Magnani R, et al. A pilot of audio computer-assisted self-interview for youth reproductive health research in Vietnam. J Adolesc Health. 2006;38(6):740.

8

Barriers to reproductive health care for migrant women

N. C. Schmidt[1*], V. Fargnoli[2], M. Epiney[1] and O. Irion[1]

Abstract

Background: Migrant mothers in developed countries often experience more complicated pregnancy outcomes and less fewer women access preventive gynecology services. To enlighten health care providers to potential barriers, the objective of this paper is to explore barriers to reproductive health services in Geneva described by migrant women from a qualitative perspective.

Methods: In this qualitative study, thirteen focus groups (FG) involving 78 women aged 18 to 66 years were conducted in seven languages. All the FG discussions were audio-recorded and later transcribed. The data was classified, after which the main themes and sub-themes were manually extracted and analyzed.

Results: Barriers were classified either into structural or personal barriers aiming to describe factors influencing the accessibility of reproductive health services vs. those influencing client satisfaction. The five main themes that emerged were financial accessibility, language barriers, real or perceived discrimination, lack of information and embarrassment.

Conclusion: Structural improvements which might meet the needs of the emergent extremely diverse population are the (1) provision of informative material that is easy to understand and available in multiple languages, (2) provision of sensitive cultural training including competence skill for all health professionals, (3) provision of specifically trained nurses or social assistance to guide migrants through the health system and (4) inclusion of monitoring and evaluation programs for the prevention of personal and systemic discrimination.

Keywords: Reproductive health, Migrant woman, Qualitative study, Focus group

Plain English summary

Migrant mothers in developed countries often experience more complicated pregnancy outcomes and fewer migrant women access preventive gynecology services. The objective of this paper was to explore barriers to services for reproductive health (RH) in Geneva described by migrant women from a qualitative perspective. The study used a qualitative approach and thirteen focus groups, involving 78 women aged 18 to 66 years, conducted in seven languages. The data was analyzed, and common themes were identified.

The five main barriers that emerged were financial accessibility, language barriers, real or perceived discrimination, lack of information and embarrassment.

In conclusion, the study suggested the following four interventions to reduce barriers for migrant women to reproductive health care services:

1. The provision of informative material that is easy to understand and available in multiple languages.
2. The mandatory provision of sensitive cultural training for health professionals.
3. The provision of specifically trained nurses or social assistance to guide migrants through the health system.

* Correspondence: nicole.schmidt@hcuge.ch
[1]Department of Obstetrics and Gynecology, University Hospitals of Geneva, Geneva, Switzerland
Full list of author information is available at the end of the article

4. The inclusion of monitoring and evaluating programs for the prevention of personal and systemic discrimination.

Background

Migration is increasing worldwide. Migrants move to high-income countries for a variety of reasons. On the one hand, individuals migrate to improve their employment opportunities (so-called labor migration), while on the other hand, individuals are forced to migrate due to conflict, human rights violations or persecution. The International Office of Migration reported in 2015 that more than one billion people in the world are migrants, among which 48% are women [1]. In Switzerland, the foreign-born population has greatly increased, and the canton of Geneva is among those with the highest migrant population. In 2016, 41% of the residents in the canton of Geneva had a nationality other than Swiss [2].

While a diverse population bears important chances for economic development, inequalities in pregnancy and childbirth outcomes and disparities in access to gynecology services between migrants and non-migrants have been reported internationally [3–5]. This finding is in accordance with studies conducted in Switzerland, which described a higher maternal and infant mortality among women with a non-Swiss nationality in comparison to their Swiss peers [6–8]. Furthermore, newborns of mothers, especially those from Africa or South East Asia, have been reported to have lower birth weights and to be more frequently transferred to the neonatal unit [6, 9]. In the field of gynecology, studies in Switzerland described more voluntary abortions among women with a non-Swiss nationality, higher numbers of unwanted pregnancies among undocumented migrants compared with women with a legal resident permit or Swiss women, as well as lower screening rates for cervical or breast cancer in some ethnic groups [10–12].

Reasons for health disparities among migrants and the population of the receiving country are multi-factorial and often difficult to disentangle. Published literature has stated, among other factors, challenges in accessing the health care system (such as language barriers, lower health literacy, and low trans-cultural proficiency of health care providers) but also socio-economic difficulties or cultural beliefs [4, 13, 14].

Engaging communities in health care interventions to reduce barriers or stigma can present a unique mode to deliver care with the potential advantage of improving individual's health. Community health programs, either in ethnic communities or in faith-based organizations, have been implemented with notable success, among others, in the United States of America [15–17].

In Switzerland, little is known about whether communities for migrant women support their members in terms of understanding and accessing the reproductive health care system. Therefore, the aim of our study was to identify barriers to access reproductive health services by migrant women in Geneva and to understand if the community played a role in addressing those barriers.

Methods
Study design

A qualitative methodology was used. Qualitative methods are commonly chosen as appropriate to capture the views of marginalized groups such as migrants or the perspectives of females [18, 19]. Between April 2014 and June 2015, thirteen focus groups (FG) were conducted to describe the experiences and perceptions of reproductive health-related events and to find commonality and identify differences with other participants. The semi-structured interview guide started in a supportive and non-judgmental way with general health topics about the comprehension of women's health, such as women's behaviors to maintain good health, and evolved to more specific topics such as negative experiences with RH services.. Core topics included i) the comprehension and promotion of women's health, ii) health-seeking behavior, iii) experience with reproductive health services in Switzerland and home country, iv) information, and v) the role of the community.

Sampling

The study used the approach of systematic, non-probabilistic sampling. According to the standards of qualitative methodology, we applied the principle of saturation and considering time and access, we aimed to recruit approximately 80 women who identified themselves as a migrant and as a member of a community.

We used multiple recruitment strategies to access the communities, including personal contact of the migrant by email or telephone, making announcements at community gatherings and using the snowball-method [20]. In some situations, a flyer in the maternal language of the targeted participants was used to provide additional information and to determine interest and eligibility. Interested communities participated in an initial meeting that supplied further information about the study. Once a community decided to participate, selected community members reviewed the FG guidelines and assisted with the translation. When interested, community members were trained to moderate the FG in the participant's language. Community members recruited the participants, and interviews were either organized in the community or in a private room provided by the hospital.

We recruited participants from communities that have been previously described as either disadvantaged or most rapidly growing foreign nationalities in Geneva city. Therefore, we included the perspective of women from Eritrea, Albania, the Philippines, the Middle East and Latin-America. Women were recruited from migrant communities that were active in different areas such as ethnically related groups, religious communities and language schools. To be eligible, participants had to identify themselves as migrants and to be aged 18 years or older. We used the concept of self-defined ethnic identity, which reflects the national identity, but also the social environment in which one interacts such as family, employment or community [21, 22].

Interview process and data collection

FGs were conducted either in French, English or the maternal language of the participants. An experienced facilitator, one out of two investigators of the research team, moderated all discussions: one medical doctor (NS) and one sociologist (VF). The investigators collaborated during the different phases of the project with the community members; for example in the translation of the study guide and interpretation of results.

Community members served as translators, or if they preferred to participate in the FG, participants identified by the group accepted a translator. All FGs were digitally audio-recorded, transcribed and translated into French (two English FG were transcribed directly into English). Translated transcripts were read through multiple times, summarized and then thematically coded using the qualitative analysis software ATLAS.ti CAQDAS. Most codes were defined in advance according to the main research questions, and additional codes emerged during the coding process itself. A snack was provided at the end of the FG, and participants received a reimbursement of a maximum of twenty Swiss Francs for their

participation, depending on the decision made by the community.

Study setting

The study was conducted in Geneva city, which is the most populous city in the French-speaking part of Switzerland. The canton of Geneva has a total of 493,706 inhabitants (2016). A large number of international organizations have their headquarters and agencies in Geneva, and in 2015 41% if the canton inhabitants were of a non-Swiss nationality. Gynecology or obstetric services are provided at the University Hospital of Geneva, a public hospital, or in private cabinets or clinics in Geneva. This study was initiated at the Department of Obstetrics at the University Hospital of Geneva and was approved by the Ethical Review Board of the Canton of Geneva (CER 14–095).

Results

Between April 2014 and June 2015, thirteen FGs in six communities were conducted (Table 1). A typical FG lasted between 90 and 150 min. The average age of the participating women was 41 years (range: 18 to 66 years), and the majority (57.7%) of the women were married. Participants were from 23 countries, and on average, the women had lived in Switzerland for nine years (range: 3 months to 25 years). Their education level was good, with 84.6% having at least a college degree. In addition, every sixth participant reported having no health insurance (15.4%). The socio-demographic characteristics are shown in Table 2.

The study had the overarching objective of exploring barriers to reproductive health services and

Table 1 Details about focus groups

Number of FGs	Number of participants	Continent of origin	Language of FG	Number Community
	3 FG test (English and French)			
1	7	Middle East	French	1
2	5	Latin-America	Spanish	2
3	7	Latin-America	Spanish	2
4	7	Middle East	Persian	1
5	6	Africa	Tigrinya	3
6	4	Latin-America	Portuguese	4
7	7	mixed (Europe, Africa, Latin-America)	French	5
8	5	mixed (Europe, Africa, Middle-East)	French	5
9	6	mixed (Europe, Africa, Middle-East)	French	5
10	5	mixed (Europe, Africa, Middle-East, Latin-America)	French	5
11	8	Europe	Albanian	5
12	5	Asia	English	6
13	4	Asia	English	6

Table 2 FG participants characteristics

	Focus group participants (n = 78)
Women 18–66 years	78 (100)
Mean age in years (SD)	40.96 (12.5)
18–39 years	33 (42.3)
>= 40 years	41 (52.6)
no answer	4 (5.1)
Religion	
christian	30 (38.5)
moslem	33 (42.3)
other	2 (2.5)
no answer	13 (16.7)
Mean years in Switzerland	9.05
<= 3 years	24 (30.8)
4–10 years	30 (38.4)
> 10 years	24 (30.8)
Martial status	
single	15 (19.2)
married or in partnership	45 (57.7)
divorced or separated	11 (14.1)
widowed	5 (6.4)
no answer	2 (2.6)
Children	
yes	57 (73.1)
no	19 (24.4)
no answer	2 (2.5)
Education	
never attended school or <= 6 years	12 (15.4)
finished secondary education	28 (35.9)
some technical school	5 (6.4)
bachelor's degree or higher	26 (33.3)
no answer	7 (9.0)
Work situation	
part or full-time work	27 (34.6)
not working	38 (48.7)
student	3 (3.8)
incapacity to work	6 (7.7)
no answer	4 (5.2)
Health insurance	
yes	63 (80.8)
no	12 (15.4)
no answer	3 (3.8)

understanding if the community played a supportive role. The results from the data analysis revealed five broad themes that had a major impact on migrant women's access to reproductive health services. The identified findings were classified according to Higginbottom and colleagues' recent paper into either factors influencing the accessibility of reproductive health services vs. factors influencing client satisfaction, and categorized as either structural or personal barriers [23].

Factors influencing the accessibility of reproductive health services

Language barrier

In all FGs, the language barrier was one of the main obstacles to accessing care. All but one woman were raised outside of Switzerland, and French was not their primary language. Nearly one-third of the participants expressed their preference for a physician speaking the same language. Esther (Middle East) explained: *My gynecologist… she is Iranian, we speak the same language, so I didn't have a problem.* Those feelings were shared by other women such as Katia (Latin America): *In my case for example, every time I go to the hospital or to a doctor, I ask for a Spanish speaking doctor. I come around with French. I am not saying that I speak very well. But for me, it is very important to express my feelings in my language because it is not the same to say it in another language that is not understood in the same way…..* Women described their inability to speak French as a major source of anxiety, and they feared misinterpretation or misunderstanding. Amanda (Latin America) explained: *She (the doctor) searched for someone who spoke Portuguese to translate for me. This was what I needed. From this moment on, I felt quieter and I started to understand.* The provision of a skilled interpreter is a service that is provided at the Geneva University hospital free of charge. However, few participants had relied on those professional interpreter services mainly due to a lack of awareness of its existence or due to the belief that costs would emerge. Mainly family members or friends served as interpreters, and most of the participants experienced the services of a family member as an interpreter as sufficient. How3ever, some women recognized the difficulties of unskilled interpreters; especially in complicated medical situation. Participants reported that family members or friends who served as interpreters were not able to correctly translate either due to difficulties in translating the medical vocabulary or due to their personal emotions. Saba from Eritrea shared her experience while in tears: *The doctor asked if I was in pain. I tried to answer but there was a huge problem of communication [then] I started to cry because I felt frustrated. I asked her to stop touching me and she called my husband. She explained things to him but he didn't* understand because medical explanations are too much for him [...]. If an interpreter were there, everything would have been easier».

In only one of the thirteen FG did the interviewees experience the interpreter as an intruder: *It's difficult to talk about gynecology issues in our culture [...]. It is a taboo, the fact that we are embarrassed. And now, on top of that, there is the interpreter. I mean, it is already difficult to talk about the problem to doctors, but we will probably not see him again. But the interpreter is part of our community. So, there is more chance to cross him again* (Solomon from East-Africa).

Lack of information

It is important to receive information to understand the health services, which are provided in the host country. Therefore, the lack of information appeared as the second main barrier expressed by participants. Two different reasons emerged: either because participants did not understand the provided information due to language barriers or because they never received any information. Several participants mentioned that they consulted with a gynecologist only in the case of medical problems, which was sometimes due to time or financial constraints (see financial acceptability), but often women were not aware of available preventive health services. Eva from Peru explained: *Only if we have a problem we start to look for a gynecologist. If we are not sick, we do not think about it.* In nearly all FGs, women shared such experiences: *I only go there [the hospital] to give birth. Otherwise, I do not know any controls (Melete from East Africa).*

Participants who migrated from countries where prevention is less known and provided stated that it would have been helpful for them to receive information about preventive services from their health care providers. Afra (East-Africa) stated: *Until today, my general practitioner didn't give me any information on preventive check-ups. I think it would be helpful if he could remind us about the controls, especially gynecology check-ups, which are available.*

Women perceived a form of information as crucial to better understand, access and utilize reproductive health care services. Several women agreed with Afra that health care providers should provide them with the essential information, especially about available preventive services such as cervical cancer screening or family planning advice. However, women also recognized the limitations with respect to the time and workload of their doctors: *I prefer it if the gynecologist explains everything to me, but sometimes he might be tired by his work and forget to do it (Woman from Kosovo).*

In addition to the information provided orally by direct contact with health or social professionals, the provision of written information material in multiple languages was rated in almost all FGs as essential to facilitate access and navigate through the Swiss health system. Participants identified different means such as the radio, the television or written information received by mail. However, the two most frequently used sources were either the Internet or health-related sessions in communities or language classes. Importantly, nearly all participants had access to a computer and identified the Internet as a valuable source of information, especially the opportunity to search for information in their maternal language.

Financial acceptability

Nearly half of the participants identified costs as the third most important barrier to health care. Even if participants had health insurance, which is mandatory in Switzerland, the costs of high deductibles or co-payments were often mentioned as a barrier to visiting the doctor, which was especially the case for preventive services. Angela (South-Asia) stated: *... going to the hospital is quite expensive. And then so, ... For two years, I have not visited a doctor.*

Embarrassment

Embarrassment emerged as a personal barrier on the participant (user) side explaining why women did not access especially preventive gynecology services such as cervical cancer or breast cancer screening. Most women perceived pelvic and vaginal examinations for cervical cancer screening as inconvenient and often painful. Juana from Latin America explained: *When they took the smear it was terrible for me. All afternoon, I had horrible pain and was bleeding.* Physical discomfort is not a barrier related specifically to immigrant women and has been mentioned by Swiss women as well [24]. However, in more than half of the FG discussions, the participants explained that they grew up experiencing the female body as taboo. Veronica from Latin America stated: *We are not taught to discover our bodies....* Elsa, a mother of two children from Africa explained: *Especially with respect to gynecological problems but also with respect to other health problems, we try to keep it [the problem] to ourselves as long as possible, and if it is a gynecological problem, we prefer to say that we have pain somewhere else because we feel very embarrassed.*

Furthermore, women experienced discomfort when health care providers were not aware of their traditions. Mahan (Middle East) expressed: *Sometimes it would be helpful if the doctor understands our traditions a little bit. For example, as a woman, we do not like to shake hands with a male doctor. But some doctors do not know this!* Similar feelings were experienced when women could not consult with a female doctor. Senobar explained (Middle-East): *They suggested to me to see a male doctor. I didn't go! In* more than half of the FGs, participants specifically mentioned a preference for a female health care provider for gynecology or obstetric consultations.

Factors influencing client satisfaction
Real or perceived discrimination
Nearly one-third of the participants expressed that they felt that they did not receive the same attendance as Swiss women. Importantly, in nearly one-third of the FGs, women expressed feelings of discrimination in their daily lives. Amanda from Latin America explained: *I would love if integration would be easier. I know that it is difficult to migrate here [to Switzerland]... But it should be easier,...., that people would have less fear. Because of the fear of losing your residence permit, everything is very complicated;* Real or perceived discrimination in the health sector was rarely mentioned with respect to the doctor-patient relationship; it was mainly expressed concerning reception at the registration desk prior to the clinical appointment: *As soon as we arrive, we feel degraded. They want our papers, for example, proof of a health insurance. Even if we have all the papers, they put us in an uncomfortable position. We do not feel welcome.* (Armani from East-Africa).

A few women expressed that waiting time as well as perceived impolite treatment by health professionals were due to their origins or language barriers. Susanna, a women from Latin-America, gave the following example: *And when I was hospitalized, I saw that the doctor spoke a lot more with women who spoke French or were Swiss. And with me, tac, tac, tac. He didn't have the time to explain to me all that I needed. This disturbed me.*

Perceived inadequate provision of health services
In addition to the perceived lack of adequate culturally competent care (see embarrassment), women experienced the process of adhering to appointments for regular obstetric or gynecology visits as very difficult. In several cases, they had to wait several weeks for their appointments, and they complained of long waiting times in the case of emergency situations. Tiba (Middle-East) explained: *I had already had to go several times to the emergency department, but even if I am dying, I will not go there again because I had to wait six hours with a fever, but no one was interested.*

Strategies to overcome barriers at the community level:
In none of the participating communities were active projects around health established. In four of six

communities, health topics, some related to RH (such as gender-based violence and access to cervical or breast cancer screening), had been discussed at least once in the past five years. However, community-based health programs that focused on a specific prevention activity such as cervical cancer screening or healthy behavior promotion over a period of several months were not available. However, importantly, health sessions organized by the community or language schools were especially appreciated by women who had recently arrived or were more illiterate. Afra from East-Africa stated: *It would be nice to have similar meetings such as those today in small groups. This would help us more than receiving letters or flyers.* Furthermore, a community group leader from the Philippines highlighted the importance of educating women from her country to foresee health problems. She recommended the conclusion of a health insurance even in the case of illegal situations to be prepared for emergency health problems as well as to access preventive services. Angelica explained: It *is our mentality that we do not want to save something for "rainy days"... It is my dream to educate women from my home country, about what will be necessary when we are getting older. It is like an old car, which might break one day. One part of this education would be that we need insurance.*

In conclusion, in the participating communities, few strategies were utilized to overcome barriers to reproductive health services.

Discussion
The current study is, to our knowledge, the first with the aim of understanding barriers to reproductive health services among migrants from a qualitative perspective. Five main themes were identified and categorized either in terms of structural or personal barriers: financial accessibility, language barriers, real or perceived discrimination, lack of information and embarrassment (Table 3). In general, our results are fairly consistent with previous national and international literature [3, 15].

However, barriers to health services might vary depending on the kind of services from country to country, but also among different migrant groups. Therefore, it is essential to study structural and personal barriers that are related to organizational behaviors.

In the following discussion, we will specifically address the nuanced findings of the structural barriers that influenced accessibility to or satisfaction with reproductive health services for migrant women because we assume that it might be relatively feasible to target those by health care organizations. Therefore, we will not address barriers such as physical discomfort, which have also been previously for women of the host country or structural barriers at the organizational level such as long

Table 3 Main barriers identified and related structural improvements

Financial accessibility

• provision of information about structures assisting patients with limited financial resources

Language barriers

• provision and information about interpreter services

Real or perceived discrimination and embarrassment

• provision of cultural competence training for professionals working in the health sector including administrative staff (might reduce embarrassment among women as they do not need to have to explain themselves or their practices)

Lack of information

• provision of information material (including in patient's maternal language)

waiting times for appointments and during visits. Because even these factors may act as a barrier to the use of such services, they can hinder migrant and Swiss patients equally [3, 24].

First, our study confirmed the recent findings by Higginbottom and colleagues who revealed that although maternity services were equally availably for all members of society, in practice the services were often not accessible to migrant women due to a lack of awareness about their existence [23]. Even if the lack of information could be interpreted as a personal barrier, it should rather be considered, in our opinion, as a structural barrier. Indeed, a health organization that is aware of this situation can provide information to their clients. The lack of information is therefore directly linked to health literacy, which has been defined by the World Health Organization as « the cognitive and social skills which determine the motivation and ability of individuals to gain access to, understand and use information in ways which promote and maintain good health » [25]. As reported previously in two separate studies in Canada and the United Kingdom, the institutional culture of maternity services has been mainly designed for those who understand and can negotiate the system. These studies demonstrated that people who recently arrived and were not familiar with the system faced a range of barriers [26, 27]. These findings are comparable to our study in which migrant women who were either undocumented or in the process of applying for asylum appreciated the system because they were guided by specifically trained nurses or social assistants. Migrants who did not benefit from those services often felt a lack of information to navigate the system and experienced the health professionals as less helpful. Legal migrant women even stated that they would also profit from those services. These positive attitudes towards social workers or migrant health nurses support the merit of including them in the system.

Furthermore, professionals who do not work specifically with asylum seekers were not provided with accurate information concerning how to help migrants and received little assistance to develop a better understanding of the constraints and barriers experienced by this specific social group.

It is also important that information material requires sufficient language proficiency among recipients. In our study, inadequate language proficiency emerged as one of the main barriers to either accession or the on-going use of services. This finding is supported by previous studies that have reported, among others, the preference of immigrants to have same-language physicians [4, 26, 27].

However, even if at the University Hospital of Geneva more than 100 different nationalities are working in the medical and nursing sector, it is an impossible task to provide a same-language physician for every participant. In all FGs, participants indicated that language barriers increased their insecurity about seeking care. Most participants sought out ad hoc interpreters to navigate the system, and our findings revealed that few participants were aware of the provision of free-of-charge skilled interpreters for clients. The few participants who used interpreter services rated the experience positively to influence its future use. Efforts should be undertaken to raise awareness of those services and to provide information about their gratuity as well as the possibility of avoiding certain translators either due to sex or cultural background.

The second structural barrier encountered in nearly all FG and which has been previously described in the literature was the financial accessibility of the system [26]. However, in contrast to other studies, the lack of insurance did not lead to a reported delay in seeking care [4]. This might be because, in 1996, the University Hospital created a health care unit that offers free or low cost medical care to undocumented migrants in Geneva. Even if uninsured migrants are referred to the general services of the University Hospital for gynecological or obstetric care, the health care unit has generated trust among the uninsured migrants over the two decades and reaches the majority of pregnant, undocumented and uninsured women [12].

One important personal barrier influencing access to health services that has been outlined by previous studies is social isolation [4, 23]. Interestingly, this barrier was not encountered frequently in our study, which might be due to two reasons. First, FGs were mainly conducted in ethnic, religious or social groups in which the women had started to create a social network. Second, most of the participants had followed either family members or friends who had already lived for several years in Switzerland. Therefore, those residing longer in the country facilitated the arrival of the new immigrants. This phenomenon also explains why the sub-theme of isolation was mentioned mainly in women who migrated as refugees due to unstable conditions in their home country and arrived in an unfamiliar country.

The last two structural barriers influenced mainly client satisfaction. Challenges in delivery services such as the provision of appointments, waiting times or turnover of health care providers can hinder women's access to services due to less satisfaction with the services and have been addressed previously [4, 23]. These barriers could be addressed at the organizational level.

One of the most important barriers influencing women's satisfaction was "real or perceived discrimination". Crush and colleagues described xenophobia, racism and discrimination as increasingly prevalent in countries that receive a large number of migrants [28]. As Geneva, is one of the cantons with the highest percentage of migrants in Switzerland, this risk might also be present. Xenophobia towards migrants might manifest itself as hostility towards migrants by authorities, neighbors, employers or service providers belonging to the host population [28]. Sometimes perceived discrimination is due to a feeling of inferiority emerging from the restricted rights and entitlements of migrants, which might be especially the case for vulnerable migrants. Furthermore, it has been reported that especially migrants who have migrated due to traumatic circumstances may be more inclined to perceive xenophobia against them [29]. However, this observation could not be confirmed in our study population because migrants with a non-refugee background also frequently expressed real or perceived discrimination. It is important for health care providers and administrative staff to be aware of real or perceived discrimination because it can influence the necessary trusts within the patient-provider relationship and can have negative effects on future health seeking behaviors [29, 30]. In the present study, it was not possible to verify if the staff intended to discriminate. However, efforts should be undertaken to include cultural competence training not only in medical education, as it is already part of the curriculum in Geneva, but also in professional practices for health care professionals as well as administrative staff. Intercultural competence training is a method that aims to enable professionals to communicate effectively and empathically while concomitantly reflecting their own culture and implicit assumptions [31]. Furthermore, it might effectively support patient-professional communications irrespective of the migration background. The inclusion of administrative staff in such training is important to lower the anxiety of participants because they are the first contact with the health system for participants. Even if some authors mentioned that training designed

to supply specific cultural knowledge about ethnic groups might risk stereotyping and obscure attention to the needs of women, other studies have also reported that such training improves the abilities of professionals in the health care sector to meet the needs of their patients [31]. In a setting such as Geneva, patient-sensitive competence training might improve patient-provider communication. Furthermore, it might strengthen understanding among health care providers for requests (such as same-sex physicians) that might cause embarrassment among women as they have to explain themselves or their practices, or have to ask for what may be regarded as special treatment.

Study limitations

While this qualitative study was among the first to explore barriers to RH services in the canton of Geneva and the role of the community, it has several limitations.

First, the qualitative approach of the FG covers the range of issues considered important by the participants. It does not describe the relative importance of the issues. Additionally, the format of the FG might have been influenced by leaders within the groups, despite the efforts of the moderators. Even if we reached thematic saturation in the thirteen-conducted FG in seven different languages, the study utilized convenience sampling for the recruitment of participants through local migrant communities in Geneva city and did not reach those living in more isolated regions who less frequently accessed the city center. Therefore, the results cannot be generalized to all migrant women, and thus future research is required.

Second, the authors of this article do not belong to an ethnic minority group. Even if we tried to reduce those barriers by discussing them and ways to influence them with stakeholders and representatives from migrant communities, the results risk interpretation from a western perspective, which leads to certain ideas about the provision of health care.

Third, the average length of time in Switzerland of our sample was nine years, and therefore this study might be susceptible to recall and temporal effect biases.

Finally, in contrast to other studies, we did not include the provider perspective [22].

Conclusions

Research examining the reduction of barriers to healthcare services is not only beneficial at the personal and institutional level, but it can also inform health policies and strategies. Especially in times during which a constant influx of new immigrants into Geneva changes the population, efforts of health care providers and public health actors must be continuously renewed and oriented to reach new arrivals. This study identified several structural and personal barriers to reproductive health services in Geneva. Even if the data from qualitative research cannot be generalized to the broader context of Switzerland, many of the findings could potentially be applicable to other countries.

Structural improvements, which might meet the needs of the heterogeneous emergent population, are as follows: (1) the provision of information material that is easy to understand and available in multiple languages, possibly using new mHealth technologies; (2) the mandatory provision of sensitive cultural training for health professionals to inform professionals about the availability of interpreter services and social services to offer appropriate care; (3) the evaluation and adaptation of the skills of nurses or social assistance to guide migrants who are not asylum seekers or who are undocumented through the Swiss health system; and, finally, (4) the inclusion of monitoring and evaluation programs for the prevention of personal and systemic discrimination.

Our study showed that migrant communities are interested in topics about health but provide few activities to support their members. Efforts should be undertaken to involve migrant communities, for example, in the distribution of information and knowledge among newcomers to ensure that they know where to find and how to use the services to which they are entitled.

Such combined efforts could, in our opinion, reduce some of the perceived or experienced barriers on the side of the user.

However, future research exploring community-based health interventions may also be beneficial.

Acknowledgements
The authors wish to acknowledge all the participating women and community organization members who dedicated their time to the project and shared their experiences and suggestions.

Funding
This study was part of a career funding financing granted by the Swiss National Foundation providing the salary of the main investigator NS and supporting part of the research costs. The salary of the main researcher NS was complemented by a research grant from Geneva University. Further research costs for sociological assistance were provided by the Federal Office of Health, Berne (Switzerland), and the foundation for population, migration and environment, Uetikon am See (Switzerland).

Authors' contributions
NS, as the main investigator, developed the main idea, helped in all phases of the research, and participated in writing the draft and finalizing the manuscript. VF conducted several FGs, participated in analyzing and interpreting the qualitative data and provided comments about the protocol and manuscript. ME, OI, and MB assisted in the development of the study protocol and provided essential comments on the final manuscript. All authors read and approved the final manuscript.

Competing interests
The authors declare that they have no competing interests.

Author details
[1]Department of Obstetrics and Gynecology, University Hospitals of Geneva, Geneva, Switzerland. [2]Department of Sociology, University of Geneva, Geneva, Switzerland.

References
1. International Organization for Mgration. Global Migration Trends Factsheet 2015. https://publications.iom.int/system/files/global_migration_trends_2015_factsheet.pdf. Accessed 4 Feb 2017.
2. Bilan et état de la population du canton de Genève en 2016. informations statistiques n° 6 – mars 2017. http://www.ge.ch/statistique/tel/publications/2017/informations_statistiques/autres_themes/is_population_06_2017.pdf. Accessed 25 Jul 2017.
3. Gagnon AJ, Zimbeck M, Zeitlin J, Alexander S, Blondel B, Buitendijk S, Desmeules M, Di Lallo D, Gagnn A, Gissler M. Migration to western industrialised countries and perinatal health: a systematic review. Soc Sci Med. 2009;69(6):934–6.
4. Scheppers E, Scheppers E, van Dongen E, Dekker J, Geertzen J, Dekker J. Potential barriers to the use of health services among ethnic minorities: a review. Fam Pract. 2006;23(3):325–48. Epub 2006 Feb 13
5. Reeske A, Rechel B. Maternal and child health – from conception to first birthday. In: Rechel B, Mladovsky P, Deville W, et al., editors. Migration and health in the European Union. Berkshire: Open University Press; 2011. p. 79–153.
6. Bollini P, Wanner P. Santé reproductive des collectivités migrantes, Etudes du SFM; 2006. p. 42.
7. Bollini P, Wanner P, Pampallona S. Trends in maternal mortality in Switzerland among Swiss and foreign nationals, 1969-2006. Int J Public Health. 2011;56(5):515–21.
8. Fässler M, Zimmermann R, Quack Lötscher KC. Maternal mortality in Switzerland 1995-2004. Swiss Med Wkly. 2010;140(1–2):25–30.
9. Merten S, Wyss C, Ackermann-Liebrich U. Caesarean sections and breastfeeding initiation among migrants in Switzerland. Int J Public Health. 2007;52(4):210–22.
10. FOPH What about the health of migrant population groups? What about the health of migrant population groups? 2007 FOPH: BAG GP 8.07 445 d 190 f 155 e 30EXT07011 178893 ISBN 3–905235-65-X.
11. Obsan Bulletin 01/2012. Population migrante et santé. Analyse des hospitalisations. In: Moreau-Gruet F, Luyet S, editors. Analyse de la statistique médicale des hôpitaux et recherche de littérature. Neuchatel: Observatoire Suisse de la Sante; 2011.
12. Wolff H, Epiney M, Lourenco AP, Costanza MC, Delieutraz-Marchand J, Andreoli N, Dubuisson JB, Gaspoz JM, Irion O. Undocumented migrants lack access to pregnancy care and prevention. BMC Public Health. 2008;8:93.
13. Heaman M, Bayrampour H, Kingston D, Blondel B, Gissler M, Roth C, Alexander S, Gagnon A. Migrant women's utilization of prenatal care: a systematic review. Matern Child Health J. 2013;17(5):816–36. https://doi.org/10.1007/s10995-012-1058-z. Review
14. Bischoff A. Caring for migrant and minority patients in European hospitals. A review of effective interventions. Swiss Forum for Migration and Population Studies: Neuchâtel; 2006.
15. Minkler M, Wallerstein N, Hall B. Community-Based Participatory Research for Health. 1st ed: Jossey-Bass; 2009.
16. Gutierrez J, Devia C, Weiss L, Chantarat T, Ruddock C, Linnell J, Golub M, Godfrey L, Rosen R, Calman N. Health, community and spirituality: evaluation of a multicultural faith-based diabetes prevention program. Diabetes Educ. 2014;40(2):214–22.
17. Fang CY, Ma GX, Handorf EA, Feng Z, Rhee J, Miller SM, Kim C, Koh HS. Addressing multilevel barriers to cervical cancer screening in Korean American women: a randomized trial of a community-based intervention. Cancer. 2017;123(6):1018 26.

18. Barbour R. Introducing qualitative research. A student guide to the craft of doing qualitative research. London: Sage; 2008.

19. Morgan DL. FGs. Ann Rev Sociol. 1996;22:129–52.

20. Ritchie J, Lewis J, Elam G. Designing and selecting samples. In: Ritchie J, Lewis J, editors. Qualitative Research Practice: A Guide for Social Science Students and Researchers. London: Sage; 2003. p. 77–108.

21. Israel BA, Checkoway B, Schluz AJ, Zimmerman MA. Health education and community empowerment: conceptualizing and measuring perceptions of individual, organizational, and community control. Health Educ Q. 1994;21: 149–70.

22. Tajfel H. Social identity and intergroup behavior. Soc Sci Inf. 1974;13:65–93. World Health Organization. 2010. Health of Migrants - The way forward. Report of a Global Consultation. 2010 Geneva: WHO.

23. Higginbottom GM, Safipour J, Yohani S, O'Brien B, Mumtaz Z, Paton P, Chiu Y, Barolia R. An ethnographic investigation of the maternity healthcare experience of immigrants in rural and urban Alberta, Canada. BMC Pregnancy Childbirth. 2016;16:20. https://doi.org/10.1186/s12884-015-0773-z.

24. Fargnoli V, Petignat P, Burton-Jeangros C. To what extent will women accept HPV self-sampling for cervical cancer screening? A qualitative study conducted in switzerland. Int J Women's Health. 2015;(7):883–8.

25. WHO. Health Promotion. Track 2: Health literacy and health behaviour. http://www.who.int/healthpromotion/conferences/7gchp/track2/en/. Accessed 25 Jul 2017.

26. Philimore J. Migrant maternity in an era of superdiversity: New migrants' access to, and experience of, antenatal care in the West Midlands, UK. Soc Sci Med. 2016;148:152–9. https://doi.org/10.1016/j.socscimed.2015.11.030.

27. Reitmanova S, Gustafson DL. "They can't understand it": maternity health and care needs of immigrant Muslim women in St. John's, Newfoundland. Matern child health. 2008;12(1):101–11. Epub 2007 26

28. Crush J, Ramachandran. Xenophobia, International Migration and Development. J Human Dev Capabilities. 2010;11:209–28.

29. Phinney JS, Horenczyk G, Liebkind K, Vedder P. Ethnic identity, immigration, and well-being: an interactional perspective. J Soc Issues. 2001;57(3):493–510.

30. Ellis BH, MacDonald HZ, Lincoln AK, Cabral HJ. Mental health of Somali adolescent refugees: the role of trauma, stress, and perceived discrimination. J Consult Clin Psychol. 2008;76(2):184–93. https://doi.org/10.1037/0022-006X.76.2.184.

31. Horvat L, Horey D, Romios P, Kis-Rigo J. Cultural competence education for health professionals. Cochrane Database Syst Rev. 2014;(5):CD009405. https://doi.org/10.1002/14651858.CD009405.pub2.

9

Disrespect and abuse of women during the process of childbirth in the 2015 Pelotas birth cohort

Marilia Arndt Mesenburg[1][*] [iD], Cesar Gomes Victora[1], Suzzane Jacob Serruya[2], Rodolfo Ponce de León[2], Andrea Homsi Damaso[1], Marlos Rodrigues Domingues[3] and Mariangela Freitas da Silveira[1]

Abstract

Background: The disrespect and abuse of women during the process of childbirth is an emergent and global problem and only few studies have investigated this worrying issue. The objective of the present study was to describe the prevalence of disrespect and abuse of women during childbirth in Pelotas City, Brazil, and to investigate the factors involved.

Methods: This was a cross-sectional population-based study of women delivering members of the 2015 Pelotas birth cohort. Information relating to disrespect and abuse during childbirth was obtained by household interview 3 months after delivery. The information related to verbal and physical abuse, denial of care and invasive and/or inappropriate procedures. Poisson regression was used to evaluate the factors associated with one or more, and two or more, types of disrespectful treatment or abuse.

Results: A total of 4275 women took part in a perinatal study. During the three-month follow-up, we interviewed 4087 biological mothers with regards to disrespect and abuse. Approximately 10% of women reported having experienced verbal abuse, 6% denial of care, 6% undesirable or inappropriate procedures and 5% physical abuse. At least one type of disrespect or abuse was reported by 18.3% of mothers (95% confidence interval [CI]: 17.2–19.5); and at least two types by 5.1% (95% CI: 4.4–5.8). Women relying on the public health sector, and those whose childbirths were via cesarean section with previous labor, had the highest risk, with approximately a three- and two-fold increase in risk, respectively.

Conclusions: Our study showed that the occurrence of disrespect and abuse during childbirth was high and mostly associated with payment by the public sector and labor before delivery. The efforts made by civil society, governments and international organizations are not sufficient to restrain institutional violence against women during childbirth. To eradicate this problem, it is essential to 1) implement policies and actions specific for this type of violence and 2) formulate laws to promote the equality of rights between women and men, with particular emphasis on the economic rights of women and the promotion of gender equality in terms of access to jobs and education.

* Correspondence: mariliaepi@gmail.com
[1]Post-Graduate Program in Epidemiology, Federal University of Pelotas, Pelotas, Brazil
Full list of author information is available at the end of the article

Plain English summary

Violence against women in health-care institutions is an emergent and global problem. In our study, we describe the prevalence of disrespect and abuse of women during childbirth among women delivering members of the 2015 Pelotas birth cohort, a large population-based study in which 4275 women participated. We also investigated the factors responsible for such disrespect and abuse. Information relating to disrespect and abuse during childbirth was obtained by household interview 3 months after delivery and included verbal and physical abuse, denial of care and invasive and/or inappropriate procedures. Approximately 10% of these women reported having experienced verbal abuse, 6% denial of care, 6% undesirable or inappropriate procedures and 5% physical abuse. At least one type of disrespect or abuse was reported by 18.3% of mothers; and at least two types, by 5.1%. Women relying on the public health sector, and those whose childbirths were via cesarean section with previous labor, presented the highest risk, with approximate three and two-fold increases in risk, respectively. Our study showed that the occurrence of disrespect and abuse during the process of childbirth was high and mostly associated to payment by the public sector and labor before delivery. To eradicate this problem, it is essential to implement policies and actions specific for this type of violence and to promote the equality of rights between women and men, with particular emphasis on women's economic rights and the promotion of gender equality with respect to access to jobs and education.

Background

Access to secure and high-quality sexual and reproductive health services is an essential right for women as these services can make an important contribution towards the reduction of maternal morbidity and mortality rates [1]. In Brazil, some major changes have occurred recently in relation to access to reproductive, maternal and child health services. Attending at least one antenatal care appointment is practically universal (98%), and 81% of all pregnant women have at least five visits [2]. Hospital deliveries are also practically universal, accounting for 98% of all births in this country [2]. Nevertheless, in spite of such impressive figures, the quality of care is not consistent across different population groups thus creating a significant matter for concern [2].

Every woman has the right to quality healthcare which is dignified, respectful, violence-free and free of discrimination. Abuse, negligence or disrespect during the process of childbirth constitute serious violations of fundamental human rights that are recognized internationally [3–5]. In Brazil, a number of public policies have been implemented over recent years aiming towards the humanization of pregnancy and delivery care, such as the Program for Humanization of Antenatal and Delivery Care implemented by the Ministry of Health in 2000 [6]. Furthermore, by law, all women are entitled to be accompanied by a person of their choice during antenatal appointments and hospitalization for delivery, including labor, childbirth and postpartum care [7].

Various forms of mistreatment and abuse of women during childbirth have been described in the literature, including physical, psychological or verbal abuse, humiliation, discrimination, denial of care and the implementation of contraindicated or improper procedures. These can occur at the level of the relationship between women and their healthcare professionals, or at the level of the healthcare service or system [1, 8, 9].

Studies published during the 1990s were the first to raise attention to the issue of obstetric violence [10–12]. Several studies conducted in Brazil [13–15], and elsewhere [1, 8, 9], have indicated that large numbers of women have become victims of this type of violence. However, violence against women during childbirth has now gained wide visibility and is acknowledged as an emerging problem, with studies reporting a prevalence of 11% to 98% [8, 9, 13, 14, 16–22]. Some of these studies have evaluated the potential relationship between disrespect or abuse during childbirth and the factors that might be associated with this practice, such as education, income, type of labor and ethnicity. However, none of the results arising from such studies have been consistent [14, 19, 23, 24], thus reinforcing the need for further studies. Most of these previous studies have relied upon qualitative methods. In particular, there are very few population-based studies, which may provide frequency estimates and identify vulnerable groups, in terms of individual and contextual factors associated with violence during childbirth [8, 9, 13].

The objective of the present study, therefore, was to evaluate the incidence of disrespect and abuse of women during the process of childbirth and to investigate factors that might be associated with this practice. Our study was based on a large population of women who gave birth in 2015 in the city of Pelotas, Brazil.

Methods

The study was based upon the 2015 Pelotas birth cohort [25], a population-based study that recruited all children born to mothers who were resident in the urban area of the municipality of Pelotas. This city is located in the extreme south of Brazil, with an urban population of 316,000 inhabitants and an annual per capita gross domestic product of approximately US$ 5390.

Women delivering in all of the city's hospitals between January 1st 2015 and December 31st 2015 were recruited and interviewed, and a follow-up home visit was carried out when each baby was 3 months of age plus or minus 7 days. Data were collected through structured questionnaires applied by trained interviewers; detailed methodology can be found in an earlier publication [25].

There are several terminologies relating to violence against women during the process of childbirth, including obstetric violence and mistreatment [26]. In our study we used the phrase "disrespect for and abuse of women during the process of childbirth", as used by the World Health Organization (WHO) [27]. At the three-month follow-up interview, four questions were used to identify disrespect and abuse: verbal abuse ("Has any professional been rude to you, cursed you or yelled at you, humiliated you or threatened not to attend to you?"); denial of care ("Has any professional refused to give you anything that you asked for, such as water or painkillers?"); physical abuse ("Has any professional ever pushed, hurt, beat or held you strongly or conducted any examinations rudely or disrespectfully?") and disrespect regarding invasive and/or inappropriate procedures ("Has any professional ever conducted any procedure against your will, without explaining the need to conduct it?"). For all questions, women were asked to consider their entire hospitalization period, from the time when they arrived until hospital discharge. Each question was coded as "yes" or "no", and positive responses were added to create a score ranging from zero to four. To identify risk factors, two dichotomous variables were constructed: a report of one or more types of disrespectful treatment or abuse, and a report of two or more types.

Socioeconomic and demographic characteristics were collected during the perinatal interview, including mother's age at delivery (up to 19 years, 20 to 29 years, 30 to 39 years or 40 years and over), self-reported skin color (white, brown or black), marital status (with or without partner), maternal education (up to 4 years, 5 to 8 years, 9 to 11 years or 12 years or more), family income (measured in Brazilian reais and divided in quintiles), type of payment for childbirth (through the public Brazilian National Health System or other, including private care and private insurance) and type of childbirth (cesarean section after the onset of labor, cesarean section before the onset of labor or vaginal delivery). Women who underwent cesarean section and answered "yes" to the question "Did you have regular contractions (at least one every ten minutes) before the cesarean section?" were considered as having gone into labor.

Quality control measures included repeating a short version of the perinatal and three-month interview to 10% of the women by means of a telephone call, or through a home visit if the woman could not be contacted by phone.

Stata 13 software was used to conduct statistical analyses (StataCorp. 2013. *Stata Statistical Software: Release 13.* College Station, TX: StataCorp LP) and the database that generated the results of this study can be accessed by contacting the corresponding author. Firstly, descriptive analyses of the characteristics of recruited women were performed and the frequencies of each type of violence, disrespect or abuse were obtained. Poisson regression was then used to conduct crude and adjusted analyses of risk factors. Poisson regression represents a more suitable alternative than logistic regression for this type of analysis because the odds ratios are overestimated in comparison to prevalence ratios, especially when estimates are low [28]. Variables that presented *p*-values lower than 0.20 in the crude analysis were then included in adjusted analyses, following a hierarchical causal model. Age, skin color, marital status, educational level and income were included as variables in the first level of this analysis. Variables relating to the type of financing used to cover hospitalization for childbirth was included in the second-level analysis while the type of childbirth was included in the third-level analysis. Because poverty and age can be strongly associated with outcome, we decided to retain family income and women's age in all models, regardless of the *p*-value in an effort to minimize potential bias.

This study was approved by the Research Ethics Committee of the Higher School of Physical Education of the Federal University of Pelotas (CAAE 26746414.5.0000.5313). All the women provided informed written consent.

Results

A total of 4333 women gave birth in the city's hospitals, of whom 4275 (98.7%) agreed to participate in this study. During the three-month follow-up period, 4110 interviews were conducted (a follow-up rate of 97.2%). Of these, 4087 interviews (95.6%) took place with the biological mothers.

Table 1 presents the socioeconomic, demographic and delivery characteristics of our study population. Nearly half of the mothers were aged 20 to 29 years (47%), and most (71%) classified their skin color as white (71%). The majority of women lived with a spouse (86%), had at least 9 years of education (65%), relied on the national health service (68%) and had cesarean sections (65%).

Table 2 describes the prevalence of each type of violence, and the disrespect and abuse scores. Approximately 10% of the mothers reported having experienced verbal abuse, 6% denial of care, and 5% reported physical abuse. In addition, 6% reported undesirable or inappropriate procedures without an explanation of why it was being conducted. The occurrence of at least one type of disrespect or abuse was reported by 18.3% of mothers (95% confidence interval [CI]: 17.2–19.5), and of at least two types by 5.1% (95% CI: 4.4–5.8).

Regarding the associations between the occurrence of at least one type of disrespect or abuse and socioeconomic, demographic, and delivery factors (Table 1), a higher

Table 1 Associated factors to disrespect or abuse during the childbirth in 2015 Pelotas Birth Cohort ($n = 4275$)

Characteristic	Number	Percent	At least one type of disrespect or abuse		At least two types of disrespect or abuse	
			Crude PR (95%CI)	Adjusted PR (95%CI)	Crude PR (95%CI)	Adjusted PR (95%CI)
Age (full years)			*< 0.001*	*< 0.001*	*< 0.056*	*0.646*
< 20	622	14.6	1.96 (1.20–3.20)	1.77 (1.06–2.96)	1.94 (0.71–5.34)	1.55 (0.55–4.41)
20 to 29	2017	47.2	1.50 (0.93–2.43)	1.39 (0.85–2.29)	1.57 (0.59–4.19)	1.36 (0.51–3.64)
30 to 39	1510	35.3	1.12 (0.68–1.82)	1.12 (0.68–1.84)	1.17 (0.43–3.17)	1.12 (0.41–3.03)
40 to 49	125	2.9	1	1	1	1
Skin color (self-reported)			*0.139*		*0.984*	
White	3024	70.8	1	–	1	–
Brown	551	13	1.11 (0.92–1.34)		1.03 (0.69–1.54)	
Black	667	15.7	1.11 (0.97–1.28)		1.03 (0.71–1.48)	
Marital status			*0.056*	*0.603*	*0.570*	–
With partner	3667	85.8	1	1	1	
Without partner	607	14.2	1.18 (1.00–1.41)	1.05 (0.87–1.26)	1.11 (0.77–1.60)	
Maternal education (years completed)			*< 0.001+*	*0.595+*	*0. < 001+*	*0.101+*
< 5	391	9.2	1.38 (1.09–1.76)	1.06 (0.80–1.40)	2.16 (1.34–3.47)	1.77 (0.99–3.13)
5 a 8	1095	25.6	1.43 (1.20–1.71)	1.02 (0.82–1.28)	1.73 (1.17–2.54)	1.41 (0.88–2.26)
9 a 11	1457	34.1	1.24 (1.04–1.47)	1.00 (0.83–1.21)	1.67 (1.16–2.41)	1.50 (1.01–2.25)
>=12	1330	31.1	1	1	1	1
Family income			*< 0.001*	*< 0.001*	*< 0.001*	*0.403*
1° quintile (poorest)	796	19.8	1.65 (1.29–2.11)	1.37 (1.02–1.82)	1.66 (1.02–2.70)	1.11 (0.63–1.96)
2° quintile	807	20.1	1.97 (1.56–2.50)	1.71 (1.31–2.23)	1.71 (1.06–2.77)	1.21 (0.72–2.04)
3° quintile	804	20.0	1.31 (1.01–1.69)	1.18 (0.89–1.55)	1.13 (0.67–1.91)	0.82 (0.47–1.41)
4° quintile	895	22.3	1.55 (1.21–1.98)	1.44 (1.12–1.85)	1.50 (0.93–2.43)	1.23 (0.75–2.02)
5° quintile (richest)	714	17.8	1	1	1	1
Type of payment for delivery care			*< 0.001*	*< 0.001*	*< 0.001*	*< 0.001*
Private care or private insurance	1302	31.7	1	1	1	1
Public sector	2801	68.3	1.88 (1.59–2.22)	1.71 (1.40–2.09)	2.98 (2.01–4.41)	3.23 (2.07–5.03)
Type of labor			*< 0.001*	*< 0.001*	*< 0.001*	*< 0.001*
C-section[a] after labor onset	1594	37.3	1	1	1	1
C-section[a] before labor onset	1189	27.8	1.67 (1.41–1.98)	1.45 (1.21–1.73)	2.79 (1.89–4.12)	2.24 (1.50–3.34)
Vaginal delivery	1488	34.9	1.63 (1.38–1.92)	1.22 (1.02–1.46)	2.83 (1.95–4.13)	1.84 (1.22–2.76)

[a]Cesarean section. The numbers in italic are the *p*-values

prevalence ratio was detected among young mothers in the second income quintile, in the public sectors, and when a cesarean section was carried out after the onset of labor. When factors associated with the occurrence of at least two types of disrespect or abuse were evaluated, mothers relying on the public health sector, and those whose childbirths were via cesarean section with previous labor, presented the highest risk, with an increased risk of three and two-fold, respectively (Table 1).

Discussion

Approximately 18% of women who delivered babies in the city of Pelotas during 2015 were victims of at least one type of disrespectful or abusive treatment during the process of childbirth. This result is similar to the findings of a previous study conducted in Kenya [23], in which 20% of women reported experiencing some type of mistreatment or abuse by healthcare professionals during labor. In a study of eight institutions in a rural area in Tanzania, Kruk et al. [21] also reported a prevalence of approximately 20%, which was slightly lower than another study conducted in the same country [18]. In the latter study, there was no significant difference in abuse when compared between human immunodeficiency virus (HIV)-positive and -negative women. These findings are in contrast with those from a study conducted in

Table 2 Prevalence of disrespect and abuse against women during childbirth, in 2015 Pelotas Birth Cohort

Disrespect or abuse	N	%	95%CI
Verbal abuse	378	9.3	8.4–10.2
Denial of care	240	5.9	5.2–6.6
Physical abuse	183	4.5	3.9–5.2
Invasive and/or inappropriate procedures	236	5.8	5.1–6.5
Score of disrespect and abuse			
None	3338	81.6	80.5–82.8
1 type	542	13.3	12.3–14.3
2 types	141	3.4	2.9–4.1
3 types	51	1.3	1.0–1.6
4 types	15	0.4	0.2–0.6

Nigeria, where Okafor et al. [19] reported that 98% of women experienced some form of disrespectful or abusive treatment among the 460 puerperal women interviewed at a child immunization clinic. The almost universal prevalence reported by that study could be explained by a detailed evaluation of the different types of disrespect and abuse, for example, episiotomy, augmentation of labor, shaving of pubic hair, sterilization, cesarean delivery and blood transfusion and aspects relating to the payment of hospital fees. The specific form of disrespectful or abusive treatment that contributed most to the observed high levels of prevalence was non-consent care, at a prevalence of 55% [19].

Some studies have reported disrespectful or abusive treatment during childbirth in Latin America. In Venezuela, a hospital study using a self-applied confidential questionnaire showed that 49.4% of women giving birth reported having experienced some form of inhumane treatment from healthcare professionals [24]. In a survey across three Mexican hospitals, 11% of mothers reported some form of mistreatment by healthcare professionals during the process of childbirth [29]. In Brazil, a study conducted in both public and private hospitals across 25 states showed that 25% of women reported having experienced some type of obstetric violence [15]. The wide range of prevalence evident in these studies, from 11% to 98%, may be related to different definitions of obstetric violence, but nevertheless there is no question that the problem is a common one.

Our present results showed that younger age, family income, type of hospitalization system for childbirth and type of childbirth were associated with the incidence of abuse or disrespect during the process of childbirth.

Several studies have been published regarding the relationship between disrespect or abuse during childbirth and a range of associated factors; however, these previous studies yielded inconsistent results. Abuya

et al. [23] found no association of any type between disrespect/abuse and maternal age, educational level, marital status and the presence of family/friends, but did show an association between parity and socioeconomic status and between detention for lack of payment and bribery requests, factors that were not included in our present analyses. In another study, Terán and colleagues [24] failed to find an association between dehumanizing treatment and educational level, but did identify a positive association with extreme age groups (adolescents and older women). These authors also showed an association between non-consented procedures with educational level and the type of childbirth. Kruk et al. further demonstrated that disrespect or abuse were associated with higher educational level, higher parity, poverty, cesarean section and depression; however, these authors failed to find an association with age, marital status and health facility factors. In another study, Okafor and colleagues [19] found no association between disrespectful or abusive care during childbirth and any other factor analyzed (maternal age, tribe, marital status, educational status and parity).

A study referred to as 'Birth in Brazil' (Nascer no Brasil), a nationally representative population-based study in which a total of 15,688 women were interviewed by telephone during the postpartum period, showed a higher chance of verbal, psychological or physical violence among women who went into labor (odds ratio [OR]: 1.79; 95% CI: 1.28–2.52), and a lower chance among those whose childbirth was privately financed (OR: 0.41; 95% CI: 0.30–0.56) and those who were accompanied by a family member throughout the childbirth process. There was no association between violence and skin color, socioeconomic position, educational level, maternal age or the type of delivery (categorized into vaginal and cesarean section only) [14].

In the Brazilian private or supplementary healthcare network, 90% of childbirths occur by means of cesarean section; of these, 78% occur without the pregnant women having gone into labor [22]. Considering that there is a greater likelihood of abuse and disrespect among women who go into labor, it might be expected that there would be a lower occurrence among those hospitalized in the private system.

Despite international recommendations suggesting that the proportion of cesarean sections should not exceed 15% [30], the levels of surgical deliveries in Brazil have reached epidemic levels and account for 55% of childbirths [22]. This reflects an over-medicalization of birth which has unfortunately accompanied public health achievements such as increased access to prenatal care and a higher proportion of childbirths in healthcare institutions [2].

The greater occurrence of violence among women who went into labor, along with the medicalization of childbirth, may be indicative of a lack of training among medical professionals in carrying out vaginal deliveries. In general terms, Brazil has adopted a highly medicalized model for obstetric care, which uses high levels of technology and little participation from the women who receive this care. During the process of childbirth, the doctor is an authority figure who holds knowledge and power, and is the protagonist of the process. In this, the woman in labor acts merely as an assistant who must obey all medical instructions and accept the procedures that are often imposed on her. In this context, disrespect and/or abuse would consist of the abusive use of power when the authority of a doctor, also represented by the team of other professionals that act under his/her orders, is directly or indirectly challenged by "disobedience", resistance or questioning [13, 31, 32]. It is also important to consider the fact that disrespect and abuse of women during the process of childbirth is permeated by issues of medicalization relating to their bodies and gender, and reflects the depreciation of their sex and the normalization of violence against women [20, 33].

Women within the Brazilian civil society have become mobilized to fight for dignified and respectful care during pregnancy and childbirth. The movement referred to as "Delivery through Principles – Women's Network for Active Maternity" (Parto do Princípio – Mulheres em Rede pela Maternidade Ativa), acts to promote women's autonomy and defend their sexual and reproductive rights, especially regarding awareness during maternity, and has denounced institutional violence during pregnancy and childbirth care to policy makers [34]. However, despite these initiatives, and the implementation of public policies such as the Program for Humanization of Labor and Childbirth, disrespectful treatment and abuse of women during childbirth still occur frequently.

In 2014, the magnitude and severity of this issue at a global level led the WHO to publish a statement [1] proposing actions to eliminate this form of violence. This statement proposed to provide greater support for research and actions, to develop programs to improve the quality of maternal healthcare, to emphasize the right for women to receive dignified and respectful care during pregnancy and childbirth and to monitor data relating to this issue and to involve all stakeholders in a concerted effort to improve the quality of care and eliminate disrespectful practices.

One possible limitation of the present study may lie in the under-reporting of disrespectful or abusive treatment, which may have reduced the magnitude of our estimates and diluted the associations observed. To minimize information bias and to avoid embarrassment and the fear of possible retaliation by the hospital or healthcare professionals, information relating to disrespect and abuse during childbirth were obtained during the three-month follow-up period. It is also important to consider the influence of women's perceptions on their reports. For example, women who had received lower levels of education and were in lower socioeconomic positions may have tended not to notice abuse because they may have considered this to be part of the normal process. On the other hand, women who presented with higher educational levels and, probably, higher levels of information relating to their rights, may have noticed more subtle forms of violence. Another important limitation is the fact that there was no individualized information on which professionals perpetrated the abuse, or whether they were doctors or nurses. Therefore, in our discussion, we considered doctors to be hierarchically superior and responsible for the team and for the decisions made during the process of childbirth.

Considering that pregnant women are in a situation of great vulnerability, and that the agents of violence against them are the ones that should be providing comprehensive care, the proportion of women who experience disrespect and abuse during the process of childbirth is absurd and unacceptable. It seems that the subjective "judgment" of permitting professionals to adopt unacceptable behavior is more tolerated in healthcare services, particularly public services. It is therefore fundamental to recognize, within the healthcare model, that obstetric care has become too medicalized and that the ethical background of the professionals involved needs to be reviewed.

Conclusion

The occurrence of disrespect and abuse during the process of childbirth in our study was high and mostly associated to payment by the public sector and labor before delivery. The efforts made by civil society, governments and international organizations are not yet sufficient to restrain institutional violence against women in childbearing. To eradicate the problem, it is essential to 1) implement policies and actions specific for this type of violence and 2) formulate laws to promote the equality of rights between women and men, with particular emphasis on women's economic rights and the promotion of gender equity with respect to access to jobs and education. In this way, it is possible to alter the social norms that strengthen and perpetuate social models that can ultimately lead to a lack of autonomy in women, and exert control over processes which relate to their own bodies and lives, and to the various forms of violence against women [29].

Acknowledgements

We wish to acknowledge the contribution of all participants, the Pelotas hospitals (Hospital Miguel Piltcher, Santa Casa de Misericórdia de Pelotas, Hospital Escola da Universidade Federal de Pelotas, Hospital Universitário São Francisco de Paula, Hospital da Beneficência Portuguesa de Pelotas) and the Municipal Secretariat of Health.

Funding

This article was based on data from the 2015 Pelotas (Brazil) Birth Cohort Study. This project was funded through a New Investigator Award (grant number 095582/Z/11/Z) from the Wellcome Trust to P.C.H. The study was conducted by the Postgraduate Program in Epidemiology of the Federal University of Pelotas, Brazil, and is currently also supported by the Brazilian National Research Council (CNPq) and Coordination for the Improvement of Higher Education Personnel (CAPES).

Authors' contributions

MAM planned the study cohort, supervised the fieldwork, conducted the analysis and wrote the manuscript. CGV worked planned the study cohort, supervised data analysis and contributed to writing and revising the manuscript. SJS and RGPL helped to write and revise the manuscript. AHD and MRD helped plan the study cohort, coordinated the fieldwork and reviewed the manuscript. MFS planned the study, coordinated the fieldwork, supervised data analysis and helped to write and revise the manuscript. All authors read and approved the final manuscript.

Competing interests

The authors declare that they have no competing interests.

Author details

[1]Post-Graduate Program in Epidemiology, Federal University of Pelotas, Pelotas, Brazil. [2]Latin American Center of Perinatology, Women and Reproductive Health, Montevideo, Uruguay. [3]Post-Graduate Program in Physical Education, Federal University of Pelotas, Pelotas, Brazil.

References

1. WHO. The prevention and elimination of disrespect and abuse during facility-based childbirth. In: World Health Organization Statment. Geneva: World Health Organization; 2014.
2. Victora CG, Aquino EM, do Carmo Leal M, Monteiro CA, Barros FC, Szwarcwald CL. Maternal and child health in Brazil: progress and challenges. Lancet. 2011;377(9780):1863–76.
3. Assembly UG: Universal declaration of human rights. In: Nova York: UN General Assembly; 1948.
4. Assembly UG: Declaration on the elimination of violence against women. In.: Nova York: UN General Assembly; 1993.
5. Assembly UG: International covenant on economic, social and cultural rights. In.: Nova York: UN General Assembly; 1976.
6. Brasil. In: Md S, editor. Programa Nacional de Humanização do Parto e Nascimento. Brasília: Ministério da Saúde; 2002. p. 27.
7. Brasil. Congresso Nacional: Lei n° 11.108, de 7 de abril de 2005. Do subsistema de acompanhamento durante o trabalho de parto, parto e pós-parto imediato. In Brasilia; 2005.
8. d'Oliveira AF, Diniz SG, Schraiber LB. Violence against women in health-care institutions: an emerging problem. Lancet. 2002;359(9318):1681–5.
9. Bohren MA, Vogel JP, Hunter EC, Lutsiv O, Makh SK, Souza JP, Aguiar C, Saraiva Coneglian F, Diniz AL, Tuncalp O, et al. The Mistreatment of Women during Childbirth in Health Facilities Globally: A Mixed-Methods Systematic Review. PLoS medicine. 2015;12(6):e1001847. discussion e1001847

10. Esposito NW. Marginalized women's comparisons of their hospital and freestanding birth center experiences: a contrast of inner-city birthing systems. Health Care Women Int. 1999;20(2):111–26.
11. Fonn S, Philpott H. Preparatory report for workshop on maternity and neonatal services policy for the PWV. Urban Health Newsl. 1995;25:38–52.
12. Jewkes R, Abrahams N, Mvo Z. Why do nurses abuse patients? Reflections from south African obstetric services. Soc Sci Med. 1998;47(11):1781–95.
13. Aguiar JM, d'Oliveira AF, Schraiber LB. Institutional violence, medical authority, and power relations in maternity hospitals from the perspective of health workers. Cadernos de saude publica. 2013;29(11):2287–96.
14. d'Orsi E, Bruggemann OM, Diniz CS, Aguiar JM, Gusman CR, Torres JA, Angulo-Tuesta A, Rattner D, Domingues RM. Social inequalities and women's satisfaction with childbirth care in Brazil: a national hospital-based survey. Cadernos de saude publica. 2014;30(Suppl 1):S1–15.
15. Venturi G, Godinho T. Mulheres brasileiras e gênero nos espaços público e privado: uma década de mudanças na opinião pública. São Paulo: Fundação Perseu Abramo: Edições SESC SP; 2013.
16. Aguiar JM. Violência institucional me maternidades públicas: hostilidade ao invés de acolhimento como uma questão de gênero. Brasil: Universidade de são Paulo; 2010.
17. McMahon SA, George AS, Chebet JJ, Mosha IH, Mpembeni RN, Winch PJ. Experiences of and responses to disrespectful maternity care and abuse during childbirth; a qualitative study with women and men in Morogoro region, Tanzania. BMC Pregnancy Childbirth. 2014;14:268.
18. Sando D, Kendall T, Lyatuu G, Ratcliffe H, McDonald K, Mwanyika-Sando M, Emil F, Chalamilla G, Langer A. Disrespect and abuse during childbirth in Tanzania: are women living with HIV more vulnerable? J Acquir Immune Defic Syndr. 2014;67(Suppl 4):S228–34.
19. Okafor II, Ugwu EO, Obi SN. Disrespect and abuse during facility-based childbirth in a low-income country. Int J Gynaecol Obstet. 2015;128(2):110–3.
20. Chadwick RJ. Obstetric violence in South Africa. S Afr Med J. 2016;106(5):423–4.
21. Kujawski S, Mbaruku G, Freedman LP, Ramsey K, Moyo W, Kruk ME. Association between disrespect and abuse during childbirth and Women's confidence in health facilities in Tanzania. Matern Child Health J. 2015; 19(10):2243–50.
22. Domingues RM, Dias MA, Nakamura-Pereira M, Torres JA, d'Orsi E, Pereira AP, Schilithz AO, Carmo Leal M. Process of decision-making regarding the mode of birth in Brazil: from the initial preference of women to the final mode of birth. Cadernos de saude publica. 2014;30(Suppl 1):S1–16.
23. Abuya T, Warren CE, Miller N, Njuki R, Ndwiga C, Maranga A, Mbehero F, Njeru A, Bellows B. Exploring the prevalence of disrespect and abuse during childbirth in Kenya. PLoS One. 2015;10(4):e0123606.
24. Terán P, Castellanos C, Blanco MG, Ramos D. Violencia obstétrica: percepción de las usuarias. Rev Obstet Ginecol Venez. 2013;73(3):171–80.
25. Hallal PC, Bertoldi AD, Domingues MR, Silveira MFD, Demarco FF, da Silva ICM, Barros FC, Victora CG, Bassani DG. Cohort profile: the 2015 Pelotas (Brazil) birth cohort study. Int J Epidemiol. 2017;0(0):1–9.
26. Savage V, Castro A. Measuring mistreatment of women during childbirth: a review of terminology and methodological approaches. Reprod Health. 2017;14(1):138.
27. WHO. Sexual and reproductive health. Available in: http://www.who.int/reproductivehealth/topics/maternal_perinatal/statement-childbirth-stakeholders/en/. Accessed 16 Mar 2018.
28. Barros AJ, Hirakata VN. Alternatives for logistic regression in cross-sectional studies: an empirical comparison of models that directly estimate the prevalence ratio. BMC Med Res Methodol. 2003;3:21.
29. Valdez RS, Solórzano EH, Iñiguez MM, Monreal LMA. Nueva evidencia a un viejo problema: el abuso de las mujeres en las salas de parto. Rev CONAMED. 2013;18(1):14–20.
30. WHO. WHO Statement on Caesarean Section Rates. Geneva: World Health Organization; 2015.
31. Souza, CM. C-sections as ideal births: the cultural constructions of beneficence and patients' rights in Brazil. Camb Q Healthc Ethics. 1994;3(3):358–66.
32. Patah LE, Malik AM. Models of childbirth care and cesarean rates in different countries. Rev Saude Publica. 2011;45(1):185–94.
33. Jewkes R, Penn-Kekana L. Mistreatment of women in childbirth: time for action on this important dimension of violence against women. PLoS Med. 2015;12(6):e1001849.
34. Parto do Princípio: Violência Obstétrica - Parirás com Dor. In.: Parto do Princípio - Mulheres em Rede pela Maternidade Ativa. 2012: 188. Brasilia.

10

Research priority-setting: reproductive health in the occupied Palestinian territory

Niveen M. E. Abu-Rmeileh[*], Rula Ghandour, Marina Tucktuck and Mohammad Obiedallah

Abstract

Background: Occupied Palestinian territory (oPt) is an authority with limited resources. Therefore, research conducted in such a setting should be prioritized and coordinated to follow a national research agenda. This study aims to produce a research agenda for reproductive health in the oPt that can be utilized by reproductive health stakeholders and contribute to the development of policy-based evidence to guide health practice.

Methods: In the current study, we followed research prioritization methods developed by the World Health Organization-Child Health and Nutrition Research Initiative. Research questions were obtained from reproductive health experts in the oPt. The questions were then grouped into thematic areas which were prioritized by the reproductive health experts. Scores were calculated and sorted to define the top priority research areas.

Results: A total of 232 research questions were prioritized by 30 reproductive health experts. Health system issues were the most addressed in the top 50 research questions. They included questions on the quality of services and health professionals' knowledge and continuous professional training. Adolescents' sexual and reproductive health and gender-based violence were rarely mentioned in the top 50 questions. The number of questions related to safe motherhood was around 50% followed by questions related to health system. Questions related to elderly women and menopause as well as reproductive system cancers were also within the top 50 ranked questions.

Conclusions: Priority research areas in reproductive health were identified for the oPt, which should be utilized by researchers with a focus on the high priority areas. Policy makers and funders should coordinate their efforts to ensure the production of research with value to the Palestinian context, in the most efficient way possible.

Key messages
- Reproductive health experts in the occupied Palestinian territory were able to identify previously unaddressed priority research areas related to reproductive health
- Future research needs to be guided by the research priority list to maximize efficient utilization of resources
- The quality of services within the health system were among the top priority research areas identified, whereas questions related to adolescents sexual and reproductive health were least prevalent

Plain English summary

Policy makers today are more reliant upon evidence-based policy planning than ever before, which increases the

demand for research production. To keep up with this increasing demand, it is especially important for countries with limited resources, such as the occupied Palestinian territory (oPt), to identify priority research areas in order to focus their resources on the needed evidence and reduce duplication of existing studies. This study aims to identify a list of the most important reproductive health research questions proposed by Palestinian health providers and experts. The participants included most of the stakeholders and experts in reproductive health service provision and research in the oPt. These experts identified research questions which were grouped by the researchers into common themes. These themes were further prioritized by the experts based on standardized methods. A list of 50 research questions were identified. Several questions related to the health system, including quality of care, health professionals' knowledge and preparedness, access to and availability of services, were among the most important questions. Questions related to high-risk

* Correspondence: nrmeileh@birzeit.edu; nrmeileh@gmail.com
Institute of Community and Public Health, Birzeit University, P.O.Box 14, BirzeitWest BankoPt, Palestine

pregnancies and maternal mortality were also within the 50 top research questions. Few questions on adolescents' sexual and reproductive health and gender-based violence were within the top 50 research questions. Future research should focus on the identified high priority areas. Policy makers and funders should work in coordination to ensure the production of research with value to the Palestinian context.

Background

Around 85% of research investment worldwide is wasted as reported by Chalmers et al. A waste in research was considered, "when the need of potential user of research evidence was ignored or when available evidence was overlooked" [1]. The reasons for waste included choosing the wrong research question, conducting studies that are poorly designed, and failing to publish unusable sections of research [1]. It thus becomes imperative to set research priorities to help maximize evidence utilization and reduce research waste, especially in low-income countries with limited research resources [2].

In the occupied Palestinian territory (oPt), research is mainly conducted by academic institutions, occasionally in collaboration with health providers. Research conducted is mainly selected based on consultation with health providers, observation, and experience of the researcher in a specific field or in response to a funder and/or health provider request [3]. The number of published papers focusing on health in Palestine/oPt has increased since 2010 compared to previous years. However, only 29% of these papers were cited more than 5 times [4], which might indicate local rather than international importance. In addition, it might indicate that these studies are not addressing the right questions.

In relation to reproductive health (RH) research, a comprehensive review on maternal and child health in the oPt described the situation with respect to the fourth and fifth Millennium Development Goals on reducing child mortality and improving maternal health, respectively. The review also identified several research areas as well as reported the type of research conducted and the quality of available data [5].

Several research priority exercises were conducted to address the global, and more specifically, low and middle-income countries needs [6–9]. However, a country-specific research priority list is imperative to help provide the needed evidence for program and intervention planning at the national level. Therefore, this study aims to build a research agenda for RH in the oPt that can be utilized by RH stakeholders and contribute to the development of policy-based evidence to guide health practice.

Methods

We used the reproductive health definition adopted by the International Conference on Population Development (ICPD) Program of Action held in Cairo in 1994. In the current study, we followed research prioritization methods developed by the World Health Organization's (WHO) Child Health and Nutrition Research Initiative (CHNRI) [10]. The prioritization exercise was implemented in three phases: (1) the generation and collection of research questions, (2) consolidation of research questions and thematic analysis, and (3) the prioritization exercise of the research questions using pre-defined scoring criteria.

Phase 1

The main stakeholders in RH in the West Bank and Gaza Strip were identified in part by consulting the stakeholders who participated in the Palestinian National Reproductive Health Strategy and Action Plan 2014–2016. These stakeholders mainly included the Palestinian Ministry of Health and other governmental ministries, the United Nations Relief and Works Agency for Palestine Refugees (UNRWA) and national non-governmental organizations as well as a number of private physicians. In addition, researchers representing Palestinian academic institutions were included, thus tapping into the clinical aspect of reproductive health alongside the academia aspect. Invitations were sent to the identified participants of 45 individuals from 21 national organizations, through email, fax, and phone. Out of those who were approached, 34 individuals from 19 organizations responded positively to the invitation (individual response rate of 75.6%). Participants were asked to propose six research questions in the field of reproductive health; each based on his/her expertise, knowledge and experience. Phase 1 was completed between December 2015 and January 2016.

Phase 2

The list of proposed research questions was independently reviewed by two researchers. A third reviewer evaluated the list of questions from the two reviewers and resolved discrepancies. A reduced and refined list of research questions was prepared for thematic analysis. Phase 2 was completed between January 28th – February 18th, 2016.

Phase 3

A total of 32 individuals from 19 organizations were invited to participate in the research priority scoring exercise, through email, phone, and fax (where appropriate). Of the total invited participants (who also participated in phase 1), 30 individuals from 16 organizations responded positively to the invitation (individual response rate of 93.8%) and four responses were received by email because of mobility issues. Phase 3 was completed between February 28th – April 1st, 2016.

The scoring criteria adopted was based on the WHO-CHNRI guidelines [11] (Table 1).

Table 1 Scoring criteria for the research priority-setting exercise in reproductive health

Criteria[a]	Definition	Score and explanation
1. Answerability	The research question can be ethically answered	0- Cannot be answered 5- Can be fully answered 0–1–2-3-4-5
2. Effectiveness	The new knowledge is likely to result in an effective intervention or program in the reproductive health field	0- Not effective 5- Very effective 0–1–2-3-4-5
3. Deliverability	The research is likely to generate new knowledge that can help in improving reproductive health in an acceptable and affordable manner	0- Cannot be delivered 5- Can be fully delivered 0–1–2-3-4-5
4. Potential impact	The results of this research will have a public health impact (improve the reproductive health from the public health perspective)	0- No Public health impact 5- High public health impact 0–1–2-3-4-5
5. Equity	The research will include and target the most vulnerable sectors of society	0- Not equitable 5- Equitable 0–1–2-3-4-5

[a]Criteria follow the World Health Organization's Child Health and Nutrition Research Initiative (WHO-CHNRI)

An excel spreadsheet with the research questions was shared with the participants. They were then instructed to score each research question against the five criteria, where each criterion had a score range of 0–5. In addition, in the case that participants were not able to make a judgment on a research question, they had the option of indicating 'I don't know' and 'not applicable' on the spreadsheet.

Data analysis

The metrics-based approach (pooling individual rankings), as employed by the WHO-CHNRI, was used for data analysis. For each research question, an unweighted mean score was calculated by summing up the individual scores of each criterion. No special weighting was applied to the criteria. 'I don't know' and 'not applicable' was treated as missing and was not included in the calculation of the average. The resulting score of each research question was obtained and the research questions were ranked and prioritized according to their score. The top 50-research questions with a total score of 85+ were reported in the results section.

Results

Figure 1 shows the study and analysis flow of the three phases. A total of 34 participants from 19 organizations responded positively to phase 1 invitation and provided 1239 research questions in reproductive health. After removing duplicate and out of scope questions and conducting thematic analysis, a total of 232 research questions emerged covering three main thematic areas (health systems, community-related and individual-related aspects within reproductive health). Out of the 34 participants, 30 individuals from 16 organizations partook in phase 3 scoring exercise (individual response rate of 93.8%). A list of 50 research questions was identified as priority research areas in reproductive health in the oPt.

Priority areas

Figure 2 presents the distribution of the top 50 research questions divided by main reproductive health areas. Eight questions out of the 50 were related to the quality of care, six were related to knowledge of health professionals about nutrition during antenatal care period, and five were related to health professionals' role division (tasks) and responsibilities. These three areas, in addition to others listed in the figure, accounted for almost 60% of the top 50 priorities, and fall under health system. Questions related to community knowledge about reproductive health areas, including school sexual and reproductive Health (SRH) programs, preconception and delivery, accounted for 15% of the top 50 questions. Moreover, the top 50 priorities included new topics such as menopause, chronic diseases and knowledge about nutrition at different stages of the reproductive life. Important topics such as reproductive system cancers were also in the list with one or two questions focusing on community and women's knowledge, preparedness and coping with cancer diseases.

Reproductive health topics

An in-depth look at the top 50 questions with the highest score following ICPD 1994 components, we found that 52% of the research questions were about safe motherhood. Within safe motherhood priority area, high-risk pregnancy received the highest number of research questions while preconception, antenatal, delivery, postnatal and maternal mortality received almost a similar number of research questions. Health system and menopause management related questions each accounted for 16% of the top 50 questions. There was

Phase I

45 individuals from 21 organizations were invited

34 individuals from 19 organizations participated

1,239 questions were generated

REMOVED duplicate questions and out of scope questions

Phase II

Reviewer 1: 228 research

Reviewer 2: 287 research

Thematic analysis

Reviewer 3: 232 research questions

Phase III

32 individuals from 19 organizations were invited

30 individuals from 16 organizations participated

A list of 50 research priority questions in reproductive health were identified and ranked

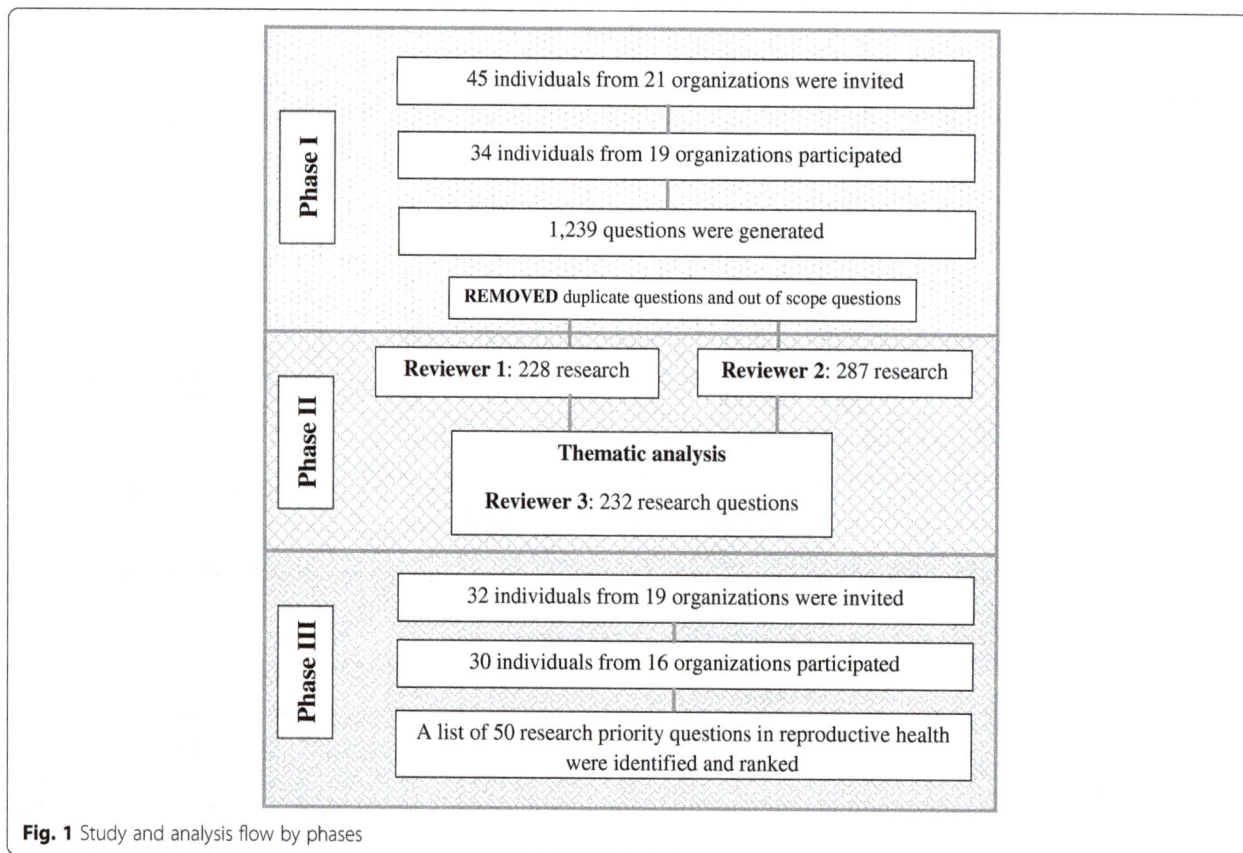

Fig. 1 Study and analysis flow by phases

only one research question on gender-based violence and two questions on adolescent reproductive health issues (Fig. 3).

Priorities by respondents

Finally, research priority areas varied among respondents. For instance, health service providers raised questions about community knowledge, attitude, and perceptions towards reproductive health services. In addition, they raised questions on specific topics, such as reproductive system cancers, abortion (and unwanted pregnancies) services and reproductive tract infections (RTIs) and sexually transmitted infections (STIs). The clinical gynecologists raised questions about the availability and affordability of

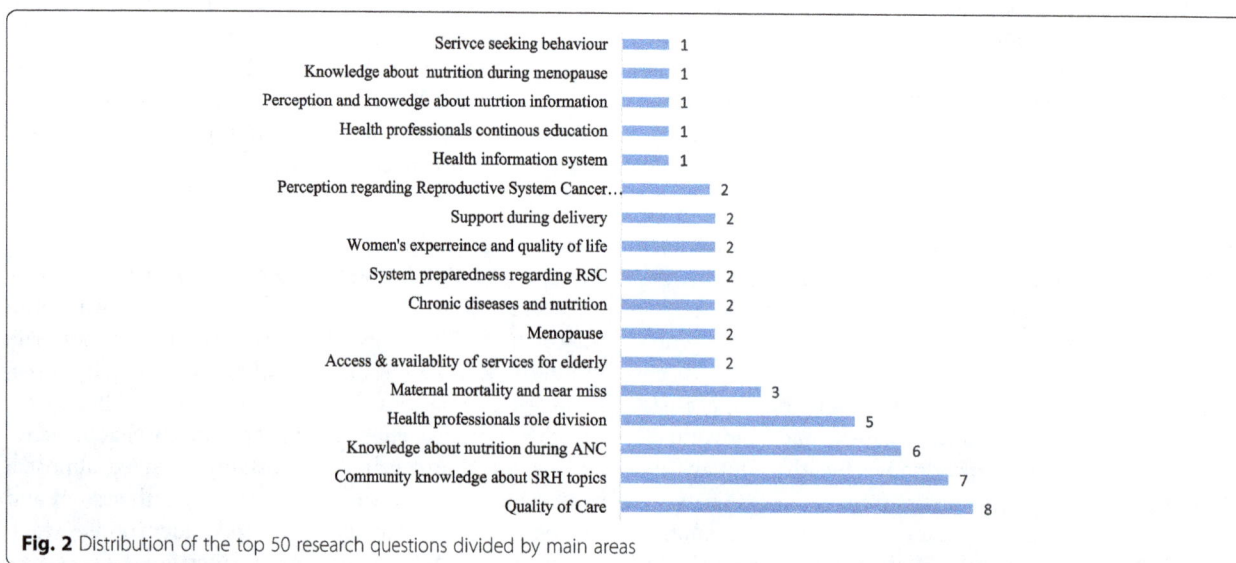

Serivce seeking behaviour — 1
Knowledge about nutrition during menopause — 1
Perception and knowedge about nutrtion information — 1
Health professionals continous education — 1
Health information system — 1
Perception regarding Reproductive System Cancer... — 2
Support during delivery — 2
Women's experreince and quality of life — 2
System preparedness regarding RSC — 2
Chronic diseases and nutrition — 2
Menopause — 2
Access & availablity of services for elderly — 2
Maternal mortality and near miss — 3
Health professionals role division — 5
Knowledge about nutrition during ANC — 6
Community knowledge about SRH topics — 7
Quality of Care — 8

Fig. 2 Distribution of the top 50 research questions divided by main areas

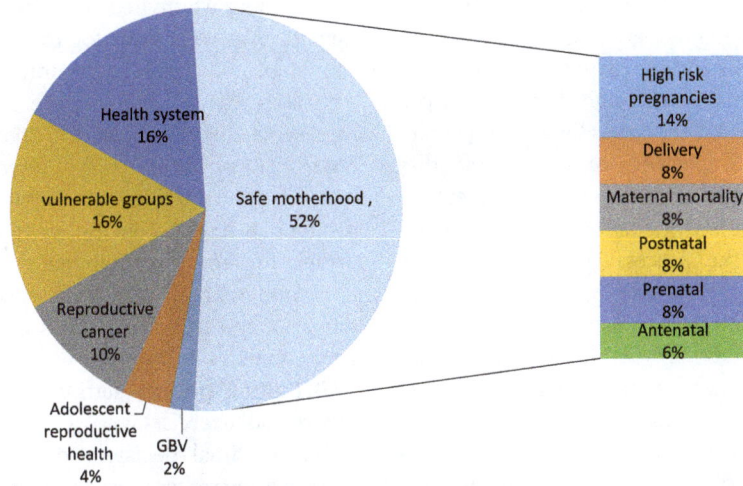

Fig. 3 The top research priority areas divided based on ICPD components

services, mainly pre-conception, infertility, abortion and miscarriages, postnatal and family planning services, and the availability of related protocols. Moreover, academia raised questions about health professionals' preparedness to work with adolescents, support for women during prenatal, delivery and postnatal, in addition to the availability, affordability, and quality of reproductive health services (Table 2).

Discussion

The current study identified the national research priority areas within reproductive health in the oPt. The list is comparable to the one identified for low and middle income countries by de Francisco et al. [12]. A wide range of questions were raised, including simple epidemiology questions, health system, and social and behavioral questions. However, the list lacked specific clinical, operational, or intervention questions. As for reproductive health topics, questions related to safe motherhood were more than 50% of the questions followed by health system related questions. Adolescents health and gender-based violence questions were least mentioned. Interestingly, a greater emphasis was given to questions related to elderly women in their menopausal phase. Usually, this group is categorized within the marginalized or vulnerable groups. It is also worth mentioning that topics such as abortion and sexually transmitted infections (STI) were neither in the top 20 nor 50 priority areas. Although they were mentioned by different local experts, they did not reach enough consensuses to be ranked highly.

The process of setting research priorities in low and middle-income countries is challenging since it requires the involvement of all stakeholders to come to a national consensus. In our study, Palestinian experts and stakeholders working in reproductive health at the governmental and non-governmental sectors, universities, gynecologists, and

Table 2 Top (highest scoring) research priority questions by reproductive health experts

Service Providers

Assess community preparedness and acceptability regarding reproductive system cancers

Evaluate the level of community knowledge, attitudes, and perceptions towards prenatal, antenatal, and postnatal services; RTI/STIs; abortion and miscarriage services; family planning and contraception; and the role of men in family planning

Evaluate the level of community knowledge, attitudes, and perceptions towards reproductive system cancers including screening and detection

Academia

Assess and evaluate the support system for women with reproductive system cancers during labor and the postnatal period

Assess and evaluate the methods adopted by health professionals in spreading awareness and education on reproductive health among adolescents

Understand the Epidemiology (prevalence/ distribution/ determinants/ associated factors) of high risk pregnancies

Evaluate the effectiveness of existing reproductive health services to prevent post-partum hemorrhage

Assess the availability of the types of services provided for family planning, postnatal care, labor, and delivery

Clinical Gynecologist

Assess the availability of the types of services provided for antenatal care, reproductive system cancers, nutrition, and infertility

Assess the protocols and guidelines implementation cycle (availability, comprehensiveness, knowledge, training, and application) regarding early marriage and teenage pregnancy

Assess the affordability and access to Antenatal care, postnatal care, labor, abortion, and miscarriage services

Other Ministries

Assess the availability of the types of services provided for antenatal care; reproductive system cancers; RTIs/STIs; menopause; infertility; GBV; early marriage and teenage pregnancies

Understand the Epidemiology (prevalence/ distribution/ determinants/ associated factors) for post-partum hemorrhage statistical offices participated in this exercise. The challenge we faced was at the beginning of this exercise because some stakeholders did not understand the process and aim of the research priority setting and they thought it is funding priorities for reproductive health services. However, once they understood the aim and importance of the exercise, they became motivated and had almost a hundred percent response rate. This is in line with Rudan's et al. main recommendation to improve the process of prioritization in health research by increasing the acceptability and popularity of such process with local policy makers [13].

The results of this study provide local and context-specific questions which cannot be compared to other countries specifically; nevertheless, they are in line with what has been reported by de Francisco et al. [12]. The results were general and not specific as reported in other studies since our study asked for general research questions while the other studies focused on interventions [7, 14] or specific governmental services [15]. In fact, research priority setting is an iterative process, and this is only the first step in a much longer process of refining the research priority areas into more specific questions. Hence this list should be reviewed and updated regularly. Based on the presented RPS findings, area specific research priority setting should be conducted for some topics, such as family planning and adolescents health, where validated methods were developed and used previously [6, 7, 16]. These areas were mentioned by different experts but did not reach consensus on specific questions.

The priorities were not similar across different respondents, perhaps because each was gearing the question toward their interest and experience. For example, the gynecologists were asking about unwanted pregnancies and abortion, health providers were interested in how to address cultural and norms barriers to family planning services, and other ministries were inquiring on how to improve family planning awareness and education, etc. Service providers in general were interested in understanding factors that are beyond their control, including cultural norms and beliefs, to improve their services. As for academics, in addition to understanding the quality of available health services, they were also interested in understanding the burden of selected topics locally that is of international importance. Although variation exists, the overall responses were complementary, and a comprehensive list of research priority was produced and agreed upon by all respondents.

Strengths and limitations

This study provides the first evidence-based research priority setting in reproductive health in the oPt. The output is a list that highlights the main areas that need to be researched to inform health policy. A slight modification to priority setting process was applied in the last phase where we invited the different stakeholders to participate in a workshop for the final scoring exercise rather than continue the communication through e-mail. This step was taken to ensure a high response rate and to receive the responses in a timely fashion. We had a high response rate at the different data collection levels which emphasizes the agreement of all experts in the reproductive health field on having national research priorities for reproductive health. We acknowledge the limitation that the study excluded neonatal health from the priority setting as these topics were not mentioned by the experts in phase 1.

Given that priority setting in health research is not a theoretical exercise with a single possible correct outcome and final decisions depend on the context [10], various approaches exist to guide the process of research priority setting [17–20]. In this study, we tried to maintain a high quality prioritization process following the CHNRI method which is a standardized method that has been used internationally and in different countries at the national level [2].

Conclusions

Priority research areas in reproductive health were identified. The research priority list should be utilized by researchers, policy makers and funders to ensure that the results of the conducted research are of value to the Palestinian population and context.

Acknowledgments
We would like to thank the Ministry of Education, the Ministry of Women Affairs, the Palestinian Central Bureau of Statistics, the Palestinian National Institute of Public Health, Health Work Committee, Juzoor for Health and Social Development, the Palestinian Medical Relief Society, An-Najah National University, Birzeit University, Al-Quds University, Bethlehem University, Ibn Sena National College, Al-Azhar University, Al-Islamic University, University College of Applied Sciences, Palestine College of Nursing, private consultants in reproductive health, and a number of health practitioners and gynecologists from Al-Makassed Charitable Hospital, the Palestine Medical Complex and the Arab Care Hospital for their participation in the research priority-setting exercise.

Funding
This work was funded by the UNDP-UNFPA-UNICEF-WHO-World Bank Special Programme of Research, Development and Research Training in Human Reproduction (HRP), a cosponsored program executed by the World Health Organization (WHO).

Authors' contributions
NMEAR conceptualized the research idea. NMEAR, MT and RG developed the study design and methods. MT, RG and MO were responsible for data collection. NMEAR, MT and RG analyzed the data. NMEAR wrote the manuscript and all authors read and approved the final draft of this manuscript.

Competing interests

The authors declare that they have no competing interests.

References

1. Chalmers I, Glasziou P. Avoidable waste in the production and reporting of research evidence. Lancet. 2009;374(9683):86–9.
2. Viergever RF, Olifson S, Ghaffar A, Terry RF. A checklist for health research priority setting: nine common themes of good practice. Health Research Policy and Systems. 2010;8(1):36.
3. Sridhar D, Batniji R. Misfinancing global health: a case for transparency in disbursements and decision making. Lancet. 2008;372(9644):1185–91.
4. Albarqouni L, Abu-Rmeileh NM, Elessi K, Obeidallah M, Bjertness E, Chalmers I. The quality of reports of medical and public health research from Palestinian institutions: a systematic review. BMJ Open. 2017;7(6)
5. Rahim HFA, Wick L, Halileh S, Hassan-Bitar S, Chekir H, Watt G, Khawaja M. Maternal and child health in the occupied Palestinian territory. Lancet, 373. (9667):967–77.
6. Hindin MJ, Christiansen CS, Jane Ferguson B. Setting research priorities for adolescent sexual and reproductive health in low-and middle-income countries. Bull World Health Organ. 2013;91(1):10–8.
7. Souza JP, Widmer M, Gülmezoglu AM, Lawrie TA, Adejuyigbe EA, Carroli G, Crowther C, Currie SM, Dowswell T, Hofmeyr J, et al. Maternal and perinatal health research priorities beyond 2015: an international survey and prioritization exercise. Reprod Health. 2014;11(1):61.
8. Dean S, Rudan I, Althabe F, Webb Girard A, Howson C, Langer A, Lawn J, Reeve ME, Teela KC, Toledano M, et al. Setting research priorities for preconception care in low- and middle-income countries: aiming to reduce maternal and child mortality and morbidity. PLoS Med. 2013;10
9. Tomlinson M, Rudan I, Saxena S, Swartz L, Tsai AC, Patel V. Setting priorities for global mental health research. Bull World Health Organ. 2009;87
10. Rudan I, Gibson JL, Ameratunga S, El Arifeen S, Bhutta ZA, Black M, Black RE, Brown KH, Campbell H, Carneiro I, et al. Setting priorities in global child Health Research investments: guidelines for implementation of the CHNRI method. Croatian Medical Journal. 2008;49(6):720–33.
11. Mendis SAA, editor. Prioritized research agenda for prevention and control of noncommunicable diseases. Geneva: World Health Organization.
12. de Francisco A dAC, Ringheim K, Liwander A, Peregoudov A, Faich HS, et al. Perceived research priorities in sexual and reproductive health for low-and middle-income countries: results from a survey. Geneva: Global Forum for Health Research; 2009.
13. Rudan I, Kapiriri L, Tomlinson M, Balliet M, Cohen B, Chopra M. Evidence-based priority setting for health care and research: tools to support policy in maternal, neonatal, and child health in Africa. PLoS Med. 2010;7
14. Dean S, Rudan I, Althabe F, Webb Girard A, Howson C, Langer A, Lawn J, Reeve M-E, Teela KC, Toledano M, et al. Setting research priorities for preconception Care in low- and Middle-Income Countries: aiming to reduce maternal and child mortality and morbidity. PLoS Med. 2013;10(9):e1001508.
15. Mayhew SH, Adjei S. Sexual and reproductive health: challenges for priority-setting in Ghana's health reforms. Health Policy Plan. 2004; 19(suppl_1):i50–61.
16. Ali M, Seuc A, Rahimi A, Festin M, Temmerman M. A global research agenda for family planning: results of an exercise for setting research priorities. Глобальный план исследований в области…. 2014;92(2):93–8.
17. Angulo A, Freij L, De Haan S, de los Rios R, Ghaffar A, Ijsselmuiden C, Janssens M, Jeenah M, Masood A, Montorzi G, et al. COHRED working paper 1. Priority setting for Health Research: toward a management process for low and middle income countries. Geneva: Council on Health Research for Development; 2006.
18. Ghaffar A, de Francisco A, Matlin S. The combined approach matrix: a priority-setting tool for health research. Geneva: Global Forum for Health Research; 2004.
19. Kaplan WA, Laing R. Priority medicines for europe and the world. Geneva: World Health Organization; 2004.
20. Rudan I, Chopra M, Kapiriri L, Gibson J, Ann LM, Carneiro I, Ameratunga S, Tsai AC, Chan KY, Tomlinson M, et al. Setting priorities in global child health research investments: universal challenges and conceptual framework. Croat Med J. 2008;49

11

Breaking bad news to antenatal patients with strategies to lessen the pain

José Atienza-Carrasco[1*] (iD), Manuel Linares-Abad[2], María Padilla-Ruiz[3,4] and Isabel María Morales-Gil[5]

Abstract

Background: To consider the thoughts and actions of healthcare personnel in situations when an adverse prenatal diagnosis must be communicated, including appropriate strategies and skills to respond to information needs and to manage the emotional responses of patients.

Methods: Descriptive qualitative study using non-participant observation and semi-structured interviews to analyse the discourses of physicians, midwives, nurses and nursing assistants who provide healthcare to obstetric patients.

Results: There may be barriers to effective communication between healthcare personnel and patients, depending on the characteristics of the persons involved, the organisation of healthcare, biotechnological progress and cultural factors.

Conclusions: The human quality of healthcare has deteriorated due to excessive workloads and to the growing role played by technology. In order to improve communication, more attention should be paid to human and spiritual dimensions, prioritising empathy, authenticity and non-judgmental listening. An appropriate model of clinical relationship should be based on shared decision making, clarifying the functions of the multidisciplinary team to alleviate a mother's suffering when a pregnancy is interrupted. To do so, protocols should be implemented to ensure the provision of comprehensive care, not only addressing biological issues but also providing psychosocial attention. Finally, training should be provided to healthcare staff to enhance their social skills and cultural competence.

This study identifies potential improvements in the interventions made by healthcare personnel and in the organisation of the institution, concerning the attention provided to pregnant women when an adverse prenatal diagnosis must be communicated.

Keywords: Communicative skills, Prenatal diagnosis, Congenital anomalies, Pregnancy, Interpersonal relations, Qualitative research

Plain English summary

Although scientific and technological progress has provided major health benefits, it can also hamper communication between healthcare personnel and patients. In modern medicine, the technical aspects of healthcare tend to prevail, in which the main focus is placed on treating the disease and less attention is paid to other aspects that are also important to the patient, such as feelings and emotions. Knowing how to communicate is an ethical and legal imperative and therefore healthcare professionals must ensure that patients are aware of everything related to their condition, to facilitate their autonomy in decision-making. If knowing how to communicate is always important, it is even more so when the content of the message is unfavourable. For example, bad news about the advance of a pregnancy can influence the mother's decision on whether to continue or to interrupt it. Professional interventions in such cases are crucial, because the psychological consequences of the situation depend on the care and support provided. Deficiencies in the communication process can generate conflicts and dissatisfaction in the professional-patient-family relationship.

* Correspondence: pepeatienzac@hotmail.com
[1]Nursing Surgery Service, Hospital Costa del Sol, Málaga, Spain
Full list of author information is available at the end of the article

Background

Technological progress and advances in the field of molecular genetics have contributed decisively to the development of prenatal diagnostics. Biotechnology offers novel, highly reliable instruments and techniques for identifying maternal risk factors, enabling the early detection of congenital malformations or defects of diverse types related to foetal formation and development [1]. However, despite this considerable progress, there is often a profound lack of interest in interpersonal communication. The ability to communicate with patients has been erroneously viewed as a lesser skill, compared to technical aspects of healthcare [2, 3], when in fact it is an essential element in the relationship between healthcare personnel and their patients, based on mutual recognition and shared decision making [4–6].

When a chromosome defect or severe foetal malformation is confirmed, the health team is obliged to inform the mother about the advisability of continuing the pregnancy, and of the prognosis and possible postpartum outcomes [7–10] respecting the patient's right to choose [4]. In many cases, healthcare personnel develop their own strategies, without taking into account the patient's holistic nature and without forming a comprehensive outlook on the health-disease binomial, capable of transforming information into a therapeutic tool [11]. Carers tend not to listen, thereby failing to obtain feedback to clarify exactly what the patient requires, and becoming emotionally distant. This inability to adapt the communication of diagnostic information to the patient's own values and preferences can generate conflicts and dissatisfaction [11–14]. Attitudes and communicative skills play a fundamental and decisive role in addressing problems, helping patients overcome psychological distress and conveying realistic expectations [15]. In prenatal preventive care programmes, the evaluation of obstetric risk, as well as ruling out biologically-based problems and identifying women at high risk of maternal and perinatal complications, should also address the patient from an inclusive perspective, because (among other reasons) the health-disease process is a multidimensional one in which biological, psychological and social factors continuously interact, in a positive or a negative sense [16].

The aim of this study is to examine the healthcare provided to pregnant women whose foetuses present congenital defects and to facilitate the design of a more personalised health model, one that responds to all their needs, rather than a limited selection. Accordingly, we have analysed the views expressed by healthcare personnel and the interventions they make when an adverse prenatal diagnosis must be communicated, including the strategies and skills employed to meet patients' information needs and to respond to their emotional responses.

Methods

This qualitative study was undertaken from a phenomenological standpoint, which enabled us to analyse specific experiences [17]. Information was collected by means of non-participant observation and semi-structured interviews, obtaining opinions from physicians, midwives, nurses and nursing assistants involved in real-life care processes relevant to the object of our study. Our analysis is based on descriptive and interpretative paradigms, which were applied to interpret the data obtained in the context of existing knowledge about the study area and in that of the participants' experiences in this respect. To maximise the scientific and methodological rigour of the study, criteria of credibility, transferability, dependence (or consistency) and confirmability were applied [17, 18].

The study was carried out at the Costa del Sol Health Agency (Marbella, Spain) from June to September 2015. During the information-compiling phase, 37 interviews were conducted, with 22 obstetricians, four midwives, three nurses and eight nursing assistants (Table 1). These healthcare personnel all worked in units within the Obstetrics service (prenatal diagnosis, perinatal medicine, hospitalisation, first, second and third-trimester pregnancy consultation and/or obstetric ambulatory care). The selection of the participants was intentional and not random, taking into account the criterion of segmentation, depending on the occupational category, hospital unit, position occupied and duration

Table 1 Sociodemographic characteristics of healthcare professionals

Professional category	Obstetrician	Midwife	Nurse	Nursing assistant
Sex				
Male				
Age				
<40	2	1		
41–45				
46–50				
>50	2			
Female				
Age				
<40	11	2	2	3
41–45	5	1		2
46–50	2		1	1
>50				2
Total	22	4	3	8
Mean age (Years)	39	38	40	44
Mean Experience (Years)	11	10	16	24

of employment at the hospital. The inclusion criteria were that participants should be physicians, midwives, nurses or nursing assistants at the hospital, have at least 1 year's experience (to acquire sufficient knowledge of the unit) and give permission for audio recording of the interview. All potential participants were sent letters indicating the purpose of the study and inviting them to take part. Participation was later confirmed by telephone.

The principal investigator[1] directly observed the interactions between patients and healthcare personnel, paying attention both to their words and to non-verbal aspects. A field diary was used to make a detailed record of all observations, after patients were informed and gave their written consent to the procedure. To avoid subjectivity, a feedback process was also applied, in which the notes made and impressions received were later shared with the same participants during the interviews.

The script for the interviews was elaborated ad hoc, taking into account our previous review of the literature and the dimensions of the study, and was examined and agreed upon by all members of the research team. The recordings were transcribed and NVivo 11 qualitative software was used to encode the information and to perform the content analysis. The qualitative data analysis was carried out using the Taylor-Bogdan system, based on data preparation, identification of emerging issues, coding, interpretation, relativisation and determination of methodological rigour [19, 20].

Both emerging issues (those arising during the interview) and predefined ones (discussion topics included in the interview design) were identified. To ensure optimum data quality, triangulation was applied, regarding both the data (using data compilation instruments such as interviews and non-participant observation) and the researchers (the analysis was performed by two researchers[1,3], first working independently and then reaching a consensus view) [21].

Data saturation was determined after analysing the number of references encoded and dimensions identified, as the point at which the reading and coding process failed to generate additional information that would require further codes or categories.

Results

Data analysis revealed the existence of three related categories: how to give bad news, communication skills in general and interactions between healthcare professionals and patients.

The following results are presented in terms of the corresponding information category, highlighting the main findings obtained for each subcategory. These findings are also shown in the tables, together with verbatim transcripts from the interviews. The occupation of the

healthcare professional is identified by a code assigned to the interview, thus ensuring anonymity and confidentiality. Finally, the data obtained are considered in the light of previous research reports in this regard.

How to give bad news
Issuers and receivers of bad news
Healthcare workers emphasise the unexpected nature of bad news and the unwanted changes they provoke in the lives of those who receive it.

Regarding who should perform this communication, there is general agreement that this should be the obstetrician, without excluding the support that other team members may provide, as long as they are well informed about the case. All accept that the pregnant woman should be the first to receive the message, that her autonomy as a human being should be recognised and that she has the right to be informed about everything related to her own health and to that of the foetus. Obstetricians stress how important it is to inform the woman's partner, too, from the outset or, if this is impossible, a person of trust who can provide support and liaison between the parties.

With respect to the medical consultation, the general opinion of the participants is that the person accompanying the mother (usually, the partner or a close relative) should have the patient's consent to hear the details about the evolution of pregnancy, as part of the clinical relationship. None of the healthcare workers believe that information should be concealed or that any pact of silence should be made with the family.

What bad news is communicated and how
Among the most frequent areas of bad news mentioned are diagnoses of miscarriage, chromosomal alteration and intrauterine foetal malformation or death. According to the participants, the early detection of congenital anomalies, in prenatal diagnosis, usually means that a decision must be taken on whether or not to interrupt the pregnancy.

Regarding how it is communicated, from the standpoint of the healthcare professionals, it is advisable to give immediate notice of the discovery of bad news and to inform the patient of the alternatives available. Whatever the prognosis, the availability of equipment to control the symptoms and to ensure the best possible quality of life and comfort should be stressed.

Most of the participants agreed that information should be transmitted gradually, and if possible in line with the patient's wish to receive it. According to healthcare workers, the patient's first reaction is often to suffer a state of shock, in which she is unable to process the information provided. A nursing assistant who works in pregnancy monitoring consultations and who, moreover, has a degree in psychology, illustrates this very well with the following comment:

AUXE01

"Gradually. I think that we should tell them everything, that the information must be complete, and not concealed or ignored, no matter how painful it may be. On the other hand, it mustn't be blurted out too abruptly. All extremes are bad; being told little by little might be agonising, but all at once can be devastating. It's important to enable feedback; you tell them the situation and, depending on the reactions you get, you know where to place more emphasis and where you need to tread lightly."

Regarding how the information should be provided, some professionals choose to prepare the ground before entering fully into the question, others prefer to convey optimism and to leave a door open to hope during the first contact with the patient. In any case, for those interviewed the communication of bad news is not a "single or isolated act" that ends here and now, but must be viewed as a process that requires time and effort. The healthcare team believes it important to inform the person affected that there will be more meetings and opportunities for her to express doubts that may arise, or simply her pain and anger.

The healthcare professionals consulted in our study consider it important to avoid the excessive use of technical terms and to adapt their verbal language to the cultural level of the patient, as detected at the time of the interview. Among the notes made in field diaries during the observation, it is significant that negative reactions were aroused among patients by certain expressions commonly used in obstetrics terminology, such as miscarriage, malformation or foetal death. In this respect, opinions among the professionals are divided: the majority consider that such terms must be used, in order to avoid ambiguity, but others prefer to use alternative expressions, in order to soften the emotional impact produced.

Within this subcategory, an aspect of some importance is that of non-verbal language in interactions with the patient. The researchers noted a reaction that was also observed by many of the obstetricians consulted, namely that the non-verbal language used by healthcare professionals during the ultrasound exploration produces expectation and concern in the women being examined.

Optimum environmental conditions when bad news must be given

Noise and interruptions are the main barriers to establishing a climate of trust during meetings with patients. The healthcare workers commented that they often have to improvise a space in which to hold these meetings, since no purpose-designed physical location is reserved for this type of communication.

These professionals agree that the ideal place for the communication of bad news should provide privacy and tranquillity, be separated from the maternity area, be comfortable and have enough natural light.

The evolution of carer-patient communication

According to the professionals interviewed, scientific-technological advances, the increasing presence of women in obstetrics and gynaecology teams and the practice of defensive medicine are the main factors underlying the evolution of communication and clinical relationships with patients.

The role of nursing staff

The obstetricians consulted acknowledge the commendable work done by nurses and auxiliaries in prenatal consultations, in perinatal medicine and during the hospital stay of women who decide to terminate their pregnancy. The support offered by these hospital workers is viewed as an essential element in achieving patients' satisfaction and collaboration.

Strategy and summary

Many healthcare workers professionals commented that when significant information must be transmitted patients should be given sufficient time to relax and to consider the situation and any doubts they may have. Accordingly, they are asked to leave the consultation during this time, to allow other patients to be attended. If this period of reflection is considerable, the patient may be offered an appointment for another day, especially if crucial decisions must be taken.

According to healthcare staff, lack of time (often caused by an overload of responsibilities) is responsible for the absence of feedback on the quality of the attention provided.

Setting of the intervention

Sometimes the suspicion or the discovery of foetal malformation arises during a routine ultrasound exploration, or the patient may be asked to attend a consultation to be given the confirmation of a previous finding. For obstetricians, the presence or absence of prior knowledge of the diagnosis and the time available are the factors that will determine the preparation or improvisation of their discourse. In this respect, healthcare workers also recognise that taking control of the situation is more complicated and that anxiety and unrest may be provoked when the diagnosis arises unexpectedly (Table 2).

Communication skills
Training in the communication of bad news

The healthcare personnel who took part in this study, especially the obstetricians, commented that their

Table 2 Category.- How to give bad news

Subcategory: issuers and receivers of bad news
Verbatim

OBST S4: *"A woman who is pregnant always expects everything to go well, that the delivery will go well and that a healthy baby will be born; anything that goes wrong is bad news".*

MID S2: *"Unexpected information that causes sadness and pain and provokes a change in your life".*

MID S1: *"Something that doesn't fit what you had expected, that spoils plans and means you have to adapt to a new situation".*

OBST S17: *"The doctor is the person who can and should communicate bad news".*

NASST S8: *"The news has to be given by the doctor and we are there to provide support".*

MID S4: *"Ideally, there should be a multidisciplinary team, including nurses and, if possible, a psychotherapist".*

NUR S3: *"Although the doctor gives the news, nurses are also involved, because the patients ask us to clarify what they don't understand".*

OBST S9: *"Obviously, you have to tell the patient and her partner, if there is one, and then assess the advisability of informing the family".*

OBST S2: *"According to the rules on patient autonomy, the patient must always be told, and we assume that whoever is with her can also receive the news".*

NUR S2: *"The patient must be informed because she is the one who is pregnant".*

MID S2: *"It is very important that the information should also be received by someone the patient trusts (…)"*

Subcategory: what bad news is communicated and how
Verbatim

NASST S6: *"(…) miscarriages, foetal malformations, syndromes, foetal heart disease, proposal to interrupt the pregnancy".*

NUR S3: *"In the ward, we have patients who decide to abort because of a diagnosis of severe malformation or chromosomal alteration".*

MID S12: *"Very often, non-viable pregnancies, anomalies detected by ultra sound scan, antepartum deaths, intrauterine growth problems".*

OBST S8: *"There is no magic formula. Usually the news is given little by little so that the information can be assimilated, but this does not always work, and for some patients it is very painful. Although for others, telling it all at once can be devastating (…)"*

OBST S13: *"(…) using the same means seen to be successful when done by more experienced colleagues".*

MID S3: *"You create your own style, by doing it over and over again".*

OBST S13: *"(…) I prefer to be totally frank. Sometimes, only when you say that the foetus is dead or that its situation is incompatible with life does the patient realise the gravity of the news".*

NUR S3: *"We try to take into account the patient's socio-cultural level, but we often forget and use too much medical jargon".*

NASST S4: *"(…) we aren't very close to the patients, we don't take their hands, we don't give them a hug, we avoid looking directly into their eyes, we focus on filling in the report, on the computer and on the ultrasound scan".*

Subcategory: optimum environmental conditions when bad news must begiven
Verbatim

NUR S1: *"Somewhere private, without interruptions, separated from the maternity area, comfortable and with sufficient natural light".*

OBST S13: *"(…) knocking at the door, people coming in and out, telephones ringing continually".*

Table 2 Category.- How to give bad news *(Continued)*

MID S2: *"The intentions are good, but there is no area specially equipped for this purpose. We try to assign a single room for a pregnancy termination, but it is not always possible".*

Subcategory: the evolution of carer-patient communication
Verbatim

OBST S8: *"We always have to bear in mind the question of the medical professional's legal defence. The social situation makes this inevitable, but it makes it very difficult to provide personalised, direct treatment".*

NUR S2: *"Consent forms, signatures in duplicate, the next appointment with another healthcare professional … all of this greatly interferes with the doctor-patient relationship".*

OBST S6: *"We pay more attention to the diagnostics, we've gained in technological capabilities and lost in human quality".*

Subcategory: the role of nursing staff, according to the physician
Verbatim

OBST S11: *"The nurses provide very important support; they help us convey the message we want the patient to receive".*

OBST S1: *"They can provide support, but diagnosis is the doctor's job and we have to communicate the message, even if we don't like it".*

OBST S12: *"(…) nurses spend many hours at the patient's bedside, so they are well aware of the patient's fears and expectations".*

Subcategory: strategy and summary
Verbatim

OBST S16: *"The extra time you give to one patient is time you're taking away from another. Ideally, an appointment should be made for another day".*

NASST S7: *"Patients are seen again at the end of the consultation, to answer their questions".*

OBST S14: *"At the end of the interview I do not have enough time for the patient to repeat everything I have explained to her and check if she has understood me".*

Subcategory: setting of the intervention
Verbatim

OBST S10: *"With experience, you usually know what to do, but patients can ask unpredictable questions that you have to address on the spot".*

OBST 16: *"Prior awareness or otherwise of the diagnosis and of the time available determines whether the talk to the patient can be prepared or must be improvised".*

OBST S13: *"Inadequate training in communication is a handicap, making it hard to adapt the discourse to meet all the patient's needs".*

OBST Obstetrician, *MID* Midwife, *NUR* Nurse, *NASST* Nursing assistant

academic training in communication and counselling was practically non-existent. They also observed that their acquisition of this type of knowledge was based solely on participation in a short course during initial training. Neither is specific postgraduate training provided; thus, most professionals define themselves as self-taught, having observed and learned from actions seen to be useful for other colleagues. However, these workers consider it extremely important to learn strategies that foster the creation of a solid and, above all, therapeutic clinical relationship.

Most of these professionals admit that a lack of communication techniques and social skills sometimes creates a barrier that can impede the development of a good clinical relationship. The kind of training that they consider appropriate to alleviate this problem, helping them to establish effective communication with patients and family members, would be based on periodic role-playing workshops, debriefing sessions and counselling by a psychologist.

The characteristics or skills that professionals believe should be possessed by those responsible for communicating bad news are proximity, empathy and assuredness.

The ability to explore psycho-social issues

Concerning the psychological aspect, we examined the extent to which healthcare professionals explore the patient's state of mind before communicating bad news. The hypothetical case was raised that the patient was experiencing considerable stress (the death of a loved one, or a recent serious diagnosis, either personal or affecting a close family member).

Within the social sphere, we considered how professionals explore the impact of bad news on patients' daily lives and on their families, social circles and work environments.

In response, the healthcare workers commented that no formal exploration is usually made of psychological questions or of the patient's social sphere, in terms of a systematic examination, and emphasised that this type of inquiry does not influence the communication of bad news. Although such an investigation might be undertaken in the private sphere, these professionals consider it very difficult to do so in the public domain since the way in which services are structured and consultations planned means that there is insufficient time to conduct a formal, regulated study.

The healthcare professionals also stated that patients' psychological and social problems should be treated in primary care and then, if appropriate, referred to a mental health clinic or to social workers.

Responding to the patient's emotions

We also inquired how healthcare professionals address the emotional responses of patients who are given bad news. In general, these workers observed that providing resources to help patients adapt to the new situation, alleviate their mental pain and reduce stress, depression or anxiety is outside their field of competence as gynaecologists and obstetricians, an area in which they lack training, and therefore that this task would be undertaken more appropriately by a psychotherapist.

The professionals who took part in our study did not consider themselves well acquainted with counselling strategies or resilience models for the effective management of patients' emotions.

Finally, the possible existence of language barriers was attributed to the cultural diversity that characterises the population of pregnant women attended at the hospital where this study was performed (Table 3).

Professional-patient interaction
Profile of the patients

The heterogeneity of the patient population at our hospital, in terms of sociocultural status and nationality, requires healthcare professionals to be especially sensitive to the need to provide culturally appropriate care. From the statements made by the participants and from the observations made by the research team, we conclude that the sociocultural characteristics of the patients are very relevant to the communication of bad news, both in how it is received (non-verbal behaviour) and in the coping strategies then adopted.

Reactions to bad news

The healthcare professionals in our study population do not find it difficult to identify the emotions aroused in patients on receiving bad news, because certain patterns tend to appear repeatedly. Moreover, the professionals consider it positive to encourage the expression of these emotions.

Demand for information

As with emotional responses, the first questions asked by women in this situation are very familiar to healthcare workers (*"Why? What did I do wrong? Now what? Does this happen often?"*). When an adverse prenatal diagnosis is made, patients are advised to request a second medical opinion before making a final decision regarding their pregnancy, and are discouraged from seeking information on the internet, because of its unreliability. Patients are warned that the only dependable information is that provided by the health team.

Influence of professionals on decision-making

The professionals realise that their opinions could affect patients' decisions about their pregnancies, depending on the communicative style employed. The way in which questions such as the prognosis and possible alternatives are addressed could facilitate or hinder a satisfactory resolution of the situation. Variability among the professionals involved in this healthcare can also make communication difficult.

Psychosocial support

Healthcare professionals are well disposed to accompany these patients and offer them support, but believe they lack training to respond adequately to the patients' grieving. The general opinion is that handling difficult situations requires the intervention and support of a psychologist specialised in providing this sort of assistance.

Table 3 Category.- Communication skills

Subcategory: training in the communication of bad news
Verbatim

OBST S14: *"In the 2nd year at university, we did workshops on doctor-patient communication, but little else in the 6 years spent in the faculty."*

OBST S12: *"During the first year of residency, we had a course on the doctor-patient relationship, in which we discussed the quality of care and the communication of bad news. But nothing since then."*

NUR S3: *"(...) I've had training in helping and in the humanisation of care, but that was a few years ago."*

MID S3: *"Every year we offer a course on how to respond to perinatal grieving, but hardly any of the medical staff take it."*

OBST S13: *"We would need to learn communicative techniques and skills through role playing and recordings of our own interventions, and then analyse them."*

MOBST S1: *"(...) we need advice from a psychotherapist, and medical team sessions to make our criteria consistent."*

➤Desirable qualities in the person who must transmit bad news:

OBST S11: *"Sensitivity and humanity, I think."*

OBST S12: *"Empathy with the patient and showing self-assuredness in what you have to convey."*

OBST S6: *"Having sufficient knowledge of pathology, of what can and can't be done, and time in which to carry out possible solutions."*

NASST S1: *"Closeness, putting yourself in the patient's place and speaking in terms that she can understand."*

Subcategory: the ability to explore psycho-social issues
Verbatim

ASST S7: *"This isn't examined. Some patients will say they've had a stressful experience, but the doctor doesn't go into this question, there isn't time."*

OBST S2: *"(...) that isn't examined. I honestly don't know what kind of inquiry might be made. If the patient has problems of this type, she usually tells you herself."*

MID S2: *"The psychological and social aspects aren't considered due to our feelings of insecurity. We make the excuse that we don't have time, but it depends to a great extent on each individual's attitude and personal interest in the matter."*

MID S4: *"Unless the patient tells you spontaneously (although you might intuitively sense it), you don't usually go into these areas, you only address the physical side."*

Subcategory: responding to the patient's emotions
Verbatim

NASST S1: *"You don't have the knowledge or skills to deal with certain problems and the easiest thing to do is to avoid them. Without specific and continuous training in the necessary areas, we can't offer patients comprehensive quality care.*

OBST S3: *"We don't have time. To respond properly we'd need a specialised consultation, with the presence of a psychologist."*

➤Counselling strategies and Models of resilience:

OBST S4: *"... yes, I'd recommend it, but to help in all these areas, right now I don't have the tools, nor do we schedule appointments to assess the patient's evolution, how she's coping with the bad news or accepting it."*

OBST S1: *"I don't know what these strategies consist of."*

MAT S4: *"What we do is listening, and little else. The patients go home, basically, with nothing."*

➤Language barriers:

OBST S2: *"There are language barriers, especially with the Chinese and Arab populations, and this makes you anxious."*

OBST Obstetrician, *MID* Midwife, *NUR* Nurse, *NASST* Nursing assistant

Influence of technology

The professionals also referred to being stressed by the bureaucratic and treatment overload they are obliged to accept in modern treatment contexts, together with the ever-greater dependence on technology. According to the professionals, these factors prevent them from dedicating sufficient time to address human concerns and to prevent the medical act from becoming increasingly impersonal (Table 4).

Discussion

As is apparent from our findings, although in health care it is frequently necessary to break bad news to patients, this obligation poses a major challenge to doctors and nurses, and can create difficult, painful situations [22, 23]. The way in which bad news is transmitted affects the patient's understanding of the information received and hence the decisions taken in this respect, the psychological adaptation to new circumstances, participation in the process and any future changes made [24–26].

Difficulties may arise from communicators' insecurity and anxiety, possibly due to inadequate training in communication techniques and care relations. Moreover, healthcare staff may lack the knowledge and skills needed to assess patients' information needs and to motivate their active participation in decision making [15, 27–29].

In this respect, intuition and/or experience are not sufficient in themselves. Communication is not a gift but a skill that can be learned [30] and for which training must be provided, because it does not necessarily improve with experience [31]. The doctors, nurses and nursing assistants who took part in this study all agree that in developing their professional competence, they learned to communicate with patients by means of trial and error and by imitation, from observing the actions of colleagues with more experience. None of the medical workers taking part in our study had received a refresher course or specific training in this respect, a shortcoming that has also been reported in previous research [32–35].

Communication skills should be included as part of the training of healthcare personnel, together with the clinical competence specific to each branch of the profession [36]. Such training can enhance empathy in carers, helping them evaluate patients' expectations, offer appropriate support, reduce emotional distress and foster compliance with clinical guidelines [26]. Indeed, good communication is an ethical and legal imperative [34, 37, 38].

In line with previous studies [33, 34, 39], we believe that other important aspects to be addressed include non-verbal language and the environment in which the bad news is to be communicated: this should be comfortable and quiet and enable privacy. However, this is

Table 4 Category.- Patient - Healthcare professional interaction

Subcategory: profile of the patients
Verbatim

OBST S13: *"Young women, between 16 and 44 years old, generally healthy for pregnancy, childbirth and postnatal care. Regarding socio-cultural level, there are all types, from low socio-cultural level to middle and high levels, immigrants, Spanish natives, Asian, European, African ... a multicultural population."*

OBST S8: *"Very heterogeneous due to the variety of races."*

OBST S7: *"Because what I say may lead to the pregnancy being interrupted, it's necessary to know that not all cultures conceive or face this prospect in the same way."*

Subcategory: reactions to bad news
Verbatim

MID S3: *"At first there is a state of shock, a sense of unreality."*

OBST S3: *"They respond with pain, crying, anguish, suffering, and the feeling of enormous disappointment."*

OBST S8: *"Although the foetus referred to in the bad news is the fruit of two people, the father and the mother, the mother's response is usually much more emotional, and the role of the father automatically becomes that of consoling the mother."*

Subcategory: demand for information
Verbatim

NASST S6: *"Why? What have I done? Is it common? Finding out the cause and trying to determine if they are responsible. Is it something I took? I made an effort (...)"*

NASST S5: *"(...) Now what? What can be done? What do you suggest? What would you do if it happened to you?"*

NUR S1: *"I think a second opinion would be a good idea, but it is very important to know who to ask."*

OBST S4: *"They resort to the internet, but they don't know how to filter the information and what information has been scientifically proven."*

MID S3: *"In the private sector, they think they are better looked after because they are given more time and attention. Perhaps we should improve things in this area."*

Subcategory: influence of professionals on decision-making
Verbatim

OBST S14: *"(...) you are often recommend what they should do. So, the way we give the news can make their decision go one way or the other."*

NUR S2: *"The lack of social skills hinders the active participation of these patients in decision making."*

OBST S13: *"I try to be as aseptic as possible, to respect their autonomy, giving them the consent form to sign ..."*

Subcategory: psychosocial support
Verbatim

OBST S10: *"(...) some patients do need it, because they collapse, they go home and for months they feel very bad and don't know who to turn to."*

MID S2: *"The psychologist should be part of the team, both to help the women and to guide staff, because burnout does happen."*

NUR S3: *"We don't know what techniques we can use to deal with conflicts that may arise during the clinical relationship."*

Subcategory: influence of technology
Verbatim

OBST S13: *"We spend more time using technology than we do listening, looking into people's eyes (...)"*

NUR S3: *"An excess of technology can dehumanise the attention we provide."*

OBST Obstetrician, *MID* Midwife, *NUR* Nurse, *NASST* Nursing assistant

not always the case, and organisational and structural problems have been identified. Consultation areas often fail to provide the above-mentioned characteristics, and noise, interruptions and lack of time due to the care burden all impede the creation of the therapeutic rapport between medical worker and patient that is necessary for successful collaboration between them.

Midwives, nurses and nursing assistants receive training in providing specific support to maternity patients, reinforcing personal qualities traditionally associated with their profession, such as closeness, kindness and sympathy. Corroborating the findings of earlier research, our results show that healthcare personnel are equipped with the necessary skills to produce a good nurse-patient relationship, although it has also been found that these capabilities are often lost if they are not refreshed during later professional practice [40].

While nurses must often play the role of communicators of bad news, many obstetricians consider this to be a function that is outside their sphere of competence. Nursing staff and midwives, however, are usually committed to working as a team, and the multidisciplinary approach has been shown to be the most effective means of communicating bad news. Indeed, if health teams do not function in a well-integrated way, the patient may receive differing or even contradictory information [33, 41].

To overcome barriers to communication, healthcare personnel should develop the ability to express empathy, closeness and solidarity with patients' emotions, and also possess active listening skills – in areas such as paying careful attention and manifesting availability to help – together with self-assuredness, transmitting a sense of security on the basis of well-grounded opinions [3, 39, 42, 43].

The lack of training in the above skills to foster effective communication is often aggravated by an absence of feedback and by insufficient time to offer more support. As a result, the relationship with the patient is very limited despite the wish to provide high quality care. A possible problem in the carer-patient relation is the tendency of carers, in some cases, to (mis)interpret the wishes and needs of patients; in consequence, the response made may not meet the patient's expectations, but correspond to what the carer believes appropriate. A good communicator should clarify matters with the patient, providing feedback to ensure that what is clear to one party is equally clear to the other [5, 6].

The acquisition of communication skills is hampered when there is no relationship between the learning process and the context in which the work must be carried out, when there is little or no flexibility in the scheduling of courses or workshops, when there is insufficient institutional recognition and when there are few opportunities for training to take place. Problems may also arise from a fear of becoming too involved when dealing with personal aspects such as feelings and emotions [44].

Health professionals may adopt different attitudes if they lack the skills to handle the emotional responses of patients who have received bad news. On the one hand, some carers believe that their responsibility is limited to addressing physical problems; in consequence, they will emphasise the development of skills related to the use of instruments developed in biomedicine, in order to provide a faster and more accurate diagnosis [1]. In monitoring the progress of a pregnancy control, such a carer's entire attention could be focused on confirming or ruling out the presence of biological problems in the foetus. Accordingly, ultrasound examinations, screening tests, the signing of consent forms and entering medical records into computer files would occupy most of the time allocated to the consultation, leaving hardly any opportunity for a face-to-face exchange of views [10]. A carer may be highly skilled in the application of certain techniques, but this will be of little use if effective communication cannot be established [31]. In fact, technology should be auxiliary to the carer's daily work [45]. Patient-centred care means understanding the human being from a biopsychosocial approach, recognising the need to consider not only the illness but also the patient's personal experience, and to understand her as a person with emotions and private concerns (the psychological sphere) in multiple aspects of life, including work, family, and the partner (social sphere) [25, 26].

On the other hand, time pressures and limitations are sometimes cited to justify the lack of attention paid to psychosocial aspects of health care [10]. In contrast to this attitude among healthcare personnel, evidence suggests that patients strongly believe there is a need to investigate their unexpressed concerns, to teach them how to evaluate the information provided and to adopt appropriate measures, on the basis of personalised recommendations [46]. Our review of the literature and our analysis of the results obtained lead us to conclude that in a context in which patients can express their concerns and fears, motivated by the health carer's open, sympathetic attitude, therapeutic communication can be established and the necessary emotional support supplied [47]. However, doctors and nurses do not usually consider the patient's mood before communicating a diagnosis, or inquire about recent stressful episodes (such as the death of a loved one, or the presence of a severe illness in the patient or in a close relative), despite research evidence that the accumulation of stress-provoking experiences shortly before a traumatic event can increase the incidence of post-traumatic stress disorders [48].

Difficulties in communication may also be due to an unexpected diagnosis, without previous indications. When a diagnosis of this type must be confirmed, the health carer often experiences anxiety, a feeling of responsibility and a fear of censure, while being pressured to supply a rapid, convincing explanation and at the same time respond to the patient's emotional reaction [8].

At other times, difficulty in transmitting an adverse diagnosis or a poor prognosis is the result of a heavy workload, together with pressing demands by patients and their families for information [49]. Studies have shown that when information is transmitted to patients and their families in sufficient quantity and quality, their anxiety is reduced and, in general, better and faster recovery is achieved and patient/carer collaboration is enhanced [23, 32].

Feelings of frustration and helplessness when the carer is unable to prevent, halt or reverse a negative outcome also hamper communication, especially when the therapeutic options are limited or non-existent. The carer must then seek to provide comfort in a situation that does not offer grounds for being hopeful [26, 50]. Feelings of frustration and powerlessness may be compounded by legal concerns, with the worry that an unsatisfied patient may present an official complaint. The judicialisation of healthcare issues may generate the notion that every human being has the right to be healed and that any failure in this respect must be due to an error, which should be punished. In the health service, more complaints are made regarding the quality of information received than any other aspect of health care [10]. Moreover, the provision of informed consent does not always guarantee the reality of bidirectional communication, but may serve only as a legal safeguard [51].

Our results also show that some healthcare professionals, due to the experience of patients' suffering and to taboos regarding death, erect barriers to communication through automated responses and patterns of avoidance, especially when there is the possibility of transferring responsibility to other carers [52]. This type of behaviour may arise due to a lack of support system for the healthcare team, or to the absence or outdated status of action protocols [50].

Language and cultural differences are the most common types of communication barrier, due to the multilingual and multicultural nature of the treatment population [53]. The two most important causes of ineffective communication are the precarity of information provided to patients and the absence of comprehension [54, 55].

The link between the principal investigator and the institution in which the study was performed may be regarded as a limitation of this study, insofar as it may have influenced the interpretation of certain professional practices. On the other hand, this association facilitated access to a wide range of scenarios in which patients and carers interact, thus providing an authentic outlook on healthcare practice.

Another potential issue is that, given the inherent properties of the qualitative method applied and the local nature of this study, the findings obtained might not be readily extrapolated to other contexts (although the method used can be transferred without difficulty). The effect of subjectivity means that a given phenomenon may be perceived, interpreted and experienced differently from one individual to another. Therefore, the interpretations of our participants, regarding the specific problem addressed in this study, will not necessarily be shared by other professionals, interacting with patients in different contexts.

Conclusions

The increasing dependence of certain diagnostic procedures on technological resources may be detrimental to interpersonal relationships, making them cold and distant. For healthcare personnel, the human quality of their profession has deteriorated, mainly due to the heavy caseloads experienced, which increasingly limit the time that can be spent with each patient. In order to improve communication, more attention should be paid to the human and spiritual dimensions of healthcare, giving greater weight to empathy, authenticity and listening (without imposing one's own interpretation). The analysis performed leads us to draw the following conclusions: a different model of clinical relationship should be promoted, based on shared decision making, and greater clarity should be granted to the functions of the multidisciplinary team with respect to the patient's grieving when a pregnancy is interrupted. To achieve these goals, protocols should be implemented to ensure comprehensive care provision, addressing not only the biological sphere but also psychosocial concerns. In this respect, too, specific training should be provided, at undergraduate and postgraduate levels, in social skills and cultural competence. In short, this study identifies possible areas of improvement related to the interventions of healthcare personnel and to the organisation of the institution itself, with particular respect to the communication to patients of an adverse prenatal diagnosis.

Acknowledgements
We thank all the staff of the Costa del Sol Health Agency who agreed to participate in this study. We also thank the research team of the Hospital of the Costa del Sol for their support. In addition, we are grateful for the contribution made to this research project by the University of Malaga.

Funding
This study was partially supported by the Costa del Sol Health Care Agency, which provided funds for the dissemination of the study results.

Authors' contributions
JAC proposed the concept for the study, conducted and transcribed the interviews, and developed the first draft of the manuscript. MLA, MPR and IMMG contributed ideas and discussed the results of the study. All the co-authors read, critically commented on and revised the successive drafts of the manuscript. They also approved the final version before submission to the journal.

Competing interests
The authors declare that they have no competing interests.

Author details
[1]Nursing Surgery Service, Hospital Costa del Sol, Málaga, Spain. [2]School of Health Sciences, Universidad de Jaén, Jaén, Spain. [3]Research Unit. Agencia Sanitaria Costa del Sol, Marbella, Spain. [4]Health Services Research on Chronic Patients Network. REDISSEC, Madrid, Spain. [5]School of Health Sciences, Universidad de Málaga, Málaga, Spain.

References
1. M. Rodriguez de Alba, A. Bustamante-Aragones, S. Perlado, M. J. Trujillo-Tiebas, J. Diaz-Recasens, J. Plaza-Arranz, y C. Ramos, Noninvasive prenatal diagnosis of monogenic disorders. Expert Opin Biol Ther, vol. 12 Suppl 1, pp. S171-S179, jun. 2012.
2. L. Butalid, J. M. Bensing, y P. F. M. Verhaak, «Talking about psychosocial problems: an observational study on changes in doctor-patient communication in general practice between 1977 and 2008.», Patient Educ Couns, vol. 94, n.º 3, pp. 314-321, mar. 2014.
3. F. A. Derksen, T. C. Olde Hartman, J. M. Bensing, y A. L. Lagro-Janssen, «Managing barriers to empathy in the clinical encounter: a qualitative interview study with GPs», The British journal of general practice : the journal of the Royal College of General Practitioners, vol. 66, n.º 653, pp. e887-e895, dic. 2016.
4. R. M. Epstein y R. L. J. Street, «Shared mind: communication, decision making, and autonomy in serious illness.», Ann Fam Med, vol. 9, n.º 5, pp. 454-461, 2011.
5. R. L. J. Street, G. Makoul, N. K. Arora, y R. M. Epstein, «How does communication heal? Pathways linking clinician-patient communication to health outcomes.», Patient Educ Couns, vol. 74, n.º 3, pp. 295-301, mar. 2009.
6. J. K. Rao, L. A. Anderson, T. S. Inui, y R. M. Frankel, «Communication interventions make a difference in conversations between physicians and patients: a systematic review of the evidence.», Med Care, vol. 45, n.º 4, pp. 340-349, abr. 2007.
7. O. Barr, H. Skirton, «Informed decision making regarding antenatal screening for fetal abnormality in the United Kingdom: a qualitative study of parents and professionals.», Nursing & health sciences, vol. 15, n.º 3, pp. 318-325, sep. 2013.
8. A. L. Greiner, J. Conklin, «Breaking bad news to a pregnant woman with a fetal abnormality on ultrasound.», Obstetrical & gynecological survey, vol. 70, n.º 1, pp. 39-44, ene. 2015.
9. J. Hodgson, P. Pitt, S. Metcalfe, J. Halliday, M. Menezes, J. Fisher, C. Hickerton, K. Petersen, y B. McClaren, «Experiences of prenatal diagnosis and decision-making about termination of pregnancy: a qualitative study.», Aust N Z J Obstet Gynaecol, vol. 56, n.º 6, pp. 605-613, dic. 2016.
10. R. Simpson y R. Bor, «'I'm not picking up a heart-beat': experiences of sonographers giving bad news to women during ultrasound scans.», The British journal of medical psychology, vol. 74 Part 2, pp. 255-272, jun. 2001.
11. R.-L. Van Keer, R. Deschepper, A. L. Francke, L. Huyghens, y J. Bilsen, «Conflicts between healthcare professionals and families of a multi-ethnic patient population during critical care: an ethnographic study.», Critical care (London, England), vol. 19, p. 441, dic. 2015.
12. K. Sweeny, J. A. Shepperd, y P. K. J. Han, «The goals of communicating bad news in health care: do physicians and patients agree?», Health expectations : an international journal of public participation in health care and health policy, vol. 16, n.º 3, pp. 230-238, sep. 2013.
13. L. Fallowfield y V. Jenkins, «Communicating sad, bad, and difficult news in medicine.», Lancet (London, England), vol. 363, n.º 9405, pp. 312-319, ene. 2004.

14. R. R. Wallace, S. Goodman, L. R. Freedman, V. K. Dalton, y L. H. Harris, «Counseling women with early pregnancy failure: utilizing evidence, preserving preference.», Patient Educ Couns, vol. 81, n.° 3, pp. 454-461, dic. 2010.

15. J. Halpern, «Empathy and patient-physician conflicts.», J Gen Intern Med, vol. 22, n.° 5, pp. 696-700, may 2007.

16. L. Martin, J. T. Gitsels-van der Wal, M. T. R. Pereboom, E. R. Spelten, E. K. Hutton, y S. van Dulmen, «Clients' psychosocial communication and midwives' verbal and nonverbal communication during prenatal counseling for anomaly screening.», Patient Educ Couns, vol. 99, n.° 1, pp. 85-91, ene. 2016.

17. M. Driessnack, V. D. Sousa, y I. A. C. Mendes, «An overview of research designs relevant to nursing: part 2: qualitative research designs.», Rev Lat Am Enfermagem, vol. 15, n.° 4, pp. 684-688, 2007.

18. Guba EG, Lincoln YS. Competing paradigms in qualitative research. Thousand Oaks: The handbook of qualitative research. CA: Sage; 1994.

19. M. Pla, "Rigor in qualitative research", Aten Primaria, vol. 24, n.° 5, pp. 295-300, 1999.

20. Taylor R, Bogdan S.J. Introduction to qualitative research methods. The search for meanings. Barcelona: Ed. Paidós; 1987.

21. N. Carter, D. Bryant-Lukosius, A. DiCenso, J. Blythe, y A. J. Neville, «The use of triangulation in qualitative research.», Oncol Nurs Forum, vol. 41, n.° 5, pp. 545-547, sep. 2014.

22. D. Meitar, O. Karnieli-Miller, y S. Eidelman, «The impact of senior medical students' personal difficulties on their communication patterns in breaking bad news.», Academic medicine : journal of the Association of American Medical Colleges, vol. 84, n.° 11, pp. 1582-1594, nov. 2009.

23. F. Delevallez, A. Lienard, A.-S. Gibon, y D. Razavi, «[Breaking bad news in oncology: the Belgian experience].», Revue des maladies respiratoires, vol. 31, n.° 8, pp. 721-728, oct. 2014.

24. C. Burgers, C. J. Beukeboom, y L. Sparks, «How the doc should (not) talk: when breaking bad news with negations influences patients' immediate responses and medical adherence intentions.», Patient Educ Couns, vol. 89, n.° 2, pp. 267-273, nov. 2012.

25. A. Gesser-Edelsburg y N. A. E. Shahbari, «Decision-making on terminating pregnancy for Muslim Arab women pregnant with fetuses with congenital anomalies: maternal affect and doctor-patient communication.», Reprod Health, vol. 14, n.° 1, p. 49, abr. 2017.

26. A. Herrera, M. Rios, J. M. Manriquez, y G. Rojas, «[Breaking bad news in clinical practice].», Rev Med Chil, vol. 142, n.° 10, pp. 1306-1315, oct. 2014.

27. N. H. M. Labrie y P. J. Schulz, «Exploring the relationships between participatory decision-making, visit duration, and general practitioners' provision of argumentation to support their medical advice: results from a content analysis.», Patient Educ Couns, vol. 98, n.° 5, pp. 572-577, may 2015.

28. J. G. Lalor, D. Devane, y C. M. Begley, «Unexpected diagnosis of fetal abnormality: women's encounters with caregivers.», Birth (Berkeley, Calif), vol. 34, n.° 1, pp. 80-88, mar. 2007.

29. M. Brann y J. J. Bute, «Communicating to promote informed decisions in the context of early pregnancy loss.», Patient Educ Couns, vol. 100, n.° 12, pp. 2269-2274, dic. 2017.

30. J. Shaw, R. Brown y S. Dunn, «The impact of delivery style on doctors' experience of stress during simulated bad news consultations.», Patient Educ Couns, vol. 98, n° 10, pp. 1255-1259, oct. 2015.

31. P. M. Moore, S. Rivera Mercado, M. Grez Artigues, y T. A. Lawrie, «Communication skills training for healthcare professionals working with people who have cancer.», The Cochrane database of systematic reviews, no. 3, p. CD003751, mar. 2013.

32. A. P. Jacques, E. J. Adkins, S. Knepel, C. Boulger, J. Miller, y D. P. Bahner, «Educating the delivery of bad news in medicine: Preceptorship versus simulation.», International journal of critical illness and injury science, vol. 1, n.° 2, pp. 121-124, jul. 2011.

33. M. L. Bascunan, «[Truth disclosure in medicine: psychological perspective].», Rev Med Chil, vol. 133, n.° 6, pp. 693-698, jun. 2005.

34. W. F. Baile, R. Buckman, R. Lenzi, G. Glober, E. A. Beale, y A. P. Kudelka, «SPIKES-A six-step protocol for delivering bad news: application to the patient with cancer.», Oncologist, vol. 5, n.° 4, pp. 302-311, 2000.

35. K. R. Monden, L. Gentry, y T. R. Cox, «Delivering bad news to patients.», Proc (Baylor Univ Med Cent), vol. 29, n.° 1, pp. 101-102, ene. 2016.

36. D. Armentrout y L. A. Cates, «Informing parents about the actual or impending death of their infant in a newborn intensive care unit.», The Journal of perinatal & neonatal nursing, vol. 25, n.° 3, pp. 261-267, 2011.

37. C. Strong, «Fetal anomalies: ethical and legal considerations in screening, detection, and management.», Clin Perinatol, vol. 30, n.° 1, pp. 113-126, mar. 2003.

38. A. Arber y A. Gallagher, «Breaking bad news revisited: the push for negotiated disclosure and changing practice implications.», Int J Palliat Nurs, vol. 9, n.° 4, pp. 166-172, abr. 2003.

39. S. Nunez, T. Marco, G. Burillo-Putze, y J. Ojeda, «[Procedures and skills for the communication of bad news in emergency units].», Med Clin, vol. 127, n.° 15, pp. 580-583, oct. 2006.

40. R. Norouzinia, M. Aghabarari, M. Shiri, M. Karimi, y E. Samami, «Communication barriers perceived by nurses and patients.», Global journal of health science, vol. 8, n.° 6, pp. 65-74, sep. 2015.

41. H. Gluyas, «Effective communication and teamwork promotes patient safety.», Nursing standard (Royal College of Nursing (Great Britain) : 1987), vol. 29, n.° 49, pp. 50-57, ago. 2015.

42. M. Omura, J. Maguire, T. Levett-Jones, T. E. Stone, «Effectiveness of assertive communication training programs for health professionals and students: a systematic review protocol.», JBI database of systematic reviews and implementation reports, vol. 14, n.° 10, pp. 64-71, oct. 2016.

43. A. Lyndon, M. G. Zlatnik, y R. M. Wachter, «Effective physician-nurse communication: a patient safety essential for labor and delivery.», Am J Obstet Gynecol, vol. 205, n.° 2, pp. 91-96, ago. 2011.

44. M. Schmid Mast, A. Kindlimann, y W. Langewitz, «Recipients' perspective on breaking bad news: how you put it really makes a difference.», Patient Educ Couns, vol. 58, n.° 3, pp. 244-251, sep. 2005.

45. F. Oflaz y H. Vural, «The evaluation of nurses and nursing activities through the perceptions of inpatients», Int Nurs Rev, vol. 57, n.° 2, pp. 232-239, jun. 2010.

46. G. Novick, «Women's experience of prenatal care: an integrative review.», Journal of midwifery & women's health, vol. 54, n.° 3, pp. 226-237, 2009.

47. E. C. Heberlein, A. H. Picklesimer, D. L. Billings, S. Covington-Kolb, N. Farber, y E. A. Frongillo, «Qualitative comparison of Women's perspectives on the functions and benefits of group and individual prenatal care.», Journal of midwifery & women's health, vol. 61, n.° 2, pp. 224-234, 2016.

48. J. C. M. Cole, J. S. Moldenhauer, K. Berger, M. S. Cary, H. Smith, V. Martino, N. Rendon, y L. J. Howell, «Identifying expectant parents at risk for psychological distress in response to a confirmed fetal abnormality.», Archives of women's mental health, vol. 19, n.° 3, pp. 443-453, jun. 2016.

49. L. T. de Beer, J. Pienaar, y S. J. Rothmann, «Work overload, burnout, and psychological ill-health symptoms: a three-wave mediation model of the employee health impairment process.», Anxiety Stress Coping, vol. 29, n.° 4, pp. 387-399, jul. 2016.

50. S. Newell y Z. Jordan, «The patient experience of patient-centered communication with nurses in the hospital setting: a qualitative systematic review protocol.», JBI database of systematic reviews and implementation reports, vol. 13, n.° 1, pp. 76-87, ene. 2015.

51. G. Ferreira Padilla, T. Ferrandez Anton, y J. Baleriola Julvez, «[Informed consent versus "communicated consent" in the need to ensure a two-way doctor-patient relationship and to improve patient and doctor satisfaction].», Aten Primaria, vol. 45, n.° 4. Spain, pp. 225-226, abr-2013.

52. F. Baena-Antequera, y E. Jurado-Garcia, «[The woman at the termination of pregnancy for fetal anomalies: clinical case].», Enferm Clin, vol. 25, n.° 5, pp. 276-281, 2015.

53. E. Paternotte, F. Scheele, C. M. Seeleman, L. Bank, A. J. J. A. Scherpbier, y S. van Dulmen, «Intercultural doctor-patient communication in daily outpatient care: relevant communication skills.», Perspectives on medical education, vol. 5, n.° 5, pp. 268-275, oct. 2016.

54. H. Harmsen, L. Meeuwesen, J. van Wieringen, R. Bernsen, y M. Bruijnzeels, «When cultures meet in general practice: intercultural differences between GPs and parents of child patients.», Patient Educ Couns, vol. 51, n.° 2, pp. 99-106, oct. 2003.

55. R. L. Sudore, C. S. Landefeld, E. J. Perez-Stable, K. Bibbins-Domingo, B. A. Williams, y D. Schillinger, «Unraveling the relationship between literacy, language proficiency, and patient-physician communication.», Patient Educ Couns, vol. 75, n.° 3, pp. 398-402, jun. 2009.

12

Women's perspectives on antenatal breast expression

Frankie J. Fair[1], Helen Watson[1], Rachel Gardner[2] and Hora Soltani[1*]

Abstract

Background: The practice of antenatal breast expression (ABE) has been proposed as a strategy to promote successful breastfeeding. Although there has been some focus on the evaluation of the effects of ABE in promotion of breastfeeding, little or no evidence exists on women's experiences of ABE or opinions on ABE, particularly amongst overweight or obese women.

Methods: This study aimed to explore women's knowledge, practices and opinions of ABE, and any differences within the overweight and obese subgroups. A cross-sectional survey was undertaken using an online questionnaire distributed by a maternity user group representative via social media. Quantitative data were analysed using Chi-square and Fisher's exact tests in SPSS. Simple thematic analysis was used for the qualitative data.

Results: A total of 688 responses were analysed; the sample represented a group of breastfeeding mothers, of whom 64.5% had heard of ABE, 8.2% had been advised to do ABE, and 14.2% had undertaken ABE. Of the women who had been advised to do ABE, 67.9% had complied. Most participants (58.6%) were unsure if ABE was a good idea; however 80.9% would consider doing ABE if it was found to be helpful to prepare for breastfeeding. Women in the overweight or obese subgroups were significantly more likely to have heard of ABE ($p < 0.001$), and positive opinion of ABE also increased with higher BMI groups. The qualitative data demonstrated participants felt ABE may be beneficial when mother or baby have medical problems, and in preparation for breastfeeding, but highlighted their concerns that it may interfere with nature and be harmful, and that they wanted more information and knowledge about ABE.

Conclusions: Amongst women who have breastfed, many have heard of ABE, compliance with advice to undertake ABE is relatively high, and ABE is considered an acceptable practice. Further investigation into the benefits and safety of ABE is warranted, to address the needs of childbearing women for evidence-based information about this practice. If the evidence base is established, overweight and obese pregnant women could be an important target group for this intervention.

Keywords: Antenatal breast expression, Maternal obesity, Breastfeeding, Survey, Opinions, Compliance

Plain English summary

It has been proposed that the manual expression of breast-milk whilst a woman is still pregnant (ABE) may promote breastfeeding. A few studies have evaluated the effects of ABE on promotion of breastfeeding but to our knowledge no study has focused on exploring women's experiences and opinions about this practice on a large scale.

This study aimed to investigate women's experiences of and opinions on this practice by undertaking a questionnaire based survey. This was distributed online and a total of 688 responses were analysed. The respondents were predominately a group of breastfeeding mothers, of whom 64.5% had heard of ABE, 8.2% had been advised to do ABE, and 14.2% had undertaken ABE. Of the women who had been advised to do ABE, 67.9% had followed this advice. Most participants (58.6%) were unsure if ABE was a good idea; however 80.9% would consider doing ABE if it was found to help prepare for breastfeeding. Overweight or obese women were more likely to have heard of ABE, and were equally as positive about undertaking it if it was found to help prepare for breastfeeding. Women felt that ABE may be beneficial when mother or baby have medical problems, and in

* Correspondence: h.soltani@shu.ac.uk
[1]Faculty of Health and Wellbeing, Sheffield Hallam University, Collegiate Crescent, Sheffield, UK
Full list of author information is available at the end of the article

preparation for breastfeeding, but had concerns that it may interfere with nature and be harmful, and said that they wanted more information about ABE. If further research finds that ABE is safe and effective, it could be developed as an intervention to promote breastfeeding, particularly for overweight and obese pregnant women.

Background

The World Health Organization recommends that infants are exclusively breastfed until 6 months of age with continued breastfeeding thereafter alongside appropriate complementary foods [1]. The health benefits of breastfeeding for both the mother and the infant are well documented [2–4]. However, the practice of breastfeeding varies extensively and identifying appropriate strategies to promote breastfeeding amongst all women are required.

Factors influencing breastfeeding

The United Kingdom (UK) Infant feeding Survey has demonstrated that the prevalence of breastfeeding is higher amongst mothers from managerial and professional occupations, those who left education aged over 18, mothers aged 30 and over, mothers from ethnic minority groups and mothers living in the least deprived areas [5].

A lower prevalence of breastfeeding and poorer breastfeeding outcomes among women who are overweight or obese is well supported by epidemiological studies [6–13]. Maternal obesity is associated with up to 13% lower breastfeeding initiation rates, and shorter duration of any breastfeeding and exclusive breastfeeding when compared to women of normal weight [13, 14]. This is of particular concern given the rising rate of overweight and obesity across the globe [15], with rates in women aged 20 years or over within the UK in 2013 standing at 57.2% with a body mass index (BMI) ≥ 25 kg/m^2 and 25.4% with a BMI ≥30 kg/m^2 [16].

Although psychosocial factors are significantly associated with the lower incidence of breastfeeding among women with a BMI over 25 kg/m^2, anatomical and physiological alterations may also play a role. Among these is that women who are overweight or obese may have mammary hypoplasia or insufficient glandular tissue as obesity in childhood negatively affects the development of breast glandular tissue [13]. Many of the characteristics experienced by women who are overweight or obese are consistent with this, including reporting stopping breastfeeding due to perceived insufficient supply [17] and being more likely to try to express in the first 2 months postpartum but less likely to have successfully expressed than women with a normal BMI [18]. A high pre-pregnancy BMI is also a predictor of delayed onset lactogenesis II [19], which is

the production of copious milk triggered by progesterone withdrawal after the removal of the placenta [13, 20]. This most critical stage of the lactation cycle [21] is more likely to be delayed (occurring more than 72 h after birth) amongst women with a high BMI than women of normal weight [22]. Various underlying physiological reasons for the increased likelihood of delayed lactogenesis II amongst women with obesity are proposed; the impact of increased oedema [13], increased likelihood of medical problems including gestational diabetes, prolonged labour, caesarean section or preterm birth [6, 23], the role of leptin released from adipose tissue which inhibits oxytocin and milk ejection [13], reduced prolactin response to infant suckling [24], and the impact of insulin imbalance [13].

Antenatal breast expression

The practice of antenatal breast expression (ABE) has been proposed as a strategy to prevent delayed lactogenesis II in both the academic and consumer literature [25, 26], and as a strategy to overcome the effects of delayed lactogenesis II by ensuring women have a store of expressed milk to prevent the use of formula milk, particularly if the mother has pre-existing or gestational diabetes [27–29]. ABE is widely recommended in UK maternity units [30–43]. A recent survey demonstrated that out of the 56 responding maternity units across 9 geographical regions in the UK, 73% offered ABE to diabetic women, 25% offered ABE to women who had risk factors for neonatal hypoglycaemia, and 19% offered ABE to all women [44]. Furthermore, the practice of ABE is promoted by some lactation support websites [29, 45].

ABE involves expressing colostrum from the breast in the antenatal period, however there is little consensus on timing of onset, frequency, duration and method of expression. Recommendations vary within the academic and consumer literature and local UK guidelines on when to commence ABE. A majority of UK maternity units recommend commencing ABE from 36 to 37 weeks (98%) with only 2% recommending commencing ABE at 35,38 or 39 weeks gestation [44], however consumer literature recommends commencing ABE from 32 to 34 weeks of pregnancy [29]. Similarly recommendations regarding how to express ABE vary, including frequency ranging from once a day [35], building up to 4 times a day [32, 34, 39] a minimum of 4 times a day [43] or as often as the woman wants [36, 40] and duration varying from 5 min [35] up to 20 min at a time [32, 38, 39].

Evidence of the effectiveness or underlying mechanism of action of ABE are still not clear, although several studies including a recent large randomised controlled trial have focused on evaluating the safety and efficacy of ABE among women with diabetes [27, 46–48]. Initial concerns raised in a retrospective cohort study about the safety of ABE in regards to influencing the timing of onset of labour if ABE was commenced prior to 37 weeks' gestation [49] have not been supported by a large randomised controlled trial of women at low risk of complications with diabetes in pregnancy [48]. This trial found no difference in gestational at birth between those randomised to ABE from 36 weeks' gestation and women randomised to standard care [48].

Given that ABE is a widely recommended practice in maternity units and on lactation support websites and that limited evaluation of the acceptability of ABE to prepare for breastfeeding has been undertaken, a wide scoping of acceptability and women's views on this practice merits a focused exploration.

This study was therefore designed to assess the general knowledge of ABE among mothers, their practices surrounding ABE and the acceptability of ABE to them should it be found to be an effective preparation for breastfeeding. It was also aimed to explore any differences in knowledge and acceptability within the overweight and obese subgroup of mothers.

Methods

A cross-sectional survey using a questionnaire was developed in consultation with maternity user group representatives; individuals representing the opinions of mothers and fathers currently expecting a baby or with a child under 1 year old. The survey questionnaire was generated using the online, cloud-based software, Survey Monkey. Applying a convenience sampling strategy, the questionnaire was distributed from December 2015 to January 2016 through a maternity service user and parenting Facebook group, which was moderated by the maternity user group representative member of the research team. This Facebook group aimed to allow parents to share stories and gain peer support, it was not focussed on method of infant feeding.

The questionnaire consisted of a mixture of question types, including free text questions and fixed response options. Demographic data was collected, including place of residence, ethnicity, age, number of pregnancies, and occupation of participants. In order to calculate BMI, the survey included a question about the participants' height and weight at the time of the survey, in either metric or imperial units.

Survey questions covered the following topics; whether participants had ever breastfed and for how long, whether they had heard of the practice of ABE, had been advised to do ABE and had undertaken ABE, and their opinion on whether ABE was a good idea and if they would consider doing ABE if it was found to be beneficial to breastfeeding.

Ethical approval was obtained from Sheffield Hallam University Research Ethics Committee, study ID: 2015-

16/ HWB-HSC-14. Consent was assumed inherent for the participants who completed the questionnaire voluntarily.

Data analysis
Logical checks and data cleaning were carried out and inconsistencies double checked for clarification. All survey data were double-entered and cleaned using SPSS 21.0. Descriptive statistics including proportions, ranges, means, standard deviation (SD), median and interquartile ranges (IQR) as appropriate were calculated for the demographic data and for closed answer questions. Categorical data were analysed using Chi-square test or Fisher's exact test where the assumptions for Chi-square test were not satisfied, such as expected count < 5 in over 20% of cells. A p value < 0.05 was regarded as indicating statistical significance.

BMI values were calculated from the reported height and weight measurements and grouped into 3 categories; BMI less than 25 kg/m^2, overweight (BMI of 25–29.9 kg/m^2) and obese (BMI of 30 kg/m^2 or more) [50]. Occupations of the participants were coded using the 3 category National Statistics Socio-economic Classification (NS-SEC) system [51].

Simple thematic analysis was used for the open ended questions by coding the data after familiarisation, and deriving categories and themes inductively.

Results
Respondent characteristics
There were 797 completed surveys. Nineteen responses were removed; eighteen repeat responses and one with implausible demographic responses. A total of 778 responses were coded and taken forward for analysis. The participants completing the survey ranged in age from 19 to 62 (mean 33.3, SD 5.7). Most of the respondents (94.8%) were living in the UK, 2.9% were in North America and a small proportion were living in other European countries or the continents of Asia, Australia and Oceania or South America (2.1%). Further analysis was limited to the 688 participants who were living in the UK, of childbearing age (16–44) and who had given birth to at least one child. Characteristics of the participants are presented in Table 1.

Most of the participants (95.5%) identified their ethnicity as White, 2.3% as Mixed ethnicity, 1.0% as Black, 1.2% as Asian. The wide geographical distribution of UK respondents can be seen in Additional file 1. The BMI of the respondents ranged from 16.7 kg/m^2 to 66.6 kg/m^2 (mean 26.8 kg/m^2, SD 6.0), 43.2% had a BMI of less than 25 kg/m^2, 32.1% were categorised as overweight and 24.7% were in the obese category.

The largest occupational group category amongst the participants was higher managerial, administrative and professional occupations (52.3%), although 21.9% of

Table 1 Characteristics of UK respondents compared to UK national values

	UK participants at time of survey (n = 688) n (%)	National values %
Age	(n = 688)	Women giving birth in England
Under 20	2(0.3%)	4.6[a]
20–24	27 (3.9%)	18.2[a]
25–29	140 (20.4%)	28.1[a]
30–34	266 (38.7%)	29.7[a]
35–39	197 (28.6%)	15.5[a]
40+	56 (8.1%)	3.9[a]
Ethnicity	(n = 683)	
White	652 (95.5%)	86.0[b]
Black	7 (1.0%)	3.3[b]
Asian	8 (1.2%)	7.5[b]
Mixed	16 (2.3%)	2.2[b]
BMI	(n = 663)	All women in England
< 25	286 (43.2%)	42.8[c]
Overweight	213 (32.1%)	33.4[c]
Obese	164 (24.7%)	23.8[c]
Occupation	(n = 683)	Female UK residents aged 16–74
Higher managerial, administrative and professional occupations	357 (52.3)	29.0[d]
Intermediate occupations	117 (17.1)	24.0[d]
Routine and manual occupations	59 (8.6)	31.0[d]
Long-term unemployed or never worked	1 (0.1)	6.0[d]
Not classified	149 (21.9)	–
Number of children birthed	(n = 681)	
1	322 (46.8)	
2	259 (37.6)	
3 or more	107 (15.6)	

[a]Age at delivery [53]; [b] [54]; [c] [55]; [d] [56]

participants' occupations fell into the NS-SEC unclassified category. A total of 46.8% of the participants had given birth to one child, 37.6% had given birth to two children and 15.6% three or more children.

Breastfeeding
A total of 677 participants had breastfed (98.4%), with 337 of these women (50.0%) mentioning that they were currently breastfeeding at the time of completing the survey. Only 650 of the participants responded to the question about longest length of time breastfeeding a child, which ranged from 0.05 months to 72 months (mean 17.3, median 15.0 (IQR = 7.7–24.0)); 95.2% reported that they were still breastfeeding at 8 weeks, 84.0% were breastfeeding at 6 months, 64.8% were breastfeeding at 12 months and 58.8% breastfed beyond 12 months.

Antenatal breast expression - awareness and experience
A total of 442 (64.5%) of the respondents had heard of ABE, 56 (8.2%) reported that they had been advised to express breastmilk during pregnancy, and 97 (14.2%) reported that they had undertaken breast expression during pregnancy (See Fig. 1).

Of the 97 participants who had expressed breastmilk during pregnancy, 38 had been advised to (39.2%), 57 (58.8%) had not been advised to and 2 (2.1%) could not remember if they had been advised to. Of the 56 women who reported that they had been advised to express breastmilk during pregnancy, 38 (67.9%) actually expressed, compared to 9.3% of women who had not been advised to express (Fig. 2).

Women who undertook ABE commenced expressing between 0 and 41 weeks of pregnancy, with a median of 36 weeks: 2 (2.2%) reported commencing ABE at 0 weeks of pregnancy, 5 (5.4%) between week 12 and 28, 43 (46.

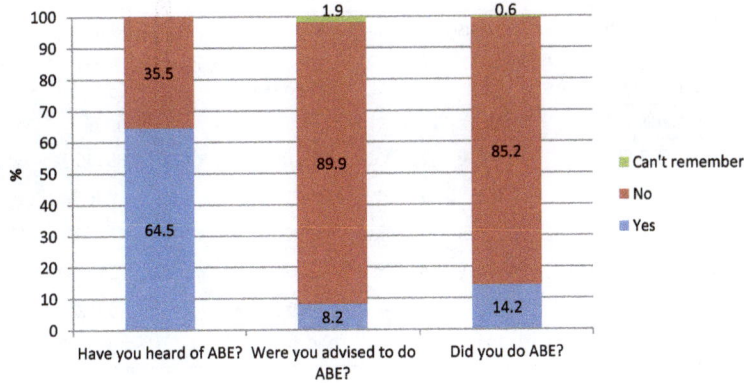

Fig. 1 Whether participants had heard of, were advised to do and if they did Antenatal Breast Expression (n = 688)

7%) between weeks 28 and 37, and 44 (45.7%) from 37 weeks onwards. Women who had practiced ABE reported giving birth at a mean of 39.7 weeks gestation in their last pregnancy, which was similar to the 39.3 weeks mean length of gestation reported by women who did not undertake ABE.

Opinions on antenatal breast expression

A majority of respondents, 398 (58.6%), were not sure if ABE was a good idea, with 233 (34.3%) of the respondents stating that they thought ABE was a good idea and 48 (7.1%) thinking ABE was not a good idea (See Table 2). Previous practice of ABE was statistically significantly associated with opinion of ABE (p < 0.001); the proportion of women who thought ABE was a good idea was highest in those who had undertaken ABE previously (78.4%), although 26.8% of those who had not previously undertaken ABE still thought ABE was a good idea.

A total of 547 (80.9%) of participants stated that they would consider doing ABE if it was found to help prepare for breastfeeding (See Table 2). Previous practice of ABE was significantly associated with whether participants would consider doing ABE in the future (p < 0.001), with only one participant (1.0%) who had previously done ABE reporting she would not consider doing ABE again if it was found to be helpful to prepare for breastfeeding.

Overweight and obese subgroups

In this sample, the proportion of women who had heard of ABE increased with increasing BMI group; 56.7% of women with a BMI of less than 25 kg/m^2 had heard of ABE compared to 63.2% of participants with a BMI within the overweight subgroup 78.7% within the obese subgroup (See Fig. 3). This association showed statistical significance (p < 0.001).

The proportion of women who thought ABE was a good idea also increased with increasing BMI group (See

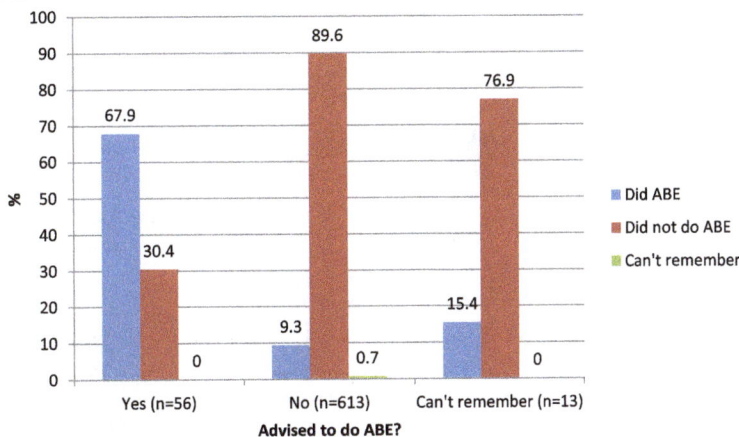

Fig. 2 Whether participants who were advised to do ABE undertook ABE (n = 682)

Table 2 Participants' opinions on ABE

		All participants	Previously undertaken ABE?				BMI			
			Yes	No	Can't remember	P value	Under 25 kg/m^2	Overweight	Obese	P value
		n (%)	n (%)	n (%)	n (%)		n (%)	n (%)	n (%)	
Is ABE a good idea?	Yes	233 (34.3)	76 (78.4)	153 (26.8)	1 (25.0)	†p < 0.001	85 (30.2)	67 (31.8)	76 (46.6)	0.007
	No	48 (7.1)	1 (1.0)	47 (8.2)	0 (0.0)		19 (6.8)	15 (7.1)	11 (6.8)	
	Not sure	398 (58.6)	20 (20.6)	372 (65.0)	3 (75.0)		177 (63.0)	129 (61.1)	76 (46.6)	
Would you consider doing ABE if it was found to help prepare for breastfeeding?	Yes	547 (80.9)	94 (96.9)	445 (78.1)	4 (100)	†p < 0.001	220 (79.4)	175 (82.6)	134 (82.2)	0.280
	No	43 (6.4)	1 (1.0)	42 (7.4)	0 (0.0)		15 (5.4)	13 (6.1)	14 (8.6)	
	Not sure	86 (12.7)	2 (2.1)	83 (14.5)	0 (0.0)		42 (15.2)	24 (11.3)	15 (9.2)	

†Fisher Exact used as expected count < 5 in over 20% of cells

Fig. 3); 46.6% of obese participants thought it was a good idea, compared with 31.8% of those who were overweight and 30.2% of those with a BMI of less than 25 kg/m^2, and this association was statistically significant (p = 0.007). However, there was no significant association between BMI group and whether participants would consider doing ABE in the future (p = 0.280).

Qualitative data - Women's opinions on antenatal breast expression

Several themes emerged from the qualitative data (See Table 3). Amongst participants who felt ABE was a good idea these were; beneficial when mother or baby have medical problems, and preparation for breastfeeding. The themes that emerged amongst participants who thought that ABE was not a good idea were; interfering with nature and harmful. For those who were unsure if ABE was a good idea the main theme was lack of knowledge.

Positive perceptions

Participants who thought that ABE was a good idea felt it would be beneficial where mother or baby have

medical problems including gestational or pre-existing diabetes, previous breast surgery, complications after birth, prematurity, low blood sugars, admission to neonatal unit or difficulties feeding;

"If there are any complications during labour which meant that you were unable to feed initially (I.e. PPH [postpartum haemorrhage], or surgery was required taking you away from baby) baby could be spoon or cup feed colostrum. Equally if baby is struggling with blood sugars, jaundice, weight loss."

"I have type 1 diabetes, antenatal expression enabled me to collect colostrum and give it to my babies at birth preventing them from having low blood sugar."

They also referred to ABE as positive preparation for successful breastfeeding, including the opportunity to become more confident with the expressing technique that they could use again after the birth, establishing a supply of colostrum, encouraging the milk supply and avoiding the use of formula milk;

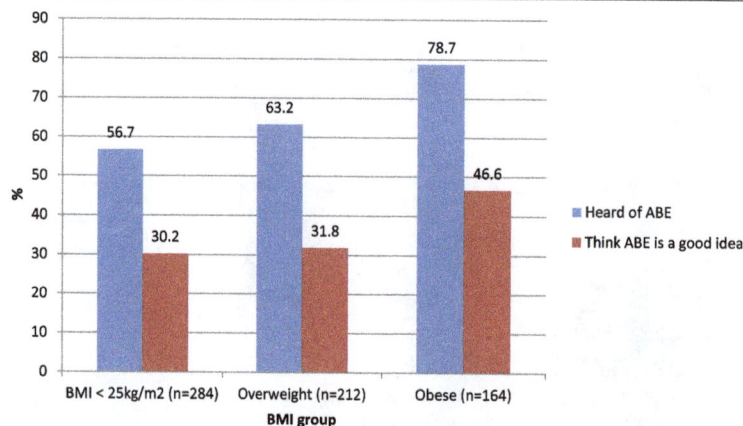

Fig. 3 BMI group and whether participants had heard of ABE and opinion on ABE

Table 3 Themes from the qualitative data

Participant opinion on ABE	Themes from qualitative data	
	Second order themes	First order themes
It's a good idea	Beneficial when mother or baby have medical problems	Helpful if mother: has gestational diabetes has pre-existing diabetes had breast surgery has low supply is unwell has complications after birth
		Beneficial if baby: has low blood sugar has to go to neonatal unit is premature has jaundice has weight loss has difficulty feeding has tongue-tie
	Preparation for successful breastfeeding	Gaining confidence with expressing technique Establishing a supply of milk Hormone stimulation Encourage milk production and supply Avoid the use of formula milk
		To promote labour
It's not a good idea	Interfering with nature	Nature gets it right Milk extraction should be after birth Using up the colostrum No need to interfere
	Harmful	May induce early labour or miscarriage Painful Stressful Bullying women to do it
I'm not sure if it's a good idea	Lack of knowledge	Never heard of it Don't know of risks/benefits

"A good idea to have some milk stored to avoid formula top ups if struggling to feed."

"I would have found it helpful...to have already got used to hand expressing as this was something I needed to do a lot once baby was born."

A few women also reported that ABE could be beneficial in promoting the onset of spontaneous labour;

"...It is used to induce labour naturally."

Negative perceptions

Participants who felt that ABE was a bad idea raised concerns that it would be harmful; causing preterm labour, painful to undertake, stressful, and result from bullying women to do it. They were also concerned that it was interfering with the natural process of initiating breastfeeding;

"I worried it would cause early labour."

"Nature gets this right, no need to interfere."

"Worried of making that [colostrum] go and turn straight into milk when baby arrives."

Uncertain perceptions

The predominant theme amongst the participants who were unsure if ABE was a good idea was their lack of knowledge; either that they had not heard of it or did not have enough information about the benefits or risks involved;

"Have never heard of it or its benefits /negatives."

"I didn't know it could be done."

"I...was never given any information."

The participants identified a number of factors that would encourage them to express breastmilk in pregnancy (See Table 4).

Table 4 rFactors that would encourage participants to express breastmilk in pregnancy

Having evidence-based information about ABE

If ABE was found to increase the likelihood of successful breastfeeding and avoiding the use of formula milk

If there were benefits to the baby

Any medical problems prior to the birth, such as diabetes

Knowing that the baby would have medical problems after birth

Reassurance of the safety of doing ABE

The support of midwives in the antenatal period

The provision of equipment to undertake ABE

Discussion

This cross-sectional study has provided insight into women's knowledge and practices surrounding ABE and the acceptability of ABE to mothers. These findings are important as implementation evidence, as this practice is already advised by midwives in many hospitals [30–43], and promoted in some lactation support literature [29, 45].

This survey demonstrated relatively high awareness, with more than half of the participants having heard of ABE. It also found relatively high compliance amongst women who had been advised to do ABE, with 67.9% of women reporting they had followed this advice. Soltani and Scott [49] found lower compliance, with less than half of women who had been advised to express actually undertaking ABE. It is not clear why 32.1% of participants who had been advised to do ABE did not follow this advice and this warrants further investigation into the decision making process for undertaking ABE. Furthermore 20.6% of those who had undertaken ABE were unsure if ABE was a good idea, and further investigation into women's sources of knowledge about ABE is needed.

Although a majority of participants (57.8%) were unsure if ABE was a good idea, ABE was found to be largely acceptable to the women. A high proportion would consider doing ABE if it was found to beneficial (79.5%), including 96.9% of women who had previously done ABE and 78.1% of those who had not previously undertaken ABE. This reflects wider evidence which demonstrated that 95% of participants who had undertaken ABE would do it again if it was found to be safe and effective [46].

Participants identified ABE as a form of preparation for breastfeeding and helpful in avoiding the use of formula milk. This reflects other findings that women who undertake ABE report increased confidence and readiness for breastfeeding, the benefit of learning the technique to use postnatally, and a reduced need for artificial milk supplementation [46].

Concerns raised by participants about the potential of ABE to cause harm included the pain of the procedure and the risk of causing preterm labour. Forster et al. [46]

reported 19.2% of women undertaking ABE experienced nipple pain and 26% experienced Braxton Hicks or contractions, although none attributed ABE to the onset of spontaneous labour. This survey did not enable us to determine if ABE had any impact on timing of the onset of labour. While a large multi-centred randomised controlled trial of women with diabetes in pregnancy who were at low risk of complications suggested no impact on gestational age at delivery from the practice of ABE [48], other smaller studies with less stringent eligibility criteria have suggested both a trend towards lower gestational age at delivery and an increased rate of special care baby admissions for babies whose mothers had undertaken ABE [46, 49]. Further evidence about the safety of ABE is therefore needed, particularly in pregnant women without diabetes. It is notable that a large proportion (54.3%) of women in this survey who undertook ABE commenced ABE prior to 37 weeks of pregnancy, and it is important to inform women if they decide to undertake ABE that commencing after 37 weeks of pregnancy will reduce the likelihood of preterm birth [49].

Women of childbearing age in this survey who were in the overweight or obese subgroups were more likely to have heard of ABE and were more likely to think that ABE was a good idea, and were no less likely, than women of normal weight, to undertaken it if it was found to be helpful for breastfeeding. This is significant as women in the overweight or obese subgroups typically have higher rates of medical problems such as diabetes [6, 23] and lower rates of successful breastfeeding outcomes [6–13]. If the safety and efficacy of ABE is established, they could therefore be considered to be an important target group for this intervention.

Strengths and limitations

This survey included a large sample of women from a wide spread of UK locations. Comparing UK participants' characteristics with national population data from England, demonstrated that this sample were more predominantly of a white ethnic group and there were a considerably lower proportion of Asian respondents. The sample was also older and of higher socioeconomic status, as indicated by occupation, than the current childbearing population, and hence some of their views and experiences may not be representative. The BMI distribution of the UK participants was very similar to that in the national population.

Undertaking this survey using online technology facilitated wide access and a high response rate that covered wide geographical areas with minimum resources. A maternity user group representative leading survey recruitment may have been an advantage to encourage such a large response rate. However, as a retrospective, self-reported questionnaire, it may have been subject to selective recall bias. The sample demonstrated a much higher breastfeeding rate than that of the national childbearing population in England; 98.4% of the participants reported they had breastfed, compared with the national breastfeeding rate of 74.3% at birth [52]. The participants had also breastfed for longer with 95.2% breastfeeding at 8 weeks compared to the national figure for England of 43.8% [52], and 84.0% reported breastfeeding at 6 months, compared to 34% of the national childbearing population [5]. This was therefore a self-selected sample of women who were highly motivated and successful breastfeeding mothers, and may not represent the opinions of the wider population. Nevertheless, even assuming a higher rate of motivation, a large proportion had concerns for implementing ABE and in depth analysis of their views are worthy of further investigation and consideration.

Conclusion

Amongst women who have breastfed, many have heard of ABE, and compliance with advice to undertake ABE is relatively high. ABE appears to be acceptable to many women, including those in overweight or obese subgroups. However, the benefit and safety of ABE needs to be established to address the needs of childbearing women for evidence-based information about this practice. If ABE is demonstrated to be beneficial in the promotion of breastfeeding, overweight and obese pregnant women could be an important target group for this intervention.

Abbreviations

ABE: Antenatal breast expression; BMI: Body mass index; IQR: Interquartile range; NS-SEC: National Statistics Socio-economic Classification; PPH: Postpartum haemorrhage; SD: Standard deviation; UK: United Kingdom

Acknowledgements

First of all, we would like to thank all the women who completed the online survey. We thank South Yorkshire Collaboration for Leadership in Applied Health Research and Care (CLAHRC-SY) for funding Helen Watson's involvement in the project, and Jo Cooke for facilitating this involvement. NIHR CLAHRC for South Yorkshire acknowledges funding from the Health Education England (HEE). The views and opinions expressed are those of the authors, and not necessarily those of the NHS, HEE, or the Department of Health. Further details can be found at http://clahrc-sy.nihr.ac.uk/. We would also like to thank Karen Kilner for her advice on the statistical analysis undertaken in this work.

Funding

No external funding was allocated to this project.

Authors' contributions

FF - study conception and survey design, cleaned and analysed the data, revised the manuscript, approved the final manuscript. HW - cleaned and analysed the data, prepared the initial manuscript draft, approved the final manuscript. RG - study conception and survey design, maternity user group liaison, lead survey distribution and promotion, approved the final manuscript. HS - study conception and survey design, revised the manuscript, approved the final manuscript.

Competing interests

The authors declare that they have no competing interests.

Author details

[1]Faculty of Health and Wellbeing, Sheffield Hallam University, Collegiate Crescent, Sheffield, UK. [2]Sheffield Maternity Services Liaison Committee and Sheffield user group charity – Forging Families, Sheffield, UK.

References

1. WHO. The optimal duration of exclusive breastfeeding. Report of the expert consultation. Geneva: WHO; 2001. http://apps.who.int/iris/bitstream/10665/67219/1/WHO_NHD_01.09.pdf?ua=1. Accessed 10 Sept 2016
2. Eidelman AI, Schanler RJ, Johnston M, et al. Breastfeeding and the use of human milk. American Academy of Pediatrics policy statement. Pediatrics. 2012;129:e827–41.
3. Salone LR, Vann WF Jr, Dee DL. Breastfeeding. An overview of oral and general health benefits. J Am Dent Assoc. 2013;144(2):143–51. https://doi.org/10.14219/jada.archive.2013.0093.
4. Lessen R, Kavanagh K. Position of the academy of nutrition and dietetics: promoting and supporting breastfeeding. J Acad Nutr Diet. 2015; https://doi.org/10.1016/j.jand.2014.12.014.
5. McAndrew F, et al. (2012) infant feeding survey 2010. Leeds: Health and Social Care Information Centre; 2012. http://content.digital.nhs.uk/catalogue/PUB08694/Infant-Feeding-Survey-2010-Consolidated-Report.pdf. Accessed 1 Oct 2016
6. Amir LH, Donath S. A systematic review of maternal obesity and breastfeeding intention, initiation and duration. BMC Pregnancy Childbirth. 2007; https://doi.org/10.1186/1471-2393-7-9.
7. Mok E, Multon C, Piguel L, Barroso E, Goua V, Christin P, et al. Decreased full breastfeeding, altered practices, perceptions, and infant weight change of prepregnant obese women: a need for extra support. Pediatrics. 2008; https://doi.org/10.1542/peds.2007-2747.
8. Krause KM, Lovelady CA, Østbye T. Predictors of breastfeeding in overweight and obese women: data from active mothers postpartum (AMP). Mater Child Health J. 2011; https://doi.org/10.1007/s10995-010-0667-7.
9. Lepe M, Bacardí Gascón M, Castañeda-González LM, Pérez Morales ME, Jiménez CA. Effect of maternal obesity on lactation: systematic review. Nutr Hosp. 2011; https://doi.org/10.1590/S0212-16112011000600012.
10. Wojcicki JM. Maternal prepregnancy body mass index and initiation and duration of breastfeeding: a review of the literature. J Women's Health. 2011; https://doi.org/10.1089/jwh.2010.2248.
11. Thompson LA, Zhang S, Black E, Das R, Ryngaert M, Sullivan S, et al. The association of maternal pre-pregnancy body mass index with breastfeeding initiation. Mater Child Health J. 2013; https://doi.org/10.1007/s10995-012-1204-7.
12. Hauff LE, Leonard SA, Rasmussen KM. Associations of maternal obesity and psychosocial factors with breastfeeding intention, initiation, and duration. Am J Clin Nutr. 2014; https://doi.org/10.3945/ajcn.113.071191.
13. Babendure JB, Reifsnider E, Mendias E, Moramarco MW, Davila YR. Reduced breastfeeding rates among obese mothers: a review of contributing factors, clinical considerations and future directions. Int Breastfeed J. 2015; https://doi.org/10.1186/s13006-015-0046-5

14. Turcksin R, et al. Maternal obesity and breastfeeding intention, initiation, intensity and duration: a systematic review. Mater Child Nutr. 2014; https://doi.org/10.1111/j.1740-8709.2012.00439.

15. Stevens G, et al. National, regional, and global trends in adult overweight and obesity prevalences. Popul Health Metrics. 2012; https://doi.org/10.1186/1478-7954-10-22.

16. Ng M, et al. Global, regional, and national prevalence of overweight and obesity in children and adults during 1980–2013: a systematic analysis for the global burden of disease study 2013. Lancet. 2014; https://doi.org/10.1016/S0140-6736(14)60460-8.

17. Guelinckx I, Devlieger R, Bogaerts A, Pauwels S, Vansant G. The effect of pre-pregnancy BMI on intention, initiation and duration of breast-feeding. Public Health Nutr. 2012; https://doi.org/10.1017/S1368980011002667.

18. Leonard SA, Labiner-Wolfe J, Geraghty SR, Rasmussen KM. Associations between high prepregnancy body mass index,breast-milk expression, and breast-milk production and feeding. Am J Clin Nutr. 2011; https://doi.org/10.3945/ajcn.110.002352.

19. Chapman DJ, Perez-Escamilla R. Maternal perception of the onset of lactation is a valid, public health indicator of lactogenesis stage II. J Nutr. 2000;130:2972–80.

20. Neville MC, Morton J. Physiology and endocrine changes underlying human lactogenesis II. J Nutr. 2001;131:3005S–8S.

21. Hartmann P, Cregan M. Lactogenesis and the effects of insulin-dependent diabetes mellitus and prematurity. J Nutr. 2001;131:3016S–20S.

22. Hilson JA, Rasmussen KM, Kjolhede CL. High prepregnant body mass index is associated with poor lactation outcomes among white, rural women independent of psychosocial and demographic correlates. J Hum Lact. 2004; https://doi.org/10.1177/0890334403261345.

23. Marchi J, Berg M, Dencker A, Olander EK, Begley C. Risks associated with obesity in pregnancy, for the mother and baby: a systematic review of reviews. Obes Rev. 2015;16:621–38.

24. Rasmussen KM, Kjolhede CL. Prepregnant overweight and obesity diminish the prolactin response to suckling in the first week postpartum. Pediatrics. 2004;113:e465–71.

25. Singh G, Chouban R, Sidhu K. Effect of antenatal expression of breastmilk at term in reducing breastfeeding failures. Med J Armed Forces of India. 2009; https://doi.org/10.1016/S0377-1237(09)80125-1.

26. West D, Marasco L. Getting your milk supply off to a good start. The breastfeeding mother's guide to making more milk. New York: McGraw-Hill; 2009.

27. East CE, Dolan WJ, Forster DA. Antenatal breast milk expression by women with diabetes for improving infant outcomes. Cochrane Database Syst Rev. 2014;7:CD010408.

28. Cox SG. Expressing and storing colostrum antenatally for use in the newborn period. Breastfeed Rev. 2006;143:11–6.

29. Britain LLLG. Antenatal expression of colostrum. Information sheet no. 2811. Nottingham, Great Britain: LaLeche League Great Britain; 2010.

30. Blackpool Teaching Hospitals NHS Foundation Trust. Antenatal Banking of Colostrum. 2012. http://www.bfwh.nhs.uk/wp-content/uploads/2015/08/PL716.pdf. Accessed 31 May 2017.

31. Buckinghamshire Healthcare NHS Trust. Antenatal hand expression. 2016. http://www.buckshealthcare.nhs.uk/Downloads/Patient-leaflets-pregnancy-labour-and-postnatal-care/Antenatal%20hand%20expression.pdf. Accessed 31 May 2017.

32. Dartford and Gravesham NHS Trust. Expressing your breastmilk in pregnancy. 2014. http://www.google.co.uk/url?sa=t&rct=j&q=&esrc=s&source=web&cd=10&cad=rja&uact=8&ved=0ahUKEwjxrLnep5rUAhWpJsAKHWV_BdcQFghiMAk&url=http%3A%2F%2Fwww.dvh.nhs.uk%2FEasySiteWeb%2FGatewayLink.aspx%3FalId%3D165903&usg=AFQjCNFc0ofNv5-rbnURq2RJmYxgQ_eL9g. Accessed 31 May 2017.

33. Derby Teaching Hospital NHS Foundation Trust. Antenatal hand expression of colostrum, draft guideline. Derby: Derby Hosital; 2007.

34. Guys and St Thomas' NHS Foundation Trust. Information about antenatal hand expressing from 37 weeks. 2016. http://www.guysandstthomas.nhs.uk/resources/patient-information/maternity/antenatal-hand-expressing-from-37-weeks.pdf. Accessed 31 May 2017.

35. Kettering General Hospital NHS Foundation Trust. Women and Child Health. Antenatal Hand Expressing. Patient information. 2015. Leaflet http://webcache.googleusercontent.com/search?q=cache:twalAGhsJK0J:www.kgh.nhs.uk/EasysiteWeb/getresource.axd%3FAssetID%3D12848%26type%3Dfull%26servicetype%3DAttachment+&cd=1&hl=en&ct=clnk&gl=uk. Accessed 31 May 2017.

36. Lancashire Teaching Hospitals. NHS Foundation Trust. Expressing your Milk Antenatally. 2015. https://www.lancsteachinghospitals.nhs.uk/download.cfm?doc=docm93jijm4n3852. Accessed 31 May 2017.

37. Royal Berkshire NHS Foundation Trust. Expressing colostrum in pregnancy 2016. http://www.royalberkshire.nhs.uk/patient-information-leaflets/maternity—expressing-colostrum.htm. Accessed 31 May 2017.

38. Royal Cornwall Hospitals. Antental hand expressing of breastmilk for type 1, type 2 or gestational diabetes. Clinical Guideline. 2016. http://www.rcht.nhs.uk/DocumentsLibrary/RoyalCornwallHospitalsTrust/Clinical/MidwiferyAndObstetrics/BreastmilkGuidelinesForAntenatalHandExpressingOf.pdf Accessed 31 May 2017.

39. Royal Surrey County Hospital NHS Foundation Trust. Expressing your breastmilk in pregnancy. 2014. http://www.royalsurrey.nhs.uk/wp-content/uploads/2015/09/PIN072_Expressing_your_breast_milk_in_pregnancy_w.pdf. Accessed 31 May 2017.

40. Sandwell and West Birmingham NHS Trust. Expressing your milk antenatally. 2014. http://www.swbh.nhs.uk/wp-content/uploads/2012/06/Expressing-your-milk-antenatally-ML4692.pdf. Accessed 31 May 2017.

41. South Devon Healthcare NHS Foundation Trust. Breatsfeeding information for women. 2015. http://www.torbayandsouthdevon.nhs.uk/uploads/25120.pdf Accessed 31 May 2017.

42. Southend University Hospital NHS Foundation Trust. Antenatal expressing and storage of your colostrum. 2015. http://www.southend.nhs.uk/media/180174/antenatal_expressing_and_storage_of_your_colostrum_sou4353_037980_0715_v1_web.pdf. Accessed 31 May 2017.

43. Wrightington, Wigan and Leigh NHS Foundation Trust. Colostrum harvesting/expressing your milk in the antenatal period. 2017. https://www.wwl.nhs.uk/Library/All_New_PI_Docs/Audio_Leaflets/Obstetrics/colostrum/obs050_colostrum_harvesting619v3.pdf. Accessed 31 May 2017.

44. Pathak S. Practice of antenatal breast expression in National Health Service in England. Int J Health Res Medico Legal Pract. 2017;3:12–4.

45. Association of Breastfeeding Mothers. Expressing your milk before your baby arrives: antenatal expression of colostrum. 2017. https://abm.me.uk/expressing-milk-baby-arrives-antenatal-expression-colostrum/. Accessed 31 May 2017.

46. Forster DA, McEgan K, Ford R, Moorhead A, Opie G, Walker S, et al. Diabetes and antenatal milk expressing: a pilot project to inform the development of a randomised controlled trial. Midwifery. 2011;27:209–14.

47. Chapman T, Pincombe J, Harris N. Antenatal breast expression: a critical review of the literature. Midwifery. 2013; https://doi.org/10.1016/j.midw.2011.12.013.

48. Forster DA, Moorhead AM, Jacobs SE, et al. Advising women with diabetes in pregnancy to express breastmilk in late pregnancy (diabetes and antenatal milk expressing [DAME]): a multicentre, unblinded, randomised controlled trial. Lancet. 2017;389:2204–13.

49. Soltani H, Scott AMS. Antenatal breast expression in women with diabetes: outcomes from a retrospective cohort study. Int Breastfeed J. 2012; https://doi.org/10.1186/1746-4358-7-18.

50. WHO. BMI Classification. 2016. http://apps.who.int/bmi/index.jsp?introPage=intro_3.html. Accessed 8 July 2016.

51. ONS. Volume 3 The National Statistics Socio-economic Classification: (Rebased on the SOC2010) User Manual. 2010. http://webarchive.nationalarchives.gov.uk/20160105160709/http://www.ons.gov.uk/ons/guide-method/classifications/current-standard-classifications/soc2010/soc2010-volume-3-ns-sec%2D-rebased-on-soc2010%2D-user-manual/index.html. Accessed 8 July 2016.

52. NHS England. NHS England statistical release breastfeeding initiation and breastfeeding prevalence 6–8 weeks. 2015. https://www.england.nhs.uk/statistics/wp-content/uploads/sites/2/2014/03/Breastfeeding-1516Q11.pdf. Accessed 29 Sept 2016.

53. HSCIC. Hospital Episode Statistics. NHS Maternity Statistics - England, 2012-13. 2015. https://digital.nhs.uk/catalogue/PUB12744. Accessed 1 Oct 2016.

54. HSCIC. NHS Maternity Statistics England 2013–14 2015 http://digital.nhs.uk/catalogue/PUB16725. Accessed 3 Oct 2016.

55. HSCIC. Statistics on obesity, physical activity and diet England. 2015. http://content.digital.nhs.uk/catalogue/pub16988/obes-phys-acti-diet-eng-2015.pdf. Accessed 3 Oct 2016.

56. ONS. 2011 Census: Key Statistics and Quick Statistics for Local Authorities in the United Kingdom. 2011. http://www.ons.gov.uk/employmentandlabourmarket/peopleinwork/employmentandemployeetypes/bulletins/keystatisticsandquickstatisticsforlocalauthoritiesintheunitedkingdom/2013-12-04#national-statistics-socio-economic-classification-ns-sec. Accessed 23 Nov 2016.

13

'Just because she's young, it doesn't mean she has to die': exploring the contributing factors to high maternal mortality in adolescents

Lucy November[*] [iD] and Jane Sandall

Abstract

Background: In Sierra Leone, 34% of pregnancies and 40% of maternal deaths are in the adolescent population. Risks are known to be higher for younger adolescents, this being borne out by a household survey in Eastern Freetown in 2015. This current qualitative study, funded by Wellbeing of Women's international midwifery fellowship, was conducted to explore the causes of this high incidence of maternal death for younger teenagers, and to identify possible interventions to improve outcomes.

Methods: This qualitative study used semi-structured interviews ($n = 19$) and focus groups ($n = 6$), with a wide range of professional and lay participants, recorded with consent. Recordings were transcribed by the first author and a Krio-speaking colleague where necessary, and Nvivo software was used to assist with theming of the data around the three main research questions.

Results: Themes from discussions on vulnerability to teenage pregnancy focused on transactional sex, especially for girls living outside of their birth family. They included sex for school fees, sex with teachers for grades, sex for food and clothes, and sex to lessen the impact of the time-consuming duties of water collection and petty trading. In addition, the criminal justice system and the availability and accessibility of contraception and abortion were included within this major theme. Within the major theme of vulnerability to death once pregnant, abandonment, delayed care seeking, and being cared for by a non-parental adult were identified. Several obstetric risks were discussed by midwives, but were explicitly related to the socio-economic factors already mentioned. A cross-cutting theme throughout the data was of gendered social norms for sexual behaviour, for both boys and girls, being reinforced by significant adults such as parents and teachers.

Conclusion: Findings challenge the notion that adolescent girls have the necessary agency to make straightforward choices about their sexual behaviour and contraceptive use. For girls who do become pregnant, risks are believed to be related more to stigma and abandonment than to physical maturity, leading to lack of family-based support and delayed care-seeking for antenatal and delivery care. Two potential interventions identified within the research are a mentoring scheme for the most vulnerable pregnant girls and a locally managed blood donation register. A feasibility study of a pilot mentoring scheme is currently underway, run by the first author and a local partner.

Keywords: Sierra Leone, Adolescent, Pregnancy, Transactional sex, Abandonment, Delayed care-seeking, Maternal death, Mentoring, Blood donation

* Correspondence: lucy.november@kcl.ac.uk
Division of Women and Children's Health, Faculty of Life Sciences and Medicine, Kings College London, St Thomas' Campus, Westminster Bridge Road, London SE1 7EH, UK

Plain English summary

In Eastern Freetown, Sierra Leone, young pregnant teenagers have a much higher risk of death than older women. This study was carried out to find out why, and what interventions might improve outcomes for this vulnerable group. The first author conducted focus groups and interviews with a wide range of professionals and lay participants, and analysed the responses and ideas generated into themes, based on the three main research questions.

Themes from discussions on 'vulnerability to teenage pregnancy' focussed on transactional sex; for school fees, sex with teachers for grades, and sex for food and clothes, as well as issues about the criminal justice system and the availability and accessibility of contraception and abortion. Under the heading 'vulnerability to death once pregnant', abandonment, delayed care-seeking, and being cared for by a non-parental adult were identified. Several risks relating to childbirth were discussed by midwives, but they were clear that these were because of the socio-economic factors already mentioned. A theme picked up throughout was that both girls and boys have behaviours modelled to them by adults such as parents and teachers which perpetuate particular ways of behaving, especially regarding sexual behaviours.

Findings challenge the notion that teenage girls have real choices regarding their sexual behaviour and contraceptive use, and suggest that risks to pregnant girls are because of stigma and abandonment, rather than physical immaturity. Two potential interventions are a mentoring scheme for the most vulnerable pregnant girls and a locally managed blood donation register. A pilot of the mentoring scheme is currently underway.

Background

Sierra Leone has an estimated maternal mortality ratio (MMR) of 1165 maternal deaths per 100,000 live births, the highest in the world [1]. It is also one of only six countries in Sub-Saharan Africa (SSA) where more than 10% of girls become mothers before the age of 16, with increased MMRs for adolescents in general, and particularly high ratios for the under-16 age group when data is disaggregated by age [2]. Overall, 34% of all pregnancies and 40% of all maternal deaths occur amongst teenage girls [1]. In response to this, in 2013, the Government of Sierra Leone (GoSL) drew together a multi-agency and cross-ministry collaboration and developed the National Strategy for the Reduction of Teenage pregnancy (hereafter referred to as 'the national strategy') with six key pillars of action [3].[1]

Sierra Leone experienced 10 years of brutal civil war which finally ended in 2001, by which time the health system was barely functional and under-used due to charges at point of care. However, in 2010, a new policy of free health care for pregnant and lactating women and children under five was introduced [4], and use of health services increased significantly; in the 5 years from 2008 to 2013, the proportion of women giving birth with a skilled birth attendant rose from 42% to 60% [1, 5]. Sadly, the Ebola Virus Disease (EVD) outbreak in 2014/15 was another devastating onslaught for the fragile health system, with 7% of health workers dying from the disease compared with 0.06% of the general population [6].

Progress in addressing the issue of teenage conception was stalled by the EVD outbreak, and during this time a combination of closed schools and increased poverty is thought to have led to a significant increase in the numbers of teenage pregnancies [7]. In the aftermath of the epidemic, the national strategy was revised and updated and was due to be relaunched in 2017, though to date has not been.

The current study came about following a local household survey conducted in 2015 in Kuntorloh, a suburb of the capital city, Freetown, by a community-based organisation (CBO), Lifeline Nehemiah Projects (LNP), due to a perception in the local community that the local MMR was significantly higher than the 1165 per 100,000 presented in the 2013 Sierra Leone demographic health survey (SLDHS). The first author had lived in Freetown and worked with LNP from 2001 to 2004 as a community health educator, and in 2015 partnered with the LNP team in a consultancy role to carry out this local survey with a team of volunteers. Data were collected on 1400 pregnancies and analysed by the first author. The overall MMR was indeed elevated, at three times the national figure. However, the data for teenagers was even more concerning, with 1 in 7 of the pregnant teenagers under 17 dying from a maternal cause (the first author's unpublished data). Despite sample-size limitations, this merited further exploration. The first author was funded by Wellbeing of Women's international midwifery fellowship to carry out this qualitative study with the aim of better understanding the factors which put younger women at greater risk of maternal death, in order to work with local people to develop and evaluate interventions to reduce these risks.

Methods
Study design

This is a qualitative study using focus groups and semi-structured interviews carried out during two field trips to Freetown in 2016/17. Groupings for focus group discussions were selected to gain the maximum insight from participants' varied perspectives, whilst working within the field trips' limited time frames. The six focus groups comprised: two groups of ten adolescent mothers, a group of nine young men (aged 19 to 29), ten midwives working in the main referral hospital, eleven health workers including midwives from two peripheral health units (PHUs), and a discussion with two secondary school teachers. Semi-structured interviews were conducted with three senior midwives (research, education and clinical), a staff-grade midwife from a PHU, two consultant advisors from UNICEF and UNFPA, three GoSL senior advisors (two from the Ministry of Health and one from the Ministry of Social Welfare), a country director and project lead for two different international non-governmental organisations (NGOs), a director of a CBO, three local women's leaders, a senior community leader, and a teenage mother who could not attend the focus groups but was keen to talk about her experience.

Recruitment and procedures

The primary inclusion criterion for the study was personal, family, or professional experience of teenage pregnancy, with purposive sampling as the first strategy. One group of young mothers was recruited within a local vocational skills training institution (not LNP); the second group of ten young mothers was recruited by invitation from a community worker; and the nine young men were recruited from the volunteers who had previously taken part in the household survey in 2015 and were known to the first author. No young mothers who were invited declined to be involved; it could be argued that this indicated coercion, however every effort was made to assure participants that participation was voluntary. This is discussed more fully within the ethical considerations.

Midwives were invited by two key informants; one within the referral hospital and one working in a local PHU. Other community participants were recruited via snowball sampling, where an existing participant suggested a new participant based on their knowledge of the circumstances or interests of the prospective participant. In the same way, some professional participants with a clear remit within the teenage pregnancy arena were contacted prior to the research visits via email request, and others were contacted and recruited by email or telephone during the research visit, having been suggested by other participating professionals. Teachers, CBO and NGO participants were recruited through personal contacts. All interviews and focus groups were conducted by the first author and her Sierra Leonean research assistant, a female LNP staff member with a master's qualification in gender studies, in either English or Krio, the commonly spoken local language with which the first author is very familiar but not fluent. Focus groups were conducted in various community settings at times when discussions could not be overheard, and no other non-participant observers were present. Interviews were conducted at settings chosen by the participant, and some interviews included the participant's junior colleagues. Most of the focus groups and interviews were between 40 and 70 min duration.

Ethical considerations

Participants were sent or given participant information sheets in the days prior to the interview or focus group where possible. Where this was not possible, the information sheet was given or read to the participant in English or in Krio prior to the interview or focus group, with opportunity to ask questions prior to giving or withholding consent. It was stressed that participating in the study was voluntary, and would not advantage or disadvantage the participant in any way. This was particularly important for the adolescent mothers and young men in the study, as they were also potential beneficiaries of various community-based provision such as LNP's vocational training, and knew of the first author's association with LNP. Where applicable, it was clearly explained that their participation was confidential and would not be disclosed to LNP staff. The information sheets included issues of anonymity, data security and that they could withdraw themselves and their data from the study within specified time frames.

Research questions

This qualitative study set out to answer three key questions about the high rate of maternal mortality amongst adolescent girls in Freetown:

- What are the factors which increase vulnerability to teenage pregnancy?
- What are the vulnerabilities which increase the risk of death from pregnancy-related causes in adolescents?
- What could be done to mitigate the risks associated with teenage pregnancy in this part of Freetown?

Data analysis

Most interviews and focus groups were recorded. Three of the government or UN agency interview participants declined to be recorded; notes were taken during these interviews which were used as personal observations. Recorded data was listened to and transcribed primarily by the first author and a Krio-speaking transcriber where applicable, who also clarified any Krio words or phrases not familiar to the first author. The data was then transferred to Nvivo which was used to assist with coding of the data into major themes categorised around the research questions. Though this study was underpinned by grounded theory, using an inductive approach to explore themes being identified from the data in an iterative manner, the time and opportunity constraints of limited field trips meant that not all the themes were entirely saturated. For example, when the subtheme 'sex for grades' was identified from a focus group with teachers, a true grounded theory approach would have led to participants in policy roles being re-interviewed to seek their views on issues such as prosecutions of teachers; unfortunately, this was not possible. In contrast, for other subthemes such as issues around blood donation, because it was identified on the first day of data collection, it was possible to hear from all subsequent participants and therefore reach the point where no new information or opinions were being expressed. Because this study used a strong partnership approach with LNP, and feedback was sought on the author's interpretation of the data, the validity of the findings is strengthened.

Results

The data from this study falls under the three major themes in line with the three key questions.

Sub-themes emerged under each major theme, and the following table summarises these. For each subtheme, the main data sources are outlined. Participant codes are given for quotations. It was not possible during transcription to identify individuals within focus groups, hence group coding rather than individual coding is given. The exception was the teachers' focus group which only had two participants (T1 and T2). FG denotes source as a focus group; I denotes source as an interview.

Major theme related to research question	Subthemes within major theme	Key informants on this subtheme
Vulnerability to teenage pregnancy	Transactional sex • 'not their own child' • 'water for water' • 'sex for school fees /grades' • the criminal justice system Contraception and abortion	• young men's focus group (YMFG) • women's leaders (WL) • teachers' focus group (T1 and T2) • Government of Sierra Leone participants (GI) • Senior NGO workers (NGO)
Vulnerability to maternal death once pregnant	Abuse and abandonment • 'just because she's young it doesn't mean she has to die' Increased birth complications • Delayed care seeking Risk of death from anaemia and PPH	• young mothers' focus groups (MFG) • hospital midwives' focus group (HMFG) • community clinic health workers focus group (HWFG) • senior midwives (SM) • senior community leader (SCL)
Possible interventions to reduce maternal death in adolescents	Mentoring Community-based blood donation • compensation • blood donation experience	• women's leaders • young men's focus group • midwives and other health workers

Vulnerability to teenage pregnancy

By definition, teenagers who do not become pregnant cannot die from maternal causes. For this reason, it is valid to include within the results, analysis and discussion, factors which lead to teenage pregnancy alongside factors which lead to maternal death in pregnant teenagers.

Transactional sex

Despite use of language such as 'being in love', the context for much of the sexual activity discussed in this study appears to define it as transactional; as a way of minimising the burden of the time-consuming duties of petty trading or water collection; for money to pay for school fees and other expenses; and as a condition proposed by school teachers for girls to pass exams or be promoted to the next school year. The lack of adult care and financial provision for girls who were living with extended family instead of their birth family seemed to exacerbate their exposure to all of these risks, although girls living within their own birth families were also under pressure to have transactional sex.

'Not their own child' Many households in Freetown include children and young people who are family relatives or unrelated to the family, as well as children born into the household. Often these additional children are sent from rural Sierra Leone to attend school or as a way of redistributing the economic burden when part of a family falls into poverty, due for example to the death of one parent.

When asked what makes some girls more vulnerable to pregnancy and maternal death, many participants proposed that living in a household other than the one into which you were born is a key vulnerability, citing 'lack of proper care' and 'no-one to guide them'. Many girls in this situation are sent out to sell goods, either for their household, or to earn money to support themselves and pay for schooling if this need is not being met for them, risking exploitation:

The other thing is the trade the girls do from house to house. When they are hawking their trade, some older men will call to them saying 'Come! I want to see or buy what you are selling'. He will call her into the house and say, 'I will buy everything you are selling if you have sex with me.' (WLI3)

And girls are faced with complex decisions with lose-lose outcomes:

Some go to school in the afternoon so in the morning they will have to do their trade before school. At a certain time before noon they will come home and get ready for school … (it can) take the whole day to sell and when a man offers to buy everything she has for sex, that can be tempting. (WLI2)

'Water for water' There are two seasons in Sierra Leone; the rainy season from around April to October, and the dry season from around November to March. Poor communities such as Kuntorloh have no water delivery infrastructure; in the rainy season water is harvested from roofs, but in the dry season water must be collected from community wells, which gradually dry up as the season progresses. Water collection is one of the time-consuming domestic duties which young people, particularly teenage girls, are responsible for; a task which can take five or six hours of queuing at the height of the dry season. Both research visits took place within the dry season, and participants were keen to talk about the risks associated with water collection, explaining that the queue can be bypassed by girls having sex with the youths who run the wells. A local expression 'water for water' was cited by several of the participants:

Teenagers get pregnant a whole lot because of the water crisis – 'if you give me water, I'll give you sex'. 'Water for water'. Especially in February, March, those two months. Oh! Very tedious – water! (WLI1)

Participants clearly viewed this sex as transactional rather than coerced or forced and it was clear that this phenomenon was not an example of the risks cited in the literature about being raped whilst walking to the water points [8].

It's an agreement, as they are in love. It's not a rape. The girls do not want to waste too much time at the stream or well. So, if the boy who controls the well or the water tap is the girl's boyfriend... even if she has twenty or even fifty containers, he will make sure her containers are filled up first. So the girls get home a little bit earlier than normal. (WLI2)

For girls who are trying to attend school and study for exams this is a real dilemma:

Interviewer: what if a girl decides that she is not going to have sex?

(WLI3): you will stand there for the rest of the day you would not be able to get the water.

This participant, an older woman, expresses her frustration at the infrastructure deterioration which has allowed this problem to develop:

The dam has got to be repaired or worked on. In days gone by here in Freetown there used to be taps at every street junction. Then we never used to have this problem of young girls getting pregnant due to water crises. (WLI3)

Clearly, the task of collecting water during the dry season can present girls with difficult choices in terms of sexual behaviour, particularly in terms of freeing up time for study and school attendance.

Sex to pay for school fees and hidden charges, and school-based financial abuse Sierra Leone does not provide free secondary school education; all families expect to pay school fees and many plan accordingly. However, it is the unpredictable, hidden costs which put additional strain on teenagers. Some of these charges are for 'extra classes', where teachers only partially cover the syllabus during regular school hours so that students are forced to pay directly to teachers to supplement normal school. Young people who have to source this money for themselves employ a range of strategies to do so, including girls engaging in transactional sex with older men, or 'sugar daddies':

The man that impregnated me was helping me a lot for my schooling, so I fell in love with him, but I was so small at the age of fourteen. (MFG).

Other more blatant financial abuse occurs when teachers require additional payments in exchange for a student passing an exam or being promoted to the next school year. This study describes a deeply entrenched system of extortion for grades and progression levied by individual teachers, both male and female:

It's just like bidding. The highest bidder has the highest grade. If you give 10 000 Leones, you will have your 10 000 Leones grade. If somebody comes with 20 000 Leones, that person will automatically have a higher grade than you! Let's say for example Salimatu comes to school, and she does not have that money. Automatically she will have to repeat (the school year). No matter how brilliant Salimatu is, she will have to repeat that class simply because she does not have that money to satisfy the teacher. You have to satisfy your teacher both in writing and in the financial aspect. (T1)

School attendance presents teenagers with a raft of financial challenges, even if their basic school fees are being paid. Having to find the extra money needed to access all of the curriculum, to ensure that assignments are graded or even to pay what are essentially bribes to teachers to pass exams and progress through school can put girls under pressure to have transactional sex with older men who can provide for them.

Sex for grades

An even more direct risk associated with schooling is the sexual abuse perpetrated by teachers whereby they arrange to have sex with female students in exchange for academic achievement [8–11]. This is identified as a pervasive issue, but one which young people are reluctant to discuss [8].

In the current study, this was borne out by the issue being discussed exclusively by professional participants rather than by the adolescents themselves. The practice appears to undermine the whole system upon which academic success is based:

Children who are not able to read or write and find it difficult to, you know, understand questions and pass exams … some male teachers exploit that situation by offering, asking them to offer sex for grades. (T2)

This seems to be a ubiquitous issue. The following refers to one of the most highly regarded girls' schools in the country:

The other day my daughter was telling me 'Mama, even when I'm submitting my assignment, my teacher is asking me for money.' If you don't give your child enough money to pay for the assignment, what happens? 'Ah Mr X, I don't get money'. 'OK, meet me at my house' … If the girl doesn't get pregnant, its infection. STI, HIV. That's why HIV is as high as it is. (NGO1)

Whilst some of the sexual activity between older girls and teachers is initiated by the girls themselves, the data also demonstrates a deliberate targeting of very young girls, with evidence of abuse of girls in very early puberty:

Even in primary school, you see these girls have grown breasts, and maybe you are thinking 'I don't want to go to bed with this girl', but your hands … you may want to like… touch her breasts, her buttocks, in that sexual way, after the class. (T1)

The evidence points towards this abuse being entrenched within the education system, with the implication that some teachers go into the profession to have easy sexual access to young girls:

One time when I was at the teacher training college, they asked us to give our names and school of choice for our teaching practice. And some of our colleagues gave their names for a female school for one reason … the reason is to have more girls you see. There are schools who are marked as 'sex schools'. Sex schools! The other day someone was telling me 'ah that school over there. If you go there, you can have women until your tire.' (T1)

The issue appears to go beyond individual teachers with reports of 'sex for grades' being accepted and even encouraged by school leaders. Participants also noted that, at times, boys are paid to investigate girls' backgrounds as potential targets for coerced sex by teachers:

Some of these teachers, they use some of these boys to investigate these girls. Like for example they will say 'Souri, I really want that girl. Go and look at the background of that girl. If they have any person that is strong in the family.' And Souri will now go to the girl, and interview the girl. If he says they are poor, then automatically the teacher will take that as an advantage. (T1)

Various methods are used by teachers to pursue and control girls such as buying the girl a mobile phone, which she is then expected to use to send sexually explicit photos. This study data would indicate that this practice is commonplace, but that the taboo around it is stronger than the 'sex for school fees' issue.

It seems apparent that for teenage girls in Sierra Leone, graduating from secondary school is not a simple matter of completing assignments on time and studying for exams. On the contrary, for some young women, pursuing an education seems to be a minefield of risk and difficult decisions where the benefits of an education have to be weighed against the risks of pregnancy, infection and the trauma of unwanted sex.

The criminal justice system

With pressure from groups such as Legal Access through Women Yearning for Equality Rights and Social Justice (LAWYERS), legislation is in place in Sierra Leone to address underage sex and child abuse, and it is the first pillar of the 2013 teenage pregnancy reduction strategy. Despite this, prosecutions, whether of family members or professionals like teachers, are rare. In the literature [8, 10], and throughout this research, two common scenarios emerge; of families negotiating a financial settlement themselves, and of families reporting the issue to the police but this process being undermined by senior community members pleading that the man be released for his 'good character'.

I think on one or two occasions, I've heard of the teacher being taken to the police. But … all the senior members of the society will come; 'Oh, let this man go, he is a teacher. He's actually doing very well in this community. Please don't let this teacher go down to prison.' (CBO1)

This senior community leader expressed frustration with the deficiencies in the legal system, proposing a zero-tolerance approach:

Even the government are unable to ... interpret and implement the law properly. When someone has done something bad they should be in prison. If someone dies in pregnancy the person responsible should be charged with murder. If this is done to one, two or three persons as a sample, the others will be afraid. But most of those who commit such offense are freed one after the other. (SCLI)

However, the picture is not entirely bleak. The national strategy is clear in laying out the legislative framework around child rights and gender-based violence, providing a common understanding of the way ahead, and some NGOs are building on this platform, providing training for community leaders on identifying and dealing with child abuse. The director of one CBO explained how he feels things are changing:

In the past, there was lots of compromising on sexual abuse cases ... but in the past three months, we have supported the prosecution of up to four or five sexual abuse cases of children between the ages of eleven and thirteen. All of them, when these cases are in court, the perpetrators have been remanded in prison. (CBOI)

There was also evidence that attitudes around abuse by professionals may be starting to change; examples were cited of recent imprisonments of policemen who had been prosecuted for child abuse. However, even though the will to implement legislation may be changing, capacity is a very real barrier; NGO and GoSL participants highlighted the lack of resources as an additional barrier in rural areas:

In certain far remote communities, where you do not have magistrates court sittings ... if a victim is staying in the community which is about 50 or 100 miles to where the court is, without all of this support, transportation, shelter, then she definitely will not come. (GI1)

Despite a legislative framework being in place to deal with sexual abuse, there currently appear to be a number of barriers to fully implementing this legislation, including a lack of political will to take the issue seriously, a lack of logistical infrastructure to facilitate trials and prosecutions, and a lack of support to girls who choose to put their heads above the parapet and challenge the inherent gender norms and power imbalances to which society generally and the education system specifically are subject.

Contraception and abortion

Access to contraception is recognised as a vital component in reducing adolescent pregnancy and maternal death [12–14], and an important part of the national strategy is to make contraceptives more accessible, available and affordable for adolescents. There is work in progress to train health workers in family planning methods, including implants, and to make government clinics adolescent-friendly by allocating trained staff to treat teenagers, with, in some clinics, a separate room to accommodate them. Marie-Stopes and other NGOs are also popular providers. Health workers made a distinction between Freetown and the provinces in regard to contraceptive services, saying that they are well stocked with contraceptives in Freetown, but this is not always the case in the more remote rural areas. Despite availability, health workers identified ongoing stigma as the major reason why girls do not access family planning in Freetown.

Though implants, known in Freetown as 'captain bands' have increased in popularity, with younger girls there is a concern about being 'found out' due to the visibility of the implant, particularly in the few days after insertion. There was also evidence of myths and taboos around contraceptive use:

They listen to the people in the street that says it gives cancer, so they're afraid. (HWFG)

However, as the midwives pointed out, child spacing for adolescents is particularly important to allow them to finish developing. A major concern amongst the midwives was that girls who were too ashamed to use the clinics often turned to unqualified suppliers whom they referred to as 'quacks'. This often also included performing unsafe abortions, which the midwives perceived to be a significant contributor to maternal mortality, although rarely counted as such:

And not only are many of them dying of childbirth, they are dying of abortion. Most of the mothers, because of the embarrassment and everything, take them for abortion. And they die, and they don't talk about it. (MWI)

Several of the young mothers described methods they had used to attempt an abortion:

In the village, when I knew that I was pregnant, I drank a lot of herbs to destroy the pregnancy. (MFG1)

I drank loads of Seven-up with blue clothes dye in it. (MFG1)

And several told of how boyfriends or parents had tried to persuade them to have an abortion, but they had refused or avoided it.

Despite significant advances in the supply and range of contraception available to women in Sierra Leone, there are persistent issues of availability in rural areas, and accessibility for stigmatised groups such as adolescents. The use of unregulated contraception and abortion put these younger women at additional risk.

Vulnerability to maternal death once pregnant

Many women in Sierra Leone have had a child in adolescence. As mentioned, the country has a very high teenage pregnancy rate, and one might reasonably conclude that this would normalise and reduce the stigma associated with teenage pregnancy. This study indicates that this is not the case, with teenage pregnancy being a significant social determinant of poor health outcomes for mother and baby. It carries a stigma which is associated with maltreatment of pregnant teenagers and low uptake of maternal and child health services in this group. Despite health workers and midwives in this study insisting that low maternal age in itself should not be a cause of maternal mortality and morbidity, there are upstream factors at work which strongly influence the likelihood of very young pregnant women surviving pregnancy and thriving as mothers.

Abuse and abandonment

A strong narrative amongst participants was that girls who find themselves pregnant are very likely to be rejected by their families. Most of the young mothers in the study had been afraid to tell their parents, particularly their fathers, fearing physical abuse:

> *So my father came home ... and said if he meets me in the home he is going to shoot me with a gun since he was a policeman. (MFG1)*

> *My elder brother was so annoyed that I was beaten and I was wounded on my back and the sore was there for a long time on my back. (MFG2)*

All girls reported being told to show the man who 'owned the pregnancy', and for those for whom the boyfriend 'denied the pregnancy', some returned home after a cooling off period, often mediated by their mother or another female family member. Where this was not possible, some remained away from home with friends or lived in abandoned buildings, often with no reliable source of support. When the baby's father was prepared to 'own the pregnancy', an arrangement was often made for financial support to the girl's family, or for the girl to live at the man's house. Girls in this situation had very mixed experiences – some were treated well, and others were made to sleep on the floor and given heavy domestic duties and very little to eat.

> *So I went to auntie Ami's parlour, and I slept there on the hard tiles until nine months and was ready to have the baby. They didn't feed me. Auntie Ami fed me once a day and let me sleep in her parlour because I did her washing and her dishes. (MFG2)*

> *They threw her out of the home and she went and stayed with the boy who was an apprentice with a taxi cab driver, so they were sleeping in cars. She was cold, anaemic, not enough blood and was not eating well. She was sharing a plate of rice with her partner. She died. (WL2)*

Other studies have found that this arrangement confers higher risk of emotional and sexual abuse for the girl, and higher risks of physical and mental health problems [8, 15].

Increased birth complications

'Just because she's young, it doesn't mean she has to die' Midwives were clear in their discussions that it is poverty and abandonment which set a girl up for maternal death rather than age per se. A strong theme which all the midwives and other health workers came back to repeatedly was 'just because she's young, it doesn't mean she has to die'. They acknowledged that young girls can be less developed and need specialist midwifery and obstetric care, but were adamant that with the right care, they should be no more destined to death than an older woman.

> *So it doesn't mean she's a teenager, she should die. (No, exactly!) If we know the risk, if she goes through the normal antenatal care, where they screen her, test the blood haemoglobin level, do head to toe assessment, palpation and all, she should receive care just as any woman who is pregnant, if we have proper, functioning systems in place. (HMFG)*

They consistently attributed adolescent maternal death to lack of care; both family care and delayed midwifery care, and were clear that one did not have to look very far upstream to discover the source of medical risks such as anaemia, malaria, pre-eclampsia and infections. Poor diet led to anaemia, and delayed care seeking meant that girls were missing out on life-saving antenatal care; blood tests for infection and haemoglobin level, antimalarial medication, iron supplements, blood pressure checks, and the health talks given at every antenatal clinic appointment:

> *And because of the inexperience, they don't know when there is a raised pressure only because they refuse to*

come to the antenatal ... and by the time they come to the hospital they come convulsing, fitting. You see them dying. (SMI1)

They reported teenagers often not registering at all with a health care provider in pregnancy, then presenting late in labour, often only accompanied by friends and lacking any adult support, and they related concealed pregnancies directly to maternal death.

Particularly for girls in rural areas, early marriage was seen by the midwives as a risk factor. For these girls, though living without stigma and in the safety of either their parents' or husband's family home, delay in care seeking was a major issue, often a result of the lack of decision-making ability of women within traditional families:

In the provinces, when the chief wants that young grownup girl, he convinces the relatives. After marrying her she becomes pregnant. Maybe she does not even attend antenatal clinic. When it comes to delivery, complication arise. To let them refer that case to the big hospital, it's a problem. Maybe the husband is not around, then the relatives do not have money and they do not have a say over that woman so they delay to make decision. So after they have made the final decision to take the woman, transportation! Maybe the road is not good, there is no ambulance for the patient to come to the hospital. So after the patient has arrived now in the big hospital ... maybe we need blood for this patient, there is no doctor to see this patient ... if she comes in with bleeding, obviously she will lose her life. (HMFG)

Clearly, teenagers who die around the time of childbirth suffer from the same obstetric conditions which befall older pregnant women, but youth in itself should not confer additional risk when considered as part of a risk assessment – a concept which the midwives clearly articulated. Obstetric risks were perceived to be magnified by delayed care seeking and the poor physical condition in which girls go into labour.

Risk of death from Anaemia and PPH

In Sierra Leone, as in many other countries in Sub-Saharan Africa, most donated blood is given by family members during an emergency. Although there were some contradictory versions of how the blood bank operates in Freetown, it was commonly reported that for a patient to be given a blood transfusion, two donors were required to donate into the blood bank. Discussions with midwives from both the peripheral clinics and the referral hospital described a clear policy for minimising the risks of anaemia and post-partum haemorrhage; all women are given iron supplements and advised on diet, and haemoglobin level is checked at 36 weeks of pregnancy, when women are urged to involve family members in identifying potential blood donors:

When the mother attends ANC, and they tell her she will need blood ... she will ask her family, saying 'look here, I've been going to ANC and they say I will need blood, so what I want you to do, as a family is to be thinking who will give blood'... it's all part of birth preparedness. (HMFG)

But with limited success:

...well most of the time they tell them but they don't comply, they don't accept that there's a problem, and then you see them running helter-skelter. (HMFG)

Where a donor cannot be found, most participants stated that non-related donors can be paid at a high premium to donate. Where people cannot afford to pay a donor, participants reported that emergency blood is given if available but that this is not always the case, to the frustration of clinicians and community leaders:

We don't have much blood in the blood bank. They end up dying. We can help but we cannot give more than what we have. (SMI3)

Someone would have to pay for blood. I have been there on about seven occasions when young girls died there. They have that problem there. There is no free blood. People do not volunteer to give blood. Unless your relative volunteers to give blood on your behalf, if not so you would have to buy. (WL3)

The severity of the situation was all too apparent when the first author donated her blood at the country's main referral hospital; it was the only unit of A+ blood in the blood bank.

Potential solutions
Mentoring

The literature from Sierra Leone consistently points to good parental communication, especially with mothers, as a protective factor for risky sexual behaviour and early pregnancy, but that parents lack confidence to discuss these issues [15, 16]. This study aligns with that; the country director of an international NGO addressing teenage pregnancy prevention in a rural area described *'overwhelming numbers of parents wanting to join in'* with their interventions to equip parents with knowledge and skills to support their children.

This was reinforced by several of the professional participants referring to their own feelings of inadequacy in this area:

We the parents also, to some extent, we are to be blamed ... because we don't make our children our friends. We have that communication barrier... some of us think that there is certain information that has to be hidden from these children, then they go astray as a result of that. You have to talk to your child! (HMFG)

Many girls reported knowing very little about sex and pregnancy before they conceived. Several girls interviewed did not know they were pregnant until a family member or relative noticed their body shape changing and took them for a test. Regarding outcomes for girls once pregnant, the ability to communicate with, and good care by family members were recognised as being protective, especially in avoiding the dangers of concealed pregnancy and abortion:

What is most dangerous thing is this abortion, because some of them are so afraid of their parents and usually it's the boyfriend who took them to non-qualified people. (MW1)

Regarding criteria for a young woman to move on positively with her life after a pregnancy, it is unsurprising that having supportive family relationships has been shown to be highly advantageous. Several professional participants referred to themselves or colleagues who had had a teenage pregnancy, but had progressed to a successful professional career due to good family support. Currently, all pregnant girls are forced to drop out of school as there is a controversial ban on 'visibly pregnant' girls attending school or sitting exams, which for some girls adds to the stigma and isolation they experience [17]. The capacity to either return to education or pursue vocational training appears to be important for mental wellbeing, avoiding rapid subsequent pregnancies, and being able to provide for their children, thus breaking the cycle of poverty. These two young mothers, enrolled at Conforti, a vocational training provider, express this:

Now that I have given birth and decided to come for that training, I have joined the PPA so I will not give birth again. (MFG1)

But I bless this institution, training us. I wasn't feeling good about myself, I just saw myself as a drop-out, I really felt it! (MFG1)

However, the additional expense of school expenses on top of providing for an additional child is often prohibitive for families. At the time of the study, LNP was providing free training in trade-based skills to local youth, and this was considered a huge community asset:

That (the Institute's graduation) was very good. Some might want to learn but are not able to pay for the education. The parents might not be rich enough to pay. But if they learn a trade they will be able to provide for themselves and their children. (SCLI))

For girls who have been abandoned by their family, or are living with the baby's father's family with little support, there is a recognised need for other adults in the community to act in the capacity of trusted adult. One participant, an older mother of five, had recognised this in her local community and been informally supporting pregnant girls for the previous five years. She described her strategy; ensuring the girl accesses health care whilst attempting to advocate for her within the family context:

I had this urge, feeling and burden for children who are thirteen, fourteen, fifteen, in schools. This was bubbling inside me so ... I started working with the girls that have been expelled from their family homes. I usually accompany them to talk to their parent, saying things like 'it's like a loaded gun - once the trigger is pulled it cannot be recalled. The only thing we can do is to take care of the girl'. I am thankful to God I have never had a victim or death... I will take the pregnant girl for check-up with a nurse making sure that everything about the pregnancy is alright then I will approach the parents. I do pray before I go to speak to the parents as some of them can be very bitter saying I would not accept the girl as she has chosen to be sexually active. Let her go and get married. I will say to them 'this child is yours, a marriage can end but the girl will be the one who look after you when you are old.' I will gather other people to help with the negotiation. Most times this is successful. (WL3)

She also described her strategy to ensure that the girls had enough money to feed themselves well and buy things for their baby; supporting them to start a small business and supervising their savings.

Considering the recent EVD epidemic in Sierra Leone which left many stigmatised orphans, and the effect of the internal migration of teenagers away from families in the provinces to Freetown, this simple community-based mentoring intervention has the potential to benefit other orphaned, abandoned or otherwise isolated adolescent mothers in Freetown.

Community-based blood donation

Blood donation in Sierra Leone is complex, with social norms around who can donate blood to whom. It is rare for a husband to donate blood for his wife, with the woman's birth family usually donating in this case:

Yes, because for example if I was pregnant, my sister would be more willing to give blood for me, or my brother, so that nothing will happen to me. Rather than my husband. (NGOI1)

It is the dads that give blood more than the husbands. (SMI1)

Whereas if a child needs blood, this will invariably be donated by the child's father:

For children, most times the father does it. The fathers are willing. But they will not give for their wife. I don't know what the issue is. (NGOI1)

This study identified altruism as a strong motivator for blood donation in Freetown:

Just because when people meet me and they explain to me 'you need to help us in this situation', I just need to do it, because that is my only way to help them. (YMFG)

But found that a significant barrier was HIV testing; either fear of discovering their status, or fear of their status being told to a family member:

Yes, I think people will be afraid to be tested, in case at the end of the day the doctor says, 'you have HIV' (YMFG)

People are afraid. People don't want to be tested because of hepatitis and HIV. So, they dodge. Some husbands they prefer to give money to donors to getting them tested, or maybe some of them know their status, they hide it from the wife, and they don't want to expose it. (NGO1)

This fear of stigma was all too fresh to participants after the recent EVD epidemic where affected people were ostracised by the community:

In this country, when I say this person has HIV, they will just run away from you, it will just turn like Ebola. (YMFG)

A further barrier was fear of the process; in a focus group of young men, there was clear lack of knowledge,

with questions asked about how much blood was taken, whether it hurt, and whether your body could recover. Lastly, some common myths were raised:

People say when you give blood you die. When you give blood, you become sick. (WLI2)

Some people think if they come and take one pint of blood from them they will die tomorrow. It is just fear. (YMFG)

Compensation All participants with whom blood donation was discussed believed that a donor should be compensated for what their body had lost in the process of donation:

Even for someone to be able to give blood they should be able to have food to eat. If not so they will be anaemic. (YMFG)

This was not considered a payment, and the donation was still classified as voluntary. For one young man who had donated blood five times to non-family members, being thanked also seemed to be an important motivator:

The one I remember was (name). I was thinking that at the end of the day, I paid my transport to go there ... I was thinking that when he got well, he would say 'hey man thank you', but ... he couldn't even look at me, but I had already done it, so I just let him forget about it. All the (other) four people, I've been happy to keep them alive, but for him, I was so angry about it, because he's my brother (non-relative), so I was thinking he would say something like 'thank you'. (YMFG)

In terms of strategies to recruit non-related volunteer donors, more overt compensation is more important. For example, health staff are offered days off in exchange for a unit of blood. It was evident that various models had been tried to recruit donors, but with limited sustainability:

There was an NGO who was paying people to donate blood. The donors were fed well. But the problem with our country we have so many groups which have been set up by so many NGOs who would come and start something, but it is for short time it does not last. (HWFG)

A potential solution was discussed with midwives and a group of young men from LNP, of having a local blood donation register, whereby a direct communication between the clinic midwife and the co-ordinator of the register would ensure that a donor could be sent to the referral hospital directly if a woman had to be referred for bleeding. This midwife felt that not having any mechanism for compensation would be a barrier as, again, being fed a meal was a minimum expectation of donors:

> *They would have to eat to replace that. We would not be able to keep this service going. It is not easy to get people to donate blood. Some people will do it once but they would make excuses the second time. They will say that they have not eaten since the morning. (MWI)*

Blood donation experience The literature also shows a clear association between the first blood donation experience and the likelihood that the donor will donate again [18], and it was clear from the young man who was a multiple donor that his experience had been positive, that he had felt well cared for and given food:

> *If you donate your blood, they will take care of you, explain to you how it's supposed to be, during the blood donation, or after the blood donation. They will explain to you 'sit down first and take a little bit of bread'. (YMFG)*

Other potential barriers to a local community register was the fear that donors might be taken for granted when there were other family members able to donate; this would need to be part of a further consultation on compensation mechanisms and eligibility.

Discussion

Vulnerability to teenage pregnancy

Transactional sex

It is evident that in Freetown, adolescent transactional sex, whether for water, money, or grades, is a social norm which is in some cases encouraged by family members, ignored by school authorities and for which legislation appears not to be effective. In many cases, expectations are placed on girls to provide for their own financial needs, and for many girls, the only option is to meet those needs with their one available resource, their bodies.

This study indicates that girls who live with extended family rather than with a parent are more vulnerable to the pressures of transactional sex and exploitation, and the literature echoes this finding [9, 15]. One 2010 study showed large anomalies between the intended reason for children being moved from rural areas to urban households and the endpoint reality for the child [15]. Sixty-seven percent of these children said they initially moved to Freetown to go to school, but only 38 % were attending school, and

60 % said they 'worked', the majority 'working in the house' [15]. Regarding pregnancy, 58 % of teenage mothers or pregnant teenagers were not living with either biological parent [15].

The more specific issue of 'sex for grades', where girls have sex with male teachers in exchange for passing exams or being promoted to the next year in school is also widely mentioned in the literature [8–11]. In Coinco's 2008 qualitative study [9] focussing on the plight of 'out-of-school' primary-aged children, the issue is discussed in some detail, with a case-study on 'teachers' sexual advances'. A 2010 joint NGO report showed that some 30% of coerced or forced sex of adolescents is by teachers [11], and a 2013 study [8] acknowledges the issue of teacher coercion, but found that participants did not talk about it, concluding that increased awareness of child rights has increased the taboo around the issue with fears of recrimination and shame acting as deterrents to fuller discussion or disclosure.

Though the issue is recognised within the literature, when policy solutions are discussed, there is little acknowledgement that the pressure for sex from teachers may hinder girls' engagement or re-engagement in education. Indeed, several narratives present the issue of sex and education as a relatively simple choice for girls; between remaining in the relationships where the transactional sex is taking place, or if support is available, returning to the school environment, with the underlying message being that school is a safe and secure environment:

> *'More targeted work is also required, for example, with regard to girls involved in sexually exploitative relationships, who need practical and personal support to exit these relationships and re-engage at school'.* (page 7) [19]

And there are even suggestions that that girls choose to pursue sex with teachers to raise their grade unfairly, rather than as an unavoidable route to completing their schooling:

> *Findings reveal that girls are also engaging in transactional sex to access a range of other amenities and merits including, for example, school grades – in the aptly termed "sexually transmitted grades"* [20] *(page 18).*

This approach seems rather simplistic in the light of key informant data in this study, which indicate that, contrary to perceptions that keeping girls in school will solve the problem of teenage pregnancy, for some girls, school is a risky environment where transactional sex is a necessary evil to ensure academic success.

Much of the messaging on early sex and teenage pregnancy appear to be presenting the issue within a 'blame frame' [21]. Girls' behaviour is perceived as the problem, with little being said about the role of men and boys, the impotence of the justice system, or the significant contributors within the structural environment such as the deficient water supply or lack of female teachers. Posters generally target girls themselves, urging them to avoid under-age sex and teenage pregnancy, with the implicit message that they are free agents, making choices around their sexuality and fertility. Whilst the 2014 communications strategy rightly proposes messages to both young men and women, to parents, carers and community leaders, some of the key messages belie the baseline premise that girls have agency and are in a position to choose their sexual behaviour: *'Abstinence is the safest way to avoid pregnancy and diseases. Young women who choose this path should be praised and encouraged'.* [16]*(Page 41).*

Some studies rightly identify that girls have transactional sex in order to access clothes and belongings which would be inaccessible without it [20]. There is a danger that this too can feed into the blame narrative, as though having sex for basic needs is more acceptable than having sex for 'luxuries'. Again, this oversimplifies the lived experiences of girls in Freetown. Seminal literature on 'the body as an asset' asserts that for a poor farmer or factory worker, the physical body is the one asset a person has to produce wealth [22]. For a girl in Freetown, her body is such an asset, and equipping herself with the right clothes, hair and accessories could be seen as a way of maximising on her potential to pay for 'necessities' such as schooling, which is widely viewed as the only exit from poverty. For example, a mobile phone could be viewed as a luxury, but with the 'body as an asset' lens, a mobile phone is to a teenage girl as a scythe is to a farmer – an essential tool to maximise one's potential to secure a livelihood.

Data suggests that sexual exploitation by teachers is not restricted to senior secondary schools, but also directed towards primary age girls in early puberty with no transaction apparent. However, the language used to discuss this issue lacks clarity, with phrases such as 'institutionalised child abuse', or even 'child abuse' not being part of the dialogue. One key participant, describing his discomfort with the situation where a teacher keeps a pubescent girl after class to 'touch her breasts and buttocks' proposed tentatively that 'this might be called abuse?' The exception to this was a child protection worker pushing for a teachers' charter and awareness-raising amongst students on the law around sexual abuse and child rights. In the recent years of the implementation of the national strategy, efforts have been made to educate communities about gender-based

violence and child rights, but there is clearly more work to be done in this area.

In many ways, this lack of conviction about what constitutes child abuse is unsurprising, since the waters are muddied by the strong gender norms which normalise early marriage and motherhood, often viewed by families as a way to prevent the risk of the stigma of teenage pregnancy outside of marriage, and boys' education is often seen as a more worthwhile investment than girls', with the expectation that early motherhood will limit educational potential. Though reported elsewhere [15], there was no evidence in this study of boys being sexually exploited by teachers. However, they are not exempt from 'money for grades' by both male and female teachers, and often do hard manual labour outside of school to pay for additional charges. All these factors undermine the education system and therefore economic growth and development. A unique finding in this study was the use of boys by teachers to scout out and groom girls, promoting and reinforcing a gendered stereotype of adult male sexual behaviour to boys through negative role modelling.

Training and employing more female teachers is recognised as important to turn the tide in this issue, but it seems that this very strategy is undermined by the issue itself; only 12% women aged 20–24 in Sierra Leone are educated to secondary level or higher, compared with 20% of men [1] and the data suggests that sex for grades is also a common barrier for women in university. This under-education of girls has serious implications for the health and economic wellbeing of the country as a whole; an international study shows that when women and girls earn income, they reinvest 90% of it into their families, compared with only 30 to 40% for a man [23].

Regarding the 'water for water' issue, the same message persists; posters encouraging girls to avoid early sex and stay in school are strategically placed near water wells [16]. The irony of this message is hard to miss when one imagines a girl considering her options of staying in the water queue and missing school, or of bypassing the queue for sex to ensure she attends school or sits an exam. A more upstream solution, to upgrade the failing water supply problem, is not mentioned as a potential strategy in policy documents.

Prevention of adolescent maternal death
Abandonment
The association between poverty and adolescent maternal death was pervasive in this study. This was particularly clear within the themes about the treatment of girls once pregnant, with clear differences between social groups. Poorer families normally see the girls as the responsibility of the father of the baby, and an

opportunity to gain some financial support, even if he is a teacher or older married man. Support deals are often brokered by community leaders for the man to support the girl during the pregnancy and pay for the child's education, even if she stays with her family. Girls who are forced to marry or to live at the man's house are often treated badly, exposed to further risks of STIs, malaria, anaemia and the additional risk of second pregnancy; compounding mortality risk.

This is in stark contrast to girls from professional families. Many of the professional women within health services, NGOs and government departments described being introduced to a colleague's son or daughter who was clearly the result of a teenage pregnancy. One participant related this phenomenon to Krios, an ethnic group within Freetown who tend towards professional occupations. She described how girls as young as eleven would be taken to a different community ('to the hills') and given caesarean sections, only to return to school without the knowledge of their peers.

This practice of the family concealing and dealing with the pregnancy and sending the girl back to school is very difficult for poorer families, yet one local woman advocated strongly for a similar mindset, articulating a view not commonly heard in poorer communities; of families continuing to treat the girl as a child, and taking the baby as a sibling of the daughter. She stressed the importance of helping girls to develop aspirations, and the need for strong role models. Much has been written about the influence of positive role models in the Sierra Leone context [8, 9, 15], and examples such as this one point to grass-roots advocacy as a powerful tool for change in tackling the inherent social inequalities of teenage pregnancy outcomes.

Delayed care seeking

The literature and current study consistently point to delayed care seeking as a key risk factor for adolescent maternal death [24]. Fear of insensitive or harsh care by health workers, lack of confidentiality and being stigmatised by other women are all cited as factors [25]. Sierra Leone has a mixture of government clinics, private clinics and a referral hospital. Several participants perceived that care in private clinics is more respectful, and women who can afford it seek out private care for this reason, despite care being generally safer within the state system.

I'm not going to go and give my money and somebody will yell at me. I will pay money where I am respected. I don't care if I don't eat for the day, but I will pay my money, as long as I'm respected and somebody speaks nicely to me. (NGO)

Well in the private hospitals, people go there for the respectful care, but also they should know that though respectful is important, the skill also is very important. Because it's the skill that will save your life. (SM)

Without the means to pay for private care, adolescents often choose to give birth with a traditional birth attendant (TBA) for similar reasons.

And even for the TBAs, right, the TBAs will never never, in as much as they have their own issues, they will never yell at a woman when they go to see them in their house. As soon as they see them, they are 'how are you?', even when they don't have all the skills. (NGO)

In addition, despite health care for pregnant and lactating women and children under five being free since 2010, there is a perception that government clinics still charge for their services, and in reality, informal charges are still common.

Viewing the situation from the health worker's point of view, training for health workers is rife with corrupt practices such as 'under the table' payments to invigilators, for forms to be processed, and for graduation, and health workers often leave their training in huge debt; this inevitably plays out in the clinics and hospitals. A key NGO participant leading a community development project aimed at reducing maternal mortality through community engagement, highlighted the importance of a strong advocate as a protective factor against these informal charges; a respected individual who could challenge disrespectful care or corrupt practices. Girls who are only supported by peers or young boyfriends are particularly vulnerable and may not return to a clinic or hospital setting if their first experience is disrespectful or corrupt, risking complications and death. One young mother who experienced abusive care in labour vowed she would never use the services again, and joked that she would protect herself with six 'captain bands'.

Midwives talked about how the combination of FGM, early marriage, polygamous households and delay in seeking care mean that girls from rural areas often arrive at the referral hospital in Freetown at the point of death. Their general feeling is that physically, girls 'shouldn't have to die just because they are young', but lack of agency means that girls have little control over their fertility or health seeking, and this makes them much more vulnerable. Midwives expressed strong emotions when talking about the helplessness they feel when girls die needlessly. One interviewee reframed the harsh treatment of women who seek health care late as an expression of frustration and helplessness as 'when they *yell at you it's because they love you and don't want these things to happen to you'.*

There were numerous examples in the data of midwives going 'above and beyond' for women, including doing a home visit to site implants for girls who were too ashamed, donating blood for a dying woman, and paying for a taxi to transport a woman to hospital who was bleeding. This is not to say that the promotion of respectful free care is unimportant, but gives another perspective to the 'disrespectful care' narrative which needs to be considered in the bigger picture of resolving the issue. Starting a career without the debt from bribes paid to move through the training process would undoubtedly affect the issue of informal charges, for example.

Potential solutions
Mentoring
Historically, sex and relationship education in school has been limited to lectures by teachers or nurses on contraception use, with little opportunity for real discussion with adults [8, 16, 19], and studies show that adolescents are strongly influenced in their attitudes to sex, and gain most of their information about sex from pornography and other media [8, 20].

Although evidence which specifically relates to mentoring of young mothers is sparse [26, 27], with most research looking at black American adolescents, limiting applicability to the African setting, there is strong evidence that connectedness with an adult, be it a parent or a non-parental adult, appears to be foundational for adolescent health and well-being more generally [26, 28], including delaying rapid second pregnancies [27]. Regarding studies in SSA, Coinco asserts that a protective factor for adolescents against risky sexual behaviour and early pregnancy in Sierra Leone is having a consistent trustworthy adult or role model involved in their lives [15], and studies in South Africa and Uganda demonstrate that AIDS-orphaned children and adolescents in a natural mentoring relationship showed significantly lower distress and mental health factors (child abuse, social discrimination, anxiety, and depression) than those not in a mentoring relationship [29, 30]. A review of the determinants of delivery service use identified low maternal age as a determinant for not accessing skilled care for delivery [31].

Within this current study, issues of abandonment leading to poor mental health, poor health-seeking behaviour and lack of knowledge about pregnancy, birth and baby care all indicate that a mentoring scheme may be effective, and evidence from other community projects indicate that having an advocate when accessing health care can mitigate against some of the barriers such as disrespectful care and informal charges (personal communication).

Following the findings of this study, a pilot mentoring scheme for younger and more vulnerable pregnant teenagers is currently underway, in order to establish feasibility to trial a scaled-up intervention. Mentors have four key roles; helping girls to re-establish family connection and support; encouraging health seeking behaviours and advocating for respectful care at clinic, in labour and in the postnatal period; providing practical advice and support with parenting; and providing support and training in a small business and to re-enter education or vocational skills training. Some outputs will be quantitative measures such as the number of antenatal visits, uptake of tetanus toxoid, uptake of prophylactic medication, sleeping under a bed net, and uptake of infant immunisations. Others will be qualitative in nature; the impact of the mentoring relationship on the young person's mental health, the impact of having an advocate on experience of antenatal care, and the impact of mentoring on family support mechanisms.

Community-based blood donation
The Guidance from the World Health Organisation (WHO) and the President's Emergency Plan for Aids Relief (PEPFAR) recommends that countries aim by 2020 for 100% blood to be donated by non-remunerated volunteers rather than family members, primarily for reasons of sustainability and safety of the service [32]. The need for an understanding of the SSA context and how this differs from the primarily European and American contexts where most of the research which underpins the guidance is carried out, was emphasised in two recent literature reviews around blood donation behaviour in SSA [33, 34]. Both reviews identify altruism as the common primary motivator for donating blood, whether to a stranger or a family member, but show that other motivators and barriers vary between countries. For example, the opportunity to have a health check and discover and treat any infections was considered a motivator in a study from South Africa, but a deterrent in studies from many of the other SSA countries. Regarding barriers to donation, a mixture of cultural and religious beliefs, myths about the dangers of donation, and lack of information about the process were all cited, and their analyses indicate the need for programming at a national or even tribal level rather than global or regional level. For example, in several of the thirty-five studies in one review, there was a belief that giving blood could cause male impotence [33]; where this is known, interventions with older repeat male donors with children as donor champions could be strategically effective.

Regarding the distinction between regular volunteer donors and those who donate to family members in an emergency, the evidence behind the rationale of safety and sustainability of the former has been challenged, with further analysis of the data showing no difference in safety and a two to five times increased cost per unit for this policy [35].

In a culture where blood is not readily available and blood donors must be brokered within the family setting, it is unsurprising that young girls in Freetown who have been rejected by their families are at higher risk of death from bleeding than women with higher levels of social capital. This is in addition to risks due to increased anaemia from poor diet and limited antenatal care. Social norms dictate that it is close relatives rather than husbands or partners who donate to women, putting young girls in an even more vulnerable situation. If a blood donor is not available, blood must be purchased which is likely to be outside the reach of more isolated teenagers.

One potential solution being considered here is to set up a local register of donors from a discreet community, linking directly to the three PHUs in that community, where donors who have already been screened are called upon in an emergency. This system would engender a sense of ownership, and allow for compensatory mechanisms between families and donors not possible within a wider donation programme. With an asset-based lens, the community in question has particular favourable assets for such a scheme; the hub of this community is a faith-based project set up during the civil war to rescue child soldiers, and which now accommodates and trains young people, based on common values such as altruism and caring for the poor. There is strong body of literature on the benefits of maximising on faith-based groups as sites for public health interventions [36], with potential for scale-up in similar communities.

In this study, compensation to eat and travel to the blood bank were considered minimum requirements to donate, with this donation still being considered voluntary and altruistic. Since paying large sums to 'professional' blood donors outside the hospital was commonplace, a system where the family 'gifts' the donor a modest amount of money to travel and eat could be reasonably considered as a sustainable model. The importance of recognition was also seen as important, and if the system was being managed within a discreet community there would be scope for developing this particular incentive.

The biggest barrier to blood donation was the fear of a positive HIV status, with the belief that this was a death sentence and would lead to social ostracization. Other barriers were fear of the process and fear that the donor would be unwell after donation. More exploration needs to be done with this community about the best ways of addressing these barriers. For example, in the focus group with young men from LNP, the fact that one young man had donated blood five times and described the process as 'like having a drip – you've all had a drip!' seemed to quickly dispel the fear in the whole group. Equally, meeting a person living with HIV, or hearing stories from community members whose lives have been saved by a voluntary donor could be important strategies for recruitment of local donors, and would need to be further explored.

Conclusion

This study has explored the causes of high maternal death in younger teenagers in Eastern Freetown, Sierra Leone using interviews and focus groups with a wide range of participants including adolescent mothers, midwives, teachers, policy makers, third sector groups and community leaders. Three main areas of discussion were vulnerability to teenage pregnancy, vulnerability to maternal death once pregnant, and possible interventions to address these vulnerabilities.

Under the more commonly explored issue of vulnerability to teenage pregnancy, it is evident that girls use transactional sex to access a range of resources including school fees, academic success, time, and money for food and clothing. Girls from poorer families, and girls cared for in a family other than their birth family appear to be particularly vulnerable. Narratives around teenage pregnancy assume a degree of agency which is not found in this data, and strategies discouraging early sex appear to emphasise giving of information and behaviour change at the expense of more upstream interventions such as improved water systems, more female teachers and better enforcement of laws on sexual abuse of children.

Regarding vulnerability to maternal death, concealing pregnancies and abortions, and being abandoned by families are significant risk factors. Midwives strongly concurred that adolescence in itself should not put girls at higher risk if maternity care is accessed in a timely manner, but in reality, the lack of adult care and supervision and lack of decision-making power put young teenagers at higher risk of death than older women who have more knowledge, social capital and agency. These factors were evident in the issue of blood donation, where delayed care seeking, lack of knowledge, and the absence of willing blood donors all put young girls at increased risk of death from bleeding.

Two potential interventions emerged from the study; a volunteer mentoring programme, and a locally managed blood donation register, neither of which have been documented previously. Of these, the pilot mentoring scheme for younger and more vulnerable pregnant teenagers is currently underway. Mentors will encourage early uptake of antenatal care and use of a trained birth attendant, will help to maintain or re-establish family support, will support moving on to training or return to school, and will support the young woman to start a small income generation activity. A feasibility study of this pilot project will use qualitative methods to determine whether the scheme is acceptable within the community, accessible to the most vulnerable girls, and whether the data collection tool is fit for purpose. This study will then form the basis of a larger trial to establish effectiveness in terms of mortality and wellbeing outcomes. If effective and scalable, this intervention has the potential to affect outcomes on a large scale for adolescents and their children across Sierra Leone and beyond.

Endnotes

[1]The six pillars are:

- Improved policy and legal environment to protect adolescents' and young people' rights
- Improvement of access to quality sexual reproductive health, protection and education services for adolescents and young people
- Comprehensive age-appropriate information and education for adolescents and young people
- Communities, adolescents and young people empowered to prevent and respond to teenage pregnancy
- Coordinating, monitoring and evaluation mechanisms in place, allowing proper management of the strategy

Abbreviations

CBO: Community Based Organisation; EVD: Ebola Virus Disease; GoSL: Government of Sierra Leone; HDI: Human Development Index; LiST: Lives Saved Tool; LNP: Lifeline Nehemiah Project; MMR: Maternal Mortality Ratio; NGO: Non-Governmental Organisation; PEPFAR: President's Emergency Plan for Aids Relief; PHU: Peripheral Health Unit; SLDHS: Sierra Leone Demographic Health Survey; SSA: Sub-Saharan Africa; TBA: Traditional Birth Attendant; WHO: World Health Organisation

Acknowledgements

Many thanks to Mangenda Kamara, my research assistant, who assisted me greatly with data collection, and to all participants who gave their time freely to take part in the study.

Funding

Lucy November was funded by Wellbeing of Women's International Midwifery Fellowship.
Jane Sandall was supported by the National Institute for Health Research (NIHR) Collaboration for Leadership in Applied Health Research and Care South London at King's College Hospital NHS Foundation Trust. The views expressed are those of the author(s) and not necessarily those of the NHS, the NIHR or the Department of Health.

Authors' contributions

LN designed the study, conducted the interviews and focus groups, analysed the data and wrote up the study with input from JS. JS contributed towards the design, execution and write up of the study. Both authors read and approved the final manuscript.

Competing interests

The authors declare that they have no competing interests.

References

1. Statistics Sierra Leone, S. S. L. and I. C. F. International. Sierra Leone Demographic and Health Survey 2013. Freetown: SSL and ICF International; 2014.
2. Neal S, et al. Childbearing in adolescents aged 12–15 years in low resource countries: a neglected issue. New estimates from demographic and household surveys in 42 countries. Acta Obstet Gynecol Scand. 2012;91(9):1114–8.
3. Government of Sierra Leone. Let girls be girls, not mothers. National strategy for the reduction of teenage pregnancy 2013 to 2015. Freetown: Government of Sierra Leone; 2013.
4. Donnelly J. How did Sierra Leone provide free health care? Lancet. 2011; 377(9775):1393–6.
5. Statistics Sierra Leone, S. S. L. and I. C. F. Macro. Sierra Leone Demographic and Health Survey 2008. Calverton: SSL and ICF Macro; 2009.
6. WHO. Health worker Ebola infections in Guinea, Liberia and Sierra Leone: a preliminary report. Geneva: World Health Organization; 2015.
7. International Labour Organization. Recovering from the Ebola Crisis. New York: UNDP; 2015.
8. De Koning K, et al. Realities of teenage pregnancy in Sierra Leone. Amsterdam: KIT publishers; 2013.
9. Coinco E. The out-of-school children of Sierra Leone. Freetown: UNICEF; 2008.
10. Wessells M. An ethnographic study of community-based child protection mechanisms and their linkage with the national child protection system of Sierra Leone. New York: The Columbia Group for Children in Adversit; 2011.
11. Mekonen Y, et al. 'Give Us a Chance': National Study on School-Related Gender-Based Violence in Sierra Leone, Concern Worldwide, Catholic Relief Services Sierra Leone Program, IBIS, Plan Sierra Leone. 2010.
12. WHO, World Health Organization guidelines on preventing early pregnancy and poor reproductive health outcomes among adolescents in developing countries. 2011.
13. Hindin MJ, Fatusi AO. Adolescent sexual and reproductive health in developing countries: an overview of trends and interventions. Int Perspect Sex Reprod Health. 2009;35(2):58–62.
14. Homer CS, et al. The projected effect of scaling up midwifery. Lancet. 2014; 384(9948):1146–57.
15. Coinco E. A glimpse into the world of teenage pregnancy in Sierra Leone. Freetown: UNICEF; 2010.
16. UNICEF, Communication strategy for the reduction of teenage pregnancy in Sierra Leone 2015–2019. Freetown: National Secretariat for the Reduction of Teenage Pregnancy; 2014.
17. Amnesty International. Shamed and blamed: pregnant girls' rights at risk in Sierra Leone. London: Amnesty International; 2015.
18. Newman BH, et al. The effect of whole-blood donor adverse events on blood donor return rates. Transfusion. 2006;46(8):1374–9.
19. Robinson B. A mountain to climb: gender-based violence and girls' right to education in Sierra Leone. Geneva: Defence for Children International; 2015.
20. Lai K. A case study exploring the relationship between mobile phone acquisition and use and adolescent girls in Freetown. Freetown: Save the Children and National Secretariat for Reducing Teenage Pregnancy in Sierra Leone; 2014.
21. Denney L, et al. Change the context not the girls: improving efforts to reduce teenage pregnancy in Sierra Leone. Freetown: Secure Livelihoods Research Consortium; 2016.
22. Narayan D, et al. Voices of the poor: crying out for change. New York: Oxford University Press for the World Bank; 2000.
23. Borges P. Women empowered: inspiring change in the emerging world. New York: Rizzoli International Publications; 2007.
24. Loaiza E, Liang M. Adolescent pregnancy, a review of the evidence. New York: UNFPA; 2013.
25. Banke-Thomas OE, Banke-Thomas AO, Ameh CA. Factors influencing utilisation of maternal health services by adolescent mothers in low-and middle-income countries: a systematic review. BMC Pregnancy childbirth. 2017;17(1):65.

26. Schaffer MA, Mbibi N. Public health nurse mentorship of pregnant and parenting adolescents. Public Health Nurs. 2014;31(5):428–37.
27. Black MM, et al. Delaying second births among adolescent mothers: a randomized, controlled trial of a home-based mentoring program. Pediatrics. 2006;118(4):e1087–99.
28. Sieving RE, et al. Youth–adult connectedness:: a key protective factor for adolescent health. Am J Prev Med. 2017;52(3, Supplement 3):S275–8.
29. Onuoha FN, Munakata T. Inverse association of natural mentoring relationship with distress mental health in children orphaned by AIDS. BMC Psychiatry. 2010;10(6):1–8.
30. Onuoha FN, et al. Negative mental health factors in children orphaned by AIDS: natural mentoring as a palliative care. AIDS Behav. 2008;13(5):980.
31. Gabrysch S, Campbell OM. Still too far to walk: literature review of the determinants of delivery service use. BMC Pregnancy Childbirth. 2009;9(1):1.
32. Ifland L. Promoting national blood systems in developing countries. Curr Opin Hematol. 2014;21(6):497–502.
33. Asamoah-Akuoko L, et al. Blood donors' perceptions, motivators and deterrents in sub-Saharan Africa – a scoping review of evidence. Br J Haematol. 2017;177:864–77.
34. Zanin TZ, et al. Tapping into a vital resource: understanding the motivators and barriers to blood donation in sub-Saharan Africa. African J Emerg Med. 2016;6(2):70–9.
35. Allain JP. Volunteer safer than replacement donor blood: a myth revealed by evidence. ISBT Sci Ser. 2010;5(n1):169–75.
36. November L. The impact of faith-based groups on public health and social capital. London: Faithaction; 2013.

14

Association of the client-provider ratio with the risk of maternal mortality in referral hospitals

Friday Okonofua[1,2,3*], Lorretta Ntoimo[2,4], Rosemary Ogu[2,3,5*] (iD), Hadiza Galadanci[6], Rukiyat Abdus-salam[7], Mohammed Gana[8], Ola Okike[9], Kingsley Agholor[10], Eghe Abe[11], Adetoye Durodola[12], Abdullahi Randawa[13] and The WHARC WHO FMOH MNCH Implementation Research StudyTeam[2]

Abstract

Background: The paucity of human resources for health buoyed by excessive workloads has been identified as being responsible for poor quality obstetric care, which leads to high maternal mortality in Nigeria. While there is anecdotal and qualitative research to support this observation, limited quantitative studies have been conducted to test the association between the number and density of human resources and risk of maternal mortality. This study aims to investigate the association between client-provider ratios for antenatal and delivery care and the risk of maternal mortality in 8 referral hospitals in Nigeria.

Methods: Client-provider ratios were calculated for antenatal and delivery care attendees during a 3-year period (2011–2013). The maternal mortality ratio (MMR) was calculated per 100,000 live births for the hospitals, while unadjusted Poisson regression analysis was used to examine the association between the number of maternal deaths and density of healthcare providers.

Results: A total of 334,425 antenatal care attendees and 26,479 births were recorded during this period. The client-provider ratio in the maternity department for antenatal care attendees was 1343:1 for doctors and 222:1 for midwives. The ratio of births to one doctor in the maternity department was 106:1 and 18:1 for midwives. On average, there were 441 births per specialist obstetrician. The results of the regression analysis showed a significant negative association between the number of maternal deaths and client-provider ratios in all categories.

Conclusion: We conclude that the maternal mortality ratios in Nigeria's referral hospitals are worsened by high client-provider ratios, with few providers attending a large number of pregnant women. Efforts to improve the density and quality of maternal healthcare providers, especially at the first referral level, would be a critical intervention for reducing the currently high rate of maternal mortality in Nigeria.

Keywords: Client-provider ratio, Maternal mortality, Nigeria, Referral hospitals

* Correspondence: feokonofua@yahoo.co.uk; vc@unimed.edu.ng; dr.ogurosemary@yahoo.com; rosemary.ogu@uniport.edu.ng
[1]University of Medical Sciences, Ondo City, Ondo State, Nigeria
[2]the Women's Health and Action Research Centre, WHO Implementation Research Group, Benin City, Nigeria
Full list of author information is available at the end of the article

Plain English summary

The considerable number of women who die during pregnancy in Nigeria is currently a critical health concern. This paper addresses the question of whether the high number of women dying in pregnancy in Nigeria's referral hospitals might be associated with the inadequate number of healthcare providers (doctors, midwives and nurses) who attend large numbers of pregnant women.

The total number of healthcare providers (doctors, specialist doctors, nurses and midwives) working in eight referral hospitals during the period was calculated. The number of women who attend antenatal and delivery care in the hospitals was also calculated. We then calculated the ratio of the number of pregnant women attending antenatal and delivery care to the number of different categories of healthcare providers (doctors, nurses, midwives and specialist doctors). Finally, we performed additional statistical analysis and examined the relationship between the number of women who died during childbirth in hospitals and the ratio of clients per available healthcare provider. The results showed that the higher the ratio of clients/patients who were managed by doctors, nurses, midwives and specialist obstetricians and gynaecologists during antenatal and delivery care, the higher the maternal mortality ratio in the hospitals.

We conclude that the number of women who die during childbirth in Nigeria's referral hospitals is associated with the low number of healthcare providers. Efforts to increase the number of trained maternal healthcare providers, especially at the first referral level, is essential for reducing the currently high rate of maternal deaths in Nigeria.

Background

The high rate of maternal mortality in Nigeria is currently one of the most critical public health concerns in the country. The available data indicate that approximately 40,000 women die each year from preventable causes, with a maternal mortality rate of 814/100,000 births [1], accounting for 15% of the annual global estimates of maternal deaths [2]. Several factors have been offered to explain the high rate of maternal mortality in Nigeria. These include high rates of unwanted and mistimed pregnancies [3, 4], delays in treatment seeking pregnancy care [5, 6], low use of skilled birth attendants [7–9], and inadequate preparedness of the healthcare system to handle emergency obstetric complications [10–13].

However, to date, the readiness and adequacy of human resources in the country to address obstetric complications that lead to maternal mortality have not been systematically investigated. It is generally believed that the paucity of human resources and lack of training and

motivation buoyed by excessive workloads are responsible for poor quality obstetric care that leads to maternal deaths in women with pregnancy complications in hospitals. While there is anecdotal and qualitative research to confirm these assertions in many parts of Africa [14–18], limited quantitative studies have been conducted to test the association between the quantum of human resources and risk of maternal mortality.

The Nigerian healthcare system established primary healthcare centres to offer Basic Emergency Obstetric Care (BEmOC) according to the recommendations of the World Health Organization and to treat simple obstetric complications that do not warrant surgical operations. By contrast, secondary and tertiary care centres were established to offer Comprehensive Emergency Obstetric Care (CEmOC) to provide additional treatments, including blood transfusions and surgical operations. If the system works well, approximately 70% of emergency complications would be handled at the level of BEmoC, while only a limited fraction would seek CEmOC. However, due to the inadequate functioning of the country's primary healthcare system, most emergencies are often referred for CEmOC in referral hospitals, thereby increasing the workloads and limiting the quality of care provided in secondary and tertiary hospitals. With this limitation in mind, the relevant question is whether increased human resource provision at referral hospitals would have a restraining effect on the rates of maternal mortality in the country.

This study was designed to investigate the association between the density of healthcare providers (doctors, nurses and midwives) and risk of maternal deaths in Nigeria's referral hospitals. We tested the null hypothesis that an increased number of healthcare providers would have no effect on the maternal mortality ratios by investigating the density of healthcare personnel in eight referral hospitals and comparing it with the maternal mortality ratios in the hospitals. We believe that the results of this study will be useful for planning the allocation of the scarce human resources available for healthcare to address the high rate of maternal mortality in Nigeria.

Methods

The data for this study were obtained as part of the formative research for a study on assessing the nature and quality of emergency obstetric care for preventing maternal and perinatal mortality in eight secondary and tertiary hospitals in Nigeria. Nigeria's healthcare system is based on a 3-tier system: Primary Health Care (PHC) as the entry point; Secondary Care (regional/general hospitals) as the first referral level; and Tertiary Care (Teaching Hospitals) as the second referral level. In this study, eight referral hospitals (two tertiary and six secondary facilities) were selected from four of six geo-political zones of Nigeria. Administratively, Nigeria has 36 states and a Federal Capital Territory (Abuja). The states are further categorized into six zones: North-central, Northeast, Northwest, Southeast, South-south, and Southwest, with each zone predominantly consisting of people of a similar culture. Two tertiary hospitals were selected from the Northwest: Ahmadu Bello University Teaching Hospital, Kaduna and Aminu Kano Teaching Hospital, Kano. Secondary care facilities were selected from three other zones: General Hospital, Ijaye, Abeokuta and Adeoyo Maternity Hospital in the Southwest; General Hospital, Minna, Niger State and Karshi Hospital, Abuja in the North-central; and Central Hospital, Benin City and Central Hospital, Warri from the South-south. We did not select any referral hospitals from the Northeast zone because it is difficult to reach these hospitals because of the ongoing insurgency in the zone. To counterbalance the selection, we also failed to sample hospitals in the contiguous southeast zone. The hospitals that we selected were selected because they are the main referral hospitals in the respective states; they attend a large population of pregnant women in the main cities of the states, with none having fewer than 4500 total deliveries per year. A large proportion of women presented in labour at the hospitals as obstetric emergencies who had intended to deliver at home, in private clinics or in the homes of traditional birth/faith-based birth attendants, but then came late to the hospitals when they experienced complications. These types of deliveries constitute approximately 50% of cases in the hospitals, accounting for an average of 150 obstetric emergencies per month per hospital. All of the hospitals are funded either by the respective states or the federal government, which means that the hospital staffing policies are also overseen by governmental departments.

Because this was a formative study leading to the design of a larger intervention, we chose pairs of states with catchment populations with similar socio-demographic characteristics to adequately represent a quasi-experimental research design. Thus, we first chose the largest referral hospitals in four states. Based on our knowledge of the ecology of the use of maternal health services, we hypothesized that secondary referral hospitals (General hospitals) have a larger uptake of obstetric emergencies, have fewer healthcare providers, and therefore have increased numbers of maternal deaths. For this reason, we sampled three secondary referral hospitals compared to only one tertiary hospital (teaching hospital). In the second stage of sampling, we chose comparative main referral hospitals in adjoining states different from the states in which the initial selections were made. The purpose was to eliminate the effect of intervention contamination if we implement the intervention at a later stage. We decided to choose teaching hospitals from the northern part of the country

because of the reported higher numbers of deliveries and maternal deaths in northern Nigeria hospitals compared to the southern part of the country. The Aminu Kano Teaching Hospital is one of the busiest teaching hospitals in Nigeria, located in Kano State, northern Nigeria, and was identified in the first stage of sampling. For comparison, we then identified the Ahmadu Bello University, Zaria, which is also a busy teaching hospital located in the contiguous state of Kaduna.

Information on the number of doctors, nurses, midwives, clients reporting for antenatal care, number of births and number of maternal deaths were obtained from each hospital for the three-year period (1 January 2011 to 31 December 2013) preceding the formative research, which was conducted between 1 January 2014 to 30 June 2014. Each participating hospital was visited, and a pre-tested study protocol was used to elicit the relevant information regarding the number of healthcare workers, deliveries, and maternal deaths during the period. The numbers of antenatal care attendees, births and maternal deaths were aggregated for the 3 years to derive the average attendees, births and maternal deaths for the period.

Ethical approval

Ethical approval for the study was obtained from the World Health Organization and the National Health Research Ethics Committee (NHREC) of Nigeria – number NHREC/01/01/2007–16/07/2014, renewed in 2015 with NHREC 01/01/20047–12/12/2015b. The Chief Medical Directors and Heads of Departments of the hospitals women were informed of the purpose of the study, and consent was obtained from the patients to conduct the study. Patients were assured that their information would be confidential. Only the hospitals that agreed to participate in the fully explained study were enlisted in the study. No names or specific contact information were obtained from the study participants.

Analytical strategy

Ratios was used to express the density of antenatal care (ANC) attendees to a provider and the number of births to a provider. Given that the quality of maternal health care provided in a hospital is a function of contributions from various departments, ratios were calculated for the following seven categories of providers: 1) all providers in the hospital consisting of all doctors in the Department of Obstetrics and Gynaecology, including specialist obstetricians, nurses/midwives, doctors and nurses in other departments in the hospital; 2) all doctors, consisting of doctors in the Department of Obstetrics and Gynaecology, specialist obstetricians, and doctors in other departments; 3) all nurses and midwives, including nurses only, nurses/midwives and midwives in the entire hospital; 4) all providers in the maternity department (mproviders), including doctors in the Department of Obstetrics and Gynaecology, specialist obstetricians, nurses/midwives and midwives; 5) all doctors in the maternity department (mdoctors), including doctors in the Obstetrics and Gynaecology Department and specialist obstetricians; 6) specialist obstetricians only; and 7) trained midwives, including nurses/midwifes and midwives. The maternal mortality ratio (MMR) was calculated per 100,000 live births. Unadjusted Poisson regression analysis was used to examine the association between the number of maternal deaths and number of providers. The Poisson regression models are best suited for count variables, such as the number of deaths. The results are presented as the incidence rate ratio (IRR), with the level of significance set at $p < 0.05$ and the marginal significance set at $p < 0.10$ because of the small sample size. A two-tailed Pearson product moment correlation was used to examine the statistical association between the births-provider ratio, ANC attendee-provider ratio and maternal mortality ratio, and the results are presented as correlation coefficients (r) with the level of significance set at $p < 0.05$. All analyses relating to maternal deaths were conducted using data from seven of eight hospitals because data on maternal deaths were not available in Karshi General Hospital, Abuja.

Results

The distribution of all providers as percentages, numbers and the average number of maternal deaths is shown in Table 1. The results of the unadjusted Poisson regression of the number of maternal deaths and number of

providers are presented in Table 2. The MMR is shown in Fig. 1. Table 3 presents the ratio of births to a provider (births-provider ratio) and average number of births, while the ANC attendees-provider ratio and average number of ANC attendees are shown in Table 4 with the associated Pearson correlation coefficients.

Distribution of healthcare providers and the average number of maternal deaths by facility

There was a total of 3754 providers in the 8 hospitals, of which 1387 (36.9%) were doctors and 2367 (63.1%) were nurses and midwives. The maternal healthcare providers (mdoctors and midwives) constituted 46.8% (1758) of all of the providers. The distribution varied widely across facilities. More than half (63.4%) of all providers were in the two teaching hospitals (Aminu Kano Teaching hospital, Kano and Ahmadu Bello University Teaching hospital, Kaduna), while Karshi General Hospital had the least number of providers. The largest number of mproviders (41.2%) was in Ahmadu Bello Teaching hospital, while Karshi General Hospital, Abuja had the smallest number of providers. There was a total of 60 specialist obstetricians in all of the facilities, with only one in Karshi General Hospital, Abuja, 2 in General Hospital Minna and 2 in State Hospital Ijaye, Abeokuta.

On average, 334,425 women received antenatal care in the 8 facilities during the three-year period (Table 4), while an average of 26,479 (Table 3) births occurred over the same period. Expressing the number of births as a percentage of the number of ANC attendees indicates that fewer than 10% of women who received ANC in the 8 facilities delivered in the facilities. However, there were

Table 1 Percentage Distribution of Health Care Providers and average maternal deaths by Facility

Facility	All providers	All doctors	All nurses & midwives	Doctors in Obs/Gyn	Specialist Obstetricians	mdoctors	Midwives	mproviders	Average mdeath
Adeoyo Maternity Hospital, Ibadan	6.5 (245)	2.9 (40)	8.7 (205)	9.0 (17)	6.7 (4)	8.4 (21)	12.9 (195)	12.3 (216)	3.8 (6)
General Hospital, Minna	9.4 (351)	3.7 (52)	12.6 (299)	4.2 (8)	3.3 (2)	4.0 (10)	11.6 (175)	10.5 (185)	27.2 (43)
Aminu Kano Teaching Hospital, Kano	26.0 (977)	28.8 (400)	24.4 (577)	26.5 (50)	28.3 (17)	26.9 (67)	6.5 (98)	9.4 (165)	13.3 (21)
Ahmadu Bello University Teaching Hospital, Zaria	37.4 (1405)	49.4 (685)	30.4 (720)	28.6 (54)	36.7 (22)	30.5 (76)	42.9 (648)	41.2 (724)	6.3 (10)
State Hospital, Ijaye Abeokuta	5.2 (195)	3.2 (45)	6.3 (150)	5.8 (11)	3.3 (2)	5.2 (13)	5.6 (85)	5.6 (98)	3.2 (5)
Karshi General Hospital, Abuja	1,9 (73)	1.2 (17)	2.4 (56)	7.4 (14)	1.7 (1)	6.0 (15)	2.7 (41)	3.2 (56)	N/A
Central Hospital, Warri	5.3 (198)	4.9 (68)	5.5 (130)	9.0 (17)	6.7 (4)	8.4 (21)	7.7 (117)	7.8 (138)	8.9 (14)
Central Hospital, Benin City	8.3 (310)	5.8 (80)	9.7 (230)	9.5 (18)	13.3 (8)	10.4 (26)	9.9 (150)	10.0 (176)	37.3 (59)
Total	100 (3754)	1387	2367	189	60	249	1509	1758	158

IRR – Incidence Rate Ratio

All providers refer to all doctors, nurses and midwives in the entire hospital; All doctors refer to all doctors in all the departments in the entire hospital; All nurses and midwives refer to all nurses and midwives in the entire hospital; mdoctors refers to doctors in Obstetrics and Gynaecology department and specialists obstetricians; mproviders refers to doctors in Obstetrics and Gynecology Departments, specialist Obstetricians and midwives; mdeath refers to maternal deaths

Table 2 Unadjusted Incidence Rate Ratios (and 95% confidence intervals) from Poisson regression analyses examining association between number of providers and number of maternal deaths

Type of provider	IRR	CI
All Providers	0.999**	0.999–1.000
All Doctors	0.998***	0.998–0.999
All Nurses & Midwives	0.999	0.999–1.000
Doctors in Obstetrics & Gynaecology Department	0.986***	0.980–0.992
Specialist Obstetricians	0.985*	0.973–0.998
Trained Midwives	0.998***	0.998–0.999
Doctors in Obstetrics & Gynaecology Department & Specialists Obstetricians	0.992***	0.988–0.996
All maternal providers	0.998***	0.998–0.999

Note: Significance-level (two-tailed): * $p < .05$, ** $p < .01$, *** $p < .001$. IRR – Incidence Rate Ratio; CI – 95% Confidence Interval

variations across the facilities. For instance, births in Adeoyo Maternity Hospital and General Hospital, Minna occurred for over 50% of the ANC attendees, whereas births in Central Hospital, Benin City occurred for 1.8% of the ANC attendees. Of the 25,587 live births in 7 facilities with a record of maternal deaths, an average of 158 maternal deaths was recorded, giving a maternal mortality ratio of 617 per 100,000 live births. The distribution across the hospitals (Fig. 1) shows that Central Hospital, Benin City recorded the highest MMR of 1469 per 100,000 live births, whereas the smallest MMR was found for Adeoyo Maternity Hospital, Ibadan (177/100,000 live births).

Unadjusted Poisson regression analysis (Table 2) showed a significant negative association between the number of maternal deaths and the number of healthcare providers. The incidence of maternal death would be expected to decrease significantly by a factor of 0.999 ($p < 0.01$) for a unit increase in the number of all providers. An increase in the number of all doctors will decrease the incidence of maternal death by a factor of 0.998 ($p < 0.001$), and an increase in the number of nurses and midwives is expected to decrease maternal death, although with marginal statistical significance (0.999 $p < 0.10$). Increasing the number of doctors in the Department of Obstetrics and Gynaecology who are not specialist obstetricians would significantly decrease the incidence of maternal death (IRR, 0.986; $p < 0.001$). With a unit increase in the number of specialist obstetricians, the IRR of maternal death would decrease (IRR, 0.985; $p < 0.05$). Increasing the number of all doctors in the maternity department, including specialist obstetricians is expected to decrease maternal death by a factor of 0.992 ($p < 0.001$), and a one-unit increase in the number of midwives will reduce maternal death (IRR, 0.998; $p < 0.001$). Increasing the number of all providers in the maternity department (mproviders) by one unit would significantly decrease maternal death (IRR, 0.998; $p < 0.001$).

Births-provider ratio

The ratio of births to all providers was 7:1, with variation across the facilities. The smallest births-all provider ratio was at the Ahmadu Bello Teaching Hospital, Zaria, where the ratio was 1:1, whereas the highest ratio was found in Central hospital, Warri, with 22 births to a provider. The ratio of births to all doctors was 19:1 and 11:1 for all nurses and midwives, respectively. Again, the smallest ratio was in Ahmadu Bello University Teaching

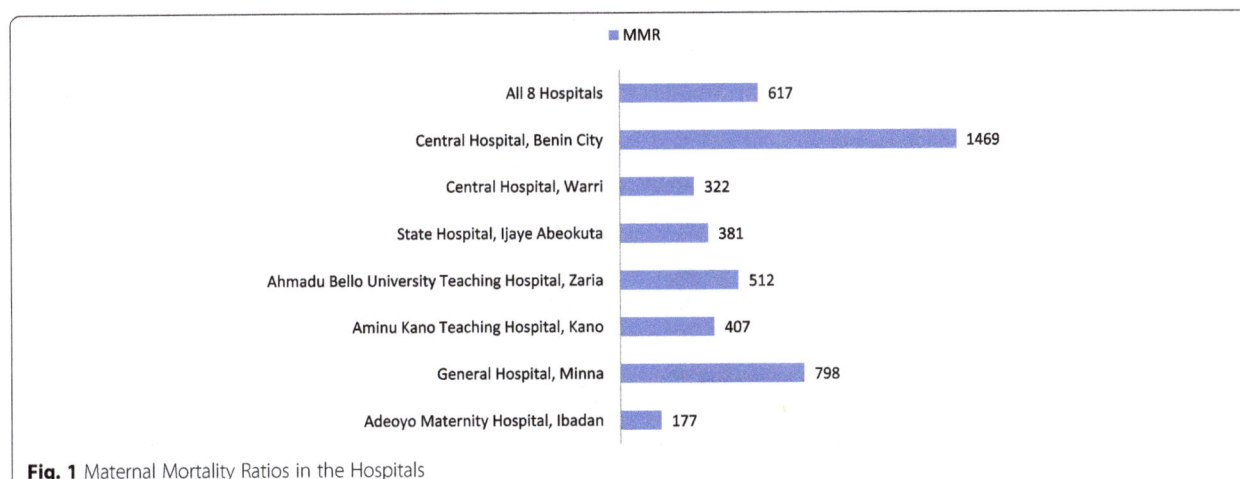

Fig. 1 Maternal Mortality Ratios in the Hospitals

Table 3 Births: Providers ratio and average number of births

Hospital	All providers	All doctors	All nurses & midwives	Specialist Obstetricians	mDoctors	Midwives	mProviders	Average births %(n)
Adeoyo Maternity Hospital, Ibadan	14	85	17	850	162	17	16	12.8 (3399)
General Hospital, Minna	15	104	18	2695	539	31	29	20.4 (5389)
Aminu Kano Teaching Hospital	5	13	9	304	77	53	31	19.5 (5164)
Ahmadu Bello University Teaching Hospital, Zaria	1	3	3	89	26	3	3	7.4 (1955)
State Hospital, Ijaye Abeokuta	7	29	9	657	101	15	13	4.9 (1314)
Karshi General Hospital, Abuja	12	52	16	892	59	22	16	3.4 (892)
Central Hospital, Warri	22	64	33	1087	207	37	32	16.4 (4349)
Central Hospital, Benin City	13	50	17	502	155	27	23	15.2 (4017)
All 8 Hospitals	7	19	11	441	106	18	15	26,479
Pearson Correlation Coefficient (r)	0.060	0.080	0.001	0.095	0.228	0.043	0.134	

All providers refer to all doctors, nurses and midwives in the entire hospital; All doctors refer to all doctors in all the departments in the entire hospital; All nurses and midwives refer to all nurses and midwives in the entire hospital; mdoctors refers to doctors in Obstetrics and Gynaecology department and specialists Obstetricians; mproviders refers to doctors in Obstetrics and Gynaecology Departments, specialist Obstetricians and midwives

Hospital, whereas the highest was in Central hospital, Warri. There were 441 births per specialist obstetrician, for a ratio of 2695:1 in General Hospital, Minna and 1087:1 in Central Hospital, Warri. The ratio of births to one doctor was 106 compared to 18:1 for midwives. Correlating the births to provider ratios to MMR showed a positive statistical association, indicating that as the birth to provider ratio increased, the number of maternal deaths increased; however, the results were not statistically significant.

ANC attendee-provider ratio

The ANC attendee to all provider ratio was 89:1, with Central Hospital, Benin City recording the highest ratio of 727 attendees to one provider. The ratio of ANC attendees to a specialist obstetrician was 5574:1; only Ahmadu Bello Teaching Hospital had a ratio below 1000:1. The ratio was 190 attendees to a provider. Disaggregating providers into doctors and midwives showed a ratio of 1343 ANC attendees to a doctor and 222 attendees to one midwife. The smallest ANC attendee-maternal healthcare provider ratio was in Ahmadu Bello Hospital, Zaria, with 14 ANC attendees to an provider, and the largest ratio was in Benin, with 1281 attendees to a provider. Although the births-provider ratio is more critical for maternal mortality, the ANC attendee-provider ratio speaks to the quality of ANC care, which is a risk factor for MMR. If the ratio is high, providers may not be able to provide optimal care, thus exposing more women to the risk of maternal death. The

Table 4 ANC Attendees: Providers ratio and average number of ANC Attendees

Hospital	All providers	All doctors	All nurses & midwives	Specialist Obstetricians	mDoctors	Midwives	mProviders	Average ANC attendees %(n)
Adeoyo Maternity Hospital, Ibadan	23	141	28	1413	269	29	26	1.7 (5651)
General Hospital, Minna	28	190	33	4939	988	56	53	2.9 (9877)
Aminu Kano Teaching Hospital	32	77	54	1821	462	316	188	9.3 (30963)
Ahmadu Bello University Teaching Hospital, Zaria	7	15	14	460	133	16	14	3.0 (10118)
State Hospital, Ijaye Abeokuta	91	396	119	8905	1370	210	182	5.3 (17810)
Karshi General Hospital, Abuja	34	145	44	2472	165	60	44	0.7 (2472)
Central Hospital, Warri	162	472	247	8017	1527	274	232	9.6 (32066)
Central Hospital, Benin City	727	2818	980	28,183	8672	1503	1281	67.4 (225467)
All 8 Hospitals	89	241	141	5574	1343	222	190	334,425
Pearson Correlation Coefficient (r)	0.851*	0.870*	0.841*	0.847*	0.890*	0.848*	0.858*	

Note: Significance-level (two-tailed): *$p < .05$
All providers refer to all doctors, nurses and midwives in the entire hospital; All doctors refer to all doctors in all the departments in the entire hospital; All nurses and midwives refer to all nurses and midwives in the entire hospital; mdoctors refers to doctors in Obstetrics and Gynaecology department and specialists Obstetricians; mproviders refers to doctors in Obstetrics and Gynaecology Departments, specialist Obstetricians and midwives

correlation coefficients were all positive and significant, indicating that the higher ANC attendee to provider ratio increased MMR.

Discussion

The study was designed to investigate the association between the client-provider ratios in Nigeria's referral hospitals and maternal deaths in the hospitals. We specifically studied how the number and density of maternal healthcare providers in hospitals predict the likelihood of maternal deaths. To the best of our knowledge, this study is one of the first to quantitatively investigate this relationship, especially in regions with high rates of maternal death. Although there is evidence in the global literature that the increased density of human resources (especially nurses, specialists and non-specialist doctors) reduces maternal, infant and child mortality [19, 20], there has been limited specific investigation in many African countries aimed at testing this relationship.

Contrary to our null hypothesis, the results of this study showed that there was a significant negative association between the number of maternal deaths and total number of providers in the hospital. We found that the incidence of maternal death significantly decreases by a factor of 0.985–0.999 with a unit increase in the number of providers of any category. This is not surprising because prevention of maternal death in a referral hospital is the responsibility of all providers working together in different departments, especially the obstetrics and gynaecology, nursing/midwifery, pathological sciences, paediatrics, medicine and surgical departments. The number of maternal deaths also showed a negative correlation with the total number of maternal healthcare providers (doctors and midwives) working in the maternal sections of the hospitals, further emphasizing the importance of a high density of providers in preventing maternal deaths in the referral hospitals.

Pregnant women receiving antenatal and intrapartum care is also a major determinant of survival. It was noteworthy that only approximately 10% of women who initially received antenatal care returned for delivery at the same hospitals. This relationship was particularly severe in the General Hospitals, especially at the Central Hospital, Benin City, fewer than 2% of women who received antenatal care returned for delivery care at the same hospital. It was not surprising, therefore, that the Central Hospital, Benin City had the highest number and ratio of maternal deaths. Although the data were not disaggregated by the booking status of women, it appears that hospitals (especially the Central Hospital) mainly attended women who had not received antenatal care, but who turned up at the time of delivery or when they experienced complications. Although a tertiary

referral hospital, the Ahmadu Bello University Teaching Hospital had only 50% of its antenatal attendees return for delivery care, which probably accounted for its lower maternal mortality ratios compared to the other hospitals. Future research is needed to address this bottleneck, especially to understand why women who received antenatal care in a particular hospital failed to return for delivery at the same hospital. Clearly, focusing on ways to retain women who receive antenatal care to deliver at the same hospital is an important intervention for preventing maternal deaths in hospitals.

The results of this study show a positive and significant correlation between a higher ANC attendee to provider ratio and increases in MMR, suggesting that higher numbers of antenatal care providers would significantly reduce the likelihood of maternal mortality. Similarly, although the results were not statistically significant, there was a positive association between higher birth to provider ratios and increases in the ratios of maternal mortality in the hospitals. Increasing women's access to skilled birth facilities has been identified as an effective intervention to reduce maternal deaths [21, 22] in developing countries. The results of this study suggest that an adequate number of healthcare providers working in referral hospitals is also important if women who seek emergency obstetric care in referral hospitals are to be offered the best chance of survival. The results of this study reveal that all of the indicators of human resources for maternal health (the number of total providers and providers and client-provider ratios) were better for the Teaching Hospitals (Ahmadu Bello University Teaching Hospital and the Aminu Kano Teaching Hospital) compared to General (Central) Hospitals. In Nigeria's healthcare system, Teaching Hospitals are the second referral level for maternal health care, while General Hospitals are supposed to function as the first referral level. Unfortunately, the system does not work this way as Teaching and General Hospitals are often used simultaneously for both primary care as well to treat complications. Although both types of hospitals perform similar tasks with respect to maternal health care, General Hospitals have not received a concomitant level of funding and human resource support, which accounts for the poorer human resource outcomes reported for these hospitals. Thus, we believe that if positive results are to be obtained for reducing maternal deaths in women referred for comprehensive emergency obstetric care in Nigerian referral hospitals, efforts must be made to improve the human resource situation in General Hospitals.

The results of this study are consistent with the findings of our previous qualitative studies [23], which reported that women attending these hospitals perceived that maternal mortality and poor obstetric outcomes in these hospitals are due to heavy workloads experienced by healthcare providers. Our recent study also reported long wait and contact times experienced by women receiving antenatal care in these hospitals [24], which is indicative of the diminished numbers of healthcare providers attending women in the hospitals. Thus, we believe that efforts focused on increasing the number of healthcare providers in maternal care centres would improve the quality of care and reduce the maternal mortality ratios.

The major strength of this study is the use of data from hospitals in four of the six geo-political zones of the country. We were unable to obtain data from the Northeast zone of the country because of the on-going insurgency, which limited our access to referral hospitals in that part of the country. We believed that the results from the Northeast zone would be difficult to compare with the other zones in the country because of the likelihood that women would be self-selective in receiving maternal health care during emergency situations as are currently being witnessed in the zone. We failed to sample women from the Southeast zone to balance the representation and ensure that equal hospitals and women from the northern and southern parts of the country were represented in the sample. Thus, the results of the study are generalizable to the entire country and can be interpreted for policymaking at the national and subnational levels. However, one major limitation of this study is the retrospective study design. Because of the poor data archival and retrieval systems in many hospitals in Nigeria, it is likely that retrospective data collection will be fraught with errors. To overcome this limitation, we used a double data collection method in which two sets of data collectors obtained data from each of the hospitals. The data were further cross-checked with the existing hospital records (in the Records Departments of the Hospitals), and specific case records were reviewed when discrepancies existed. Thus, we believe that the data are substantially accurate and are useful for investigating and resolving the research question.

Conclusions

We conclude that the maternal mortality ratios in Nigeria's referral hospitals are worsened by high client provider ratios, with few providers attending a large number of pregnant women experiencing complications. This situation is more severe in General Hospitals (first referral hospitals) compared to Teaching Hospitals (second referral hospitals). Efforts to improve the quantum of maternal healthcare providers, especially at the first referral level, and build their capacity to deliver effective care represents a critical intervention for reducing the currently high rate of maternal mortality in Nigeria.

Abbreviations

ANC: Antenatal care; BEmOC: Basic Emergency Obstetric Care; CEmOC: Comprehensive Emergency Obstetric Care; FMOH: Federal Ministry of Health; MMR: Maternal Mortality Ratio; MNCH: Maternal Newborn Child Health; NHREC: National Health Research Ethics Committee of Nigeria; PHC: Primary Health Care; WHARC: The Women's Health and Action Research Centre; WHO: World Health Organization

Acknowledgements

We are grateful to Dr. Taiwo Oyelade and Dr. Mariana Widmer of the Nigeria and Geneva offices of the WHO for their support of the study.

Funding

The project was funded, in part, by the Alliance for Health Policy and Systems Research, World Health Organization (WHO), Geneva through its program on improving implementation research on maternal health in developing countries, Protocol ID A65869. The WHO had no role in the design of the study and in the collection, analysis, and interpretation of data and in the writing of the manuscript.

Authors' contributions

FO conceived the research, supervised all phases of the study, and drafted the manuscript. LN coordinated the data analysis. RO coordinated the research at the 8 study sites; HG, RA, MG, OO, KA, AE, AD, and AR were the individual site supervisors. All of the authors participated in the design and implementation of the study. All of the authors meet the 3 ICMJE authorship criteria. All of the authors have read and approved the final manuscript.

Competing interests

The authors declare that they have no competing interests.

Author details

[1]University of Medical Sciences, Ondo City, Ondo State, Nigeria. [2]the Women's Health and Action Research Centre, WHO Implementation Research Group, Benin City, Nigeria. [3]Centre of Excellence in Reproductive Health Innovation, University of Benin, Benin City, Nigeria. [4]Department of Demography and Social Statistics, Federal University Oye-Ekiti, Oye, Ekiti State, Nigeria. [5]Department of Obstetrics and Gynaecology, University of Port Harcourt, Port Harcourt, Rivers State, Nigeria. [6]Aminu Kano Teaching Hospital, Kano, Nigeria. [7]Adeoyo Maternity Hospital, Ibadan, Oyo State, Nigeria. [8]General Hospital, Minna, Niger State, Nigeria. [9]Karshi General Hospital, Federal Capital Territory, Abuja, Nigeria. [10]Central Hospital, Warri, Delta State, Nigeria. [11]Central Hospital, Benin City, Edo State, Nigeria. [12]General Hospital, Ijaye Abeokuta, Ogun State, Nigeria. [13]Ahmadu Bello University, Zaria, Kaduna State, Nigeria.

References

1. Alkema L, Zhang S, Chou D, Gemmill A, Moller A-B, Fat DM, et al. A Bayesian approach to the global estimation of maternal mortality. ArXiv151103330 Stat [Internet]. 2015 Nov 10 [cited 2016 Aug 15]; Available from: http://arxiv.org/abs/1511.03330.

2. World Health Organization. WHO | Trends in maternal mortality: 1990 to 2015 [Internet]. WHO. 2015 [cited 2017 Jul 29]. Available from: http://www.who.int/reproductivehealth/publications/monitoring/maternal-mortality-2015/en/.

3. Say L, Chou D, Gemmill A, Tunçalp Ö, Moller A-B, Daniels J, et al. Global causes of maternal death: a WHO systematic analysis. Lancet Glob Health. 2014 Jun 1;2(6):e323–33.

4. Bauserman M, Lokangaka A, Thorsten V, Tshefu A, Goudar SS, Esamai F, et al. Risk factors for maternal death and trends in maternal mortality in low- and middle-income countries: a prospective longitudinal cohort analysis. Reprod Health. 2015;12(Suppl 2):S5.

5. Okonofua F, Ogu R, Agholor K, Okike O, Abdus-salam R, Gana M, et al. Qualitative assessment of women's satisfaction with maternal health care in referral hospitals in Nigeria. Reprod Health. 2017;14:44.

6. Okonofua FE, Abejide A, Makanjuola RA. Maternal mortality in Ile-Ife, Nigeria: a study of risk factors. Stud Fam Plan. 1992;23(5):319–24.

7. Anastasi E, Borchert M, Campbell OMR, Sondorp E, Kaducu F, Hill O, et al. Losing women along the path to safe motherhood: why is there such a gap between women's use of antenatal care and skilled birth attendance? A mixed methods study in northern Uganda. BMC Pregnancy Childbirth. 2015;15:287.

8. Adegoke A, Utz B, Msuya SE, van den Broek N. Skilled birth attendants: who is who? A descriptive study of definitions and roles from nine sub Saharan African countries. PLoS One. 2012;7(7):e40220.

9. Okonofua F, Ogu R. Traditional versus birth attendants in provision of maternity care: call for paradigm shift. Afr J Reprod Health. 2014 Mar;18(1):11–5.

10. Okonofua F, Randawa A, Ogu R, Agholor K, Okike O, Abdus-salam RA, et al. Views of senior health personnel about quality of emergency obstetric care: a qualitative study in Nigeria. PLoS One. 2017 Mar 27;12(3):e0173414.

11. Hussein J, Hirose A, Owolabi O, Imamura M, Kanguru L, Okonofua F. Maternal death and obstetric care audits in Nigeria: a systematic review of barriers and enabling factors in the provision of emergency care. Reprod Health. 2016;13(1):47.

12. Oladapo OT, Adetoro OO, Ekele BA, Chama C, Etuk SJ, Aboyeji AP, et al. When getting there is not enough: a nationwide cross-sectional study of 998 maternal deaths and 1451 near-misses in public tertiary hospitals in a low-income country. BJOG Int J Obstet Gynaecol. 2016 May;123(6):928–38.

13. Akeju DO, Oladapo OT, Vidler M, Akinmade AA, Sawchuck D, Qureshi R, et al. Determinants of health care seeking behaviour during pregnancy in Ogun state, Nigeria. Reprod Health. 2016 Jun 8;13(Suppl 1):32.

14. Abawi K, Chandra-Mouli V, Toskin I, Festin MP, Gertiser L, Idris R, et al. E-learning for research capacity strengthening in sexual and reproductive health: the experience of the Geneva Foundation for Medical Education and Research and the Department of Reproductive Health and Research, World Health Organization. Hum Resour Health. 2016;14:76.

15. Crofts JF, Ellis D, Draycott TJ, Winter C, Hunt LP, Akande VA. Change in knowledge of midwives and obstetricians following obstetric emergency training: a randomised controlled trial of local hospital, simulation centre and teamwork training. BJOG. 2007;114:1534.

16. Cometto G, Tulenko K, Muula AS, Krech R. Health workforce brain drain: from denouncing the challenge to solving the problem. PLoS Med. 2013 Sep 17;10(9):e1001514.

17. Onyango-Ouma W, Laisser R, Mbilima M, Araoye M, Pittman P, Agyepong I. An evaluation of Health Workers for Change in seven settings: a useful management and health system development tool. Health Policy Plan [Internet]. 2001;16. Available from: https://doi.org/10.1093/heapol/16.suppl_1.24.

18. Uzondu CA, Doctor HV, Findley SE, Afenyadu GY, Ager A. Female health Workers at the Doorstep: a pilot of community-based maternal, newborn, and child health service delivery in northern Nigeria. Glob Health Sci Pract. 2015 Mar 2;3(1):97–108.

19. Murphy GT, Goma F, MacKenzie A, Bradish S, Price S, Nzala S, et al. A scoping review of training and deployment policies for human resources for health for maternal, newborn, and child health in rural Africa. Hum Resour Health. 2014 Dec 16;12:72.

20. Gupta N, Maliqi B, França A, Nyonator F, Pate MA, Sanders D, et al. Human resources for maternal, newborn and child health: from measurement and planning to performance for improved health outcomes. Hum Resour Health 2011 Jun 24;9:16.

21. Gülmezoglu AM, Lawrie TA, Hezelgrave N, Oladapo OT, Souza JP, Gielen M, et al. Interventions to Reduce Maternal and Newborn Morbidity and Mortality. In: Black RE, Laxminarayan R, Temmerman M, Walker N, editors. Reproductive, Maternal, Newborn, and Child Health: Disease Control Priorities, Third Edition (Volume 2) [Internet]. Washington (DC): The International Bank for Reconstruction and Development/The World Bank; 2016 [cited 2017 Jul 29]. Available from: http://www.ncbi.nlm.nih.gov/books/NBK361904/.

22. Dumont A, Fournier P, Abrahamowicz M, Traore M, Haddad S, Fraser WD. Quality of care, risk management, and technology in obstetrics to reduce hospital-based maternal mortality in Senegal and Mali (QUARITE): a cluster-randomised trial. Lancet [Internet]. 2013;382. Available from: https://doi.org/10.1016/S0140-6736(13)60593-0.

23. Ogu RN, Ntoimo LF, Okonofua FE. Perceptions of Nigerian women on workloads in maternity hospitals and its effect on maternal health care. Midwifery. 2017;55(12):1–6.

24. Okonofua FE, Ogu RN, Ntoimo LF, Gana M, Okike O, Durodola A, et al. Where do delays occur when women receive antenatal care in referral hospitals in Nigeria? A client flow multi-site study. Ghana Med. J. nn51(3):In press.

15

Too afraid to go: fears of dignity violations as reasons for non-use of maternal health services

Sumit Kane[1,2]* [iD], Matilda Rial[3], Maryse Kok[1], Anthony Matere[4], Marjolein Dieleman[1,5] and Jacqueline E. W. Broerse[5]

Abstract

Background: South Sudan has one of the worst health and maternal health situations in the world. Across South Sudan, while maternal health services at the primary care level are not well developed, even where they exist, many women do not use them. Developing location specific understanding of what hinders women from using services is key to developing and implementing locally appropriate public health interventions.

Methods: A qualitative study was conducted to gain insight into what hinders women from using maternal health services. Focus group discussions (5) and interviews (44) were conducted with purposefully selected community members and health personnel. A thematic analysis was done to identify key themes.

Results: While accessibility, affordability, and perceptions (need and quality of care) related barriers to the use of maternal health services exist and are important, women's decisions to use services are also shaped by a variety of social fears. Societal interactions entailed in the process of going to a health facility, interactions with other people, particularly other women on the facility premises, and the care encounters with health workers, are moments where women are afraid of experiencing dignity violations. Women's decisions to step out of their homes to seek maternal health care are the results of a complex trade-off they make or are willing to make between potential threats to their dignity in the various social spaces they need to traverse in the process of seeking care, their views on ownership of and responsibility for the unborn, and the benefits they ascribe to the care available to them.

Conclusions: Geographical accessibility, affordability, and perceptions related barriers to the use of maternal health services in South Sudan remain; they need to be addressed. Explicit attention also needs to be paid to address social accessibility related barriers; among others, to identify, address and allay the various social fears and fears of dignity violations that may hold women back from using services. Health services should work towards transforming health facilities into social spaces where all women's and citizen's dignity is protected and upheld.

Keywords: Maternal Health Services, South Sudan, Service Utilization, Dignity, Social Fears, Social Accessibility

Plain language summary

Years of conflict have led to South Sudan having one of the worst health and maternal health situations in the world. While health services are being slowly rebuilt, many people, including pregnant women, do not use the available services. This study shows that women's decisions to use available services were not merely about whether they were aware of risks involved in pregnancy and childbirth, or about whether the services were reachable, affordable or of good quality. We found that in South Sudan, the social norm is that a pregnant woman is expected to be well taken care of, and should be seen to be well taken care of, by her man and his family; the appearance of being well taken care of, socially dignifies the woman's pregnancy. In view of this, a woman's decision to seek care during pregnancy and childbirth also depended upon whether in the process of stepping out of her home to go and use services, her

* Correspondence: Sumit.Kane@unimelb.edu.au
[1]KIT Royal Tropical Institute, Mauritskade 63, Amsterdam 1092 AD, The Netherlands
[2]Nossal Institute for Global Health, Melbourne School of Population and Global Health, University of Melbourne, Level 5, 333 Exhibition Street, Melbourne, VIC 3010, Australia
Full list of author information is available at the end of the article

dignity as a pregnant woman could be maintained and protected - from the judging eyes of society, from other women in the health facility, and while interacting with health workers. Her decision thus also depended upon a complex trade-off she was willing to make between the benefits she thought the care would bring to her, and the potential risks to her social dignity. Explicit attention also needs to be paid to identify, address and allay the fears of dignity violations that may hold women back from using maternal health services in South Sudan.

Background

South Sudan has one of the world's worst population health indicators; for instance, the maternal mortality ratio stands at 789/100,000 live births [1], less than 30% of women are attended to by a skilled health worker; and the rate of institutional delivery assisted by a skilled birth attendant is less than 20% [2]. In post-conflict contexts, healthcare provision and improving population health outcomes is particularly difficult because of poor infrastructure, limited human resources, and weak stewardship [3–5]. In South Sudan too, the long drawn conflict has weakened the health system, and there are severe shortages of health workers and few well-functioning health facilities [2, 8]. De Francisco A et al. [6], drawing on the International Covenant on Economic, Social and Cultural Rights [7], argue that for public health programs to be useful to and to be used by the people they mean to serve, one "requires location-specific investigations" ([6], pg.19–20). In a recent review of maternal and child health policies in South Sudan, Mugo et al. [8] noted that "Informing policy with evidence requires acute sensitivity to local context"; in a subsequent paper, they further emphasize the need to "address the socio-economic factors that prevent women from using maternal health services" in South Sudan [9]. This paper presents the findings of such an investigation from South Sudan; it complements the recent work by Mugo et al. [10], Wilunda et al. [11], Lawry et al. [12] on barriers to maternal health in South Sudan.

This paper reports findings from a study done within the context of a project designed to support the Ministry of Health (MoH) of Western Bahr el Ghazal (WBeG) state of South Sudan to improve sexual and reproductive health (SRH) service delivery. There is robust evidence that "A health centre, intrapartum-care strategy can be justified as the best bet to bring down high rates of maternal mortality" [13]; the project, among other things, explicitly focused on improving access to and use of maternal health services. Within the operational research component of the project, a range of questions regarding SRH related behaviors and decision making were identified and studied; one of them being 'why inspite of

having maternal health services in the vicinity, many women still do not use the maternal health services?'

Findings from the broader study are reported in earlier papers which report how social norms and gender norms shape procreation decisions, birth spacing and family planning related decisions in South Sudan [14, 15]. Wilunda et al. [11] and Lawry et al. [12] in their recently published papers, elaborate upon geographical, financial, security and cultural barriers to the use of maternity services in South Sudan. These barriers also featured prominently in our study findings; however, we also identified other 'social' reasons why many women, do not use, or hesitate to use, the maternal health services currently on offer in Wau county of WBeG state of South Sudan. In this paper we focus on these 'social accessibility' [16] related barriers. We do so to highlight the importance of this important dimension of health services accessibility; in the process, we propose the notion of 'social accessibility' and contribute to extend the understanding of what all 'health services accessibility' should entail.

Methods

A qualitative study was conducted; data was collected through focus group discussions (FGDs) and semi-structured interviews (SSIs) conducted with a variety of purposefully selected informants, as detailed in Table 1. Following sections further explain the sampling and recruitment principles and processes.

Topic guides for FGDs and SSIs were developed using de Francisco et al.'s (6) conceptual framework. According to the framework, individuals and social groups occupy positions of relative advantage or disadvantage with respect to their access to resources (social and material), within overlapping spheres of influence: the household, community, larger society, and the political environment. Individual's and social groups' position and relations in these overlapping spheres of influence shape their SRH related decisions and actions. Topic guides for community members included questions exploring people's expectations from, and reasons for (non-)use of maternal health services. The topic guides for health and other workers included questions on the same lines, but with a view to explore their perspectives on the (non-)use of maternal health services. The FGD and SSI topic guides for community members were prepared in English and translated into the local language, Wau Arabic. The topic guides were defined further during the initial stakeholder workshops, pre-tested in the study site, and were adapted iteratively as the study progressed.

Study sites

The study was conducted in Wau County of WBeG State of South Sudan. While South Sudan is home to more than 50 ethnic groups, in WBeG, the Fertit, an

Table 1 Overview of study participants and data collection

Method	Profiles of study participants	Number of activities (number of participants)
FGD	Community members: Female 18–35 years (Not in union[a])	1 (8)
	Community members: Female 18–35 years (In union)	1 (8)
	Community members: Male > 35 years	1 (8)
	Community members: Male 18–35 years	1 (8)
	Health workers	1 (6)
SSI with community members	Community member: Female 18–35 years (Not in union)	5
	Community member: Female 18–35 years (In union)	6
	Community member: Male 18–35 years	6
	Community member: Female > 35 years	6
	Community member: Male > 35 years	4
SSI with key informants	Traditional birth attendants	4
	Traditional leaders	3
	Health facility personnel	5
	State SRH managers	2
	NGO representatives	3

[a]Participants were either In Union or Not In Union at the time of the study. Relationship status is presented this way because in Wau people say they are married only if the relationship was formalised either in a traditional ceremony, or in the church – even if they cohabit. For convenience we use the terms married/unmarried in the paper

agriculturalist people, predominate. Two locations in Wau County were selected based on the homogeneity of the residents (all Fertit). Both locations were within walking distance of functioning maternal health services - this was important as health service coverage (geographical) is poor in many parts of WBeG. In both the locations, maternal health services were provided in a primary care facility staffed by one clinical officer, one nurse, 1–2 midwives and a pharmacist. In both facilities, the staff were a mix of locals, and returnees who originally hailed from WBeG. The two locations represented two different settings in Wau County – Wau town and the other a rural area. However, in both settings the socioeconomic situation was similar, with most people engaged in subsistence farming or informal manual labour. The assumption behind choosing these two locations was that perhaps within the same ethnic group, depending on the setting, the decisions and decision-making processes around whether or not to use maternal health services, might be moderated differently.

Sampling, recruitment of study participants and data collection

Details of study participants are presented in Table 1. Community members were purposefully selected with the assistance of village elders, health workers from a local NGO and the county health department. The assistance was limited to guiding the researchers to the village and to making introductions; the actual selection was done by the researchers themselves. Amongst community members, only those of age 18 years and above

were included in this study. We purposefully categorized participants into those between 18 and 35 years and those above 35 years with the assumption that the two age groups might have different health seeking behaviors.

Data collection began with FGDs amongst community members, followed by SSIs to obtain more in-depth understanding. FGD participants were homogenous in terms of ethnicity, age and marital status, yet diversity was sought in terms of social and economic status (criteria included ownership of assets like bicycles, and level of education). Health facility personnel responsible for maternal health in facilities close to the study sites were included as participants. Individuals with active maternal health related role within the county and state health system i.e. traditional leaders, traditional birth attendants, SRH service managers, and representatives of NGOs working on maternal health, were also included as key informants.

Data were collected from October 2014 to April 2015, over 3 visits to Wau. FGDs and interviews with community members, traditional leaders and traditional birth attendants were conducted by research team members who hailed from the study area, were fluent in Wau Arabic, and had experience with conducting qualitative research. Data were collected till analytical saturation was reached, and no new insight emerged; this was possible to assess, as at the end of each day of data collection, the research team debriefed and discussed the emerging findings. In total 5 FGDs (with 38 participants) and 44 SSIs were conducted.

Data analysis

SSIs and FGDs were digitally recorded, translated from Wau Arabic into English (where applicable) and transcribed verbatim. An inductive thematic analysis of the transcripts was conducted [17]. Analysis began with an initial thorough reading of transcripts by three researchers (SK, MR, MK) to identify broad themes about the reasons for use or not of maternal health services. The guiding principle in this process was to identify the various reasons that were important to participants and to ascertain that the chosen themes captured the main aspects of participants' reasons behind using or not using SRH services. The next step involved moving from these themes to an interpretation of the broader significance of and meanings attached to these themes, and the implications of these themes; in parallel, and iteratively through this process, the identified themes were reviewed, refined, and named. The NVivo 11 software was used to code all transcripts and to run queries on the dataset. Findings from the preliminary analysis were refined through follow up interviews with 2 participants in each study site ($n = 4$), one traditional leader, one local resource person, and through a workshop involving community health workers, health facility personnel and SRH services managers ($n = 13$).

Ethical considerations

Informed consent was given by all study participants; for those who could not read, the consent form was read out to them and their consent was recorded. Confidentiality was maintained throughout, and steps were taken to anonymise the data and to minimise risk of accidental disclosure and access by unauthorized third parties. Since the study included questions about the local health services and the responsiveness of providers, special care was taken to ensure that identities of participants were not revealed to the local health workers. All participants were explicitly informed of their right to refuse to participate and to not answer questions they might find to be intrusive. Keeping in mind the possibility of some participants being reminded of traumatic experiences, medical referral services and counselling support were made available. No such situation requiring referral emerged during data collection or in the period after the study.

Results

While the study did not dwell into the details of level and nature of knowledge about SRH matters, all community members – women and men across age groups, and all traditional leaders, recognized the benefits of modern maternity care, and were aware about the importance of antenatal care, institutional delivery, and to

some extent, post-natal care. Reliable, state and county level data on availability, accessibility and utilization of maternal health services is not available in South Sudan. However, in the study area, services were available and accessible; and study participants indicated that they appreciated the presence of these services, and used these services. Issues related to geographical access, financial access, and perceived quality of care were reported as being important barriers to the use of services by our study participants. These barriers are important, however they are not the focus of this paper, and hence not presented and discussed here.

This section presents other social reasons why inspite of being knowledgeable about and having maternal health services in their vicinity, many women still did not use these services. Findings are presented as themes; three major themes emerged. The first theme presents how various social fears shape women's care seeking. The second theme presents how women's social expectations and social interactions around the act of visiting a health facility shape their care seeking behavior. In the third theme, women's and society's views about pregnancy are presented with a view to locate the findings of the first two themes in the local context, and to better explain them.

Social fears

Women, both young and old, talked of fear and of 'being afraid' in some form or the other. They often did so without probing, indicating that the experience probably had wide relevance, and was an important feature of women's interaction with the maternal health services, specifically of why women, used the maternal health services, or not. The importance of this cognitive process was acknowledged by professional informants too; although their observations were limited to and primarily referred to fears related to painful medical procedures and to the insecurity involved in the act of travelling to health facilities.

Fear of being embarrassed

Women were afraid of being embarrassed during the care encounter; in our study, this feeling had two broad facets. One related to not having enough money to cover the expenses incurred, and another related to not having one's husband by one's side.

Maternal health services in South Sudan are free in primary care facilities, although some user fees are levied in hospitals. However, the facilities in the study area often did not have enough supplies and drugs; patients were asked to buy these from private pharmacies. In Wau, people had to spend money to buy goods (soap, cloth, cotton, medicines etc) that are needed when delivering in a health facility, for transport, for stay if one were from another place (as is often the case around Wau), and also to pay for fees (including for informal payments to health workers). Not having enough money was clearly cited as a reason for not using services by both men and women. As the following quote illustrates, one of the underlying mechanisms through which not having money also shaped care seeking decisions, was that women were afraid that if they were to be asked to pay, and they did not have enough money on them, they would be shamed or even be belittled.

"It might be money, some things go back to the economy, maybe there is no money and she is afraid that when she goes they will charge her a lot of money." [Woman under 35, Not In Union].

Another underlying mechanism through which not having money affected care seeking decisions, was that women were afraid that if they did not have enough money to pay for the expenses incurred at the hospital, they might not be allowed to return home. This led some to not only not use the hospital facilities, it also led them to turn to (and often to prefer) the services offered by traditional birth attendants (TBAs). Unlike hospitals, TBAs were flexible; they did not necessarily expect cash, and could be paid in instalments, over a longer period of time.

"TBAs can wait even for a year for the women to pay them, but if you go to the hospital and you don't pay they won't let you go home, so women fear." [FGD, Women above 35].

Women who were widowed, or did not have a husband, or whose husband was away, or had been abandoned the husband, or had no family to support them, were afraid that health workers would ask them about their husbands, and would insist that their husbands be present. In South Sudan, a pregnancy is a matter of pride, and it is important that it is dignified by and seen to be valued by the man and his family. It is deeply embarrassing to women if they are seen to be on their own, and with no man to dignify their pregnancy. Women fear this embarrassment, and instead of going to health facilities, prefer to stay at home to avoid the embarrassment.

"She is also afraid that they might tell her to bring her husband ... and the man is not there. Because of fear they stay at home" [Woman under 35, Not in Union].

For such women, as was often the case, not having enough money, further amplified the problem. They were particularly worried that if they did not have enough money on their person, the health workers might ask them to bring their husband, further exposing them to embarrassment.

Fear of being ill-treated

There is a large body of literature from low and middle-income countries which documents ill-treatment of patients by workers in health facilities. To some extent, and linked to the fear of being embarrassed, women in the study community were also afraid of the midwives being rude to them. In the following quote, a young woman points out how some women are so afraid, that they would rather deliver at home, inspite of knowing well that to do so, is dangerous.

"The people who do not want to go to the hospital are people who are afraid. They fear delivery, and fear that the midwives will be rude to them. So that is why they don't go to the hospital but still deliver at home .. (even when they know that it).. is dangerous." [Woman under 35, Not in Union].

Senior health workers and SRH service managers, recognised this situation. They were well aware of, and felt ashamed about the poor attitudes of some of their staff. Privately, some expressed frustration at the situation – pointing out that the shortage of health workers in the area meant that hey had very little room to reprimand and discipline errant health workers.

"Yes I do agree, this situation is very embarrassing ... some midwives are verbally abusive and have bad attitudes. Some women will prefer not to come back to the hospital because of the maltreatment." [Health Facility Personnel - Manager].

Fear of being denied services

Many steps are being taken to improve maternal health services in South Sudan; for instance, to improve the continuity of care, a paper card is issued to every pregnant woman. In this card, health workers record the progress of the pregnancy and the pregnant woman's medical situation. We found that health workers diligently use these cards, and impress upon women the importance of carrying these cards when they visit health facilities; most women also understood the importance of these cards. However, it was these very cards that paradoxically appeared to hinder the use of maternal health services. Some women could not afford these cards (approximate price = 0.25 EUR), and therefore hesitated to visit the health centres. We found that many women lost their cards, had their cards torn, or soiled; as the following quotes show, women in such situations were afraid of being reprimanded by the health workers, and denied services.

"This will affect you, if you have a child (are in the process of delivery) and you do not have a follow up card no one will accept you even the trained midwives they will not assist you. Even the hospital will not accept you."[Woman under 35, Not in Union].

"If the midwife finds that you do not have a hospital card, she will tell you that she cannot go to you because you did not go for checkups. If a crime comes to me, what will I say? I will not go to you. We have this kind of situations here." *[FGD, Women over 35].*

These quotes also illustrate how the way these check-ups and cards related processes were implemented in practice; perhaps unwittingly, these service delivery improvement processes, paradoxically gave some women the impression that not carrying these cards, or not attending earlier antenatal check-ups, was akin to committing a crime. An impression that seemed to be enough to make some women afraid, and to not use maternal health services.

Insecurity related fear

Poor rule of law is a problem in much of South Sudan. The state apparatus is unable to protect people from antisocial elements, including but not limited to ethnic militias. The prevailing insecurity featured prominently in both men and women's explanations for not using health facilities. People were afraid of being accosted on the way to the health facilities at night, but also during the day.

"If labour pains start at around 2 am, and there is no way to go to the hospital, and there is no transport, and you fear criminals on the way." *[Woman under 35, Not in Union].*

"There is no transport, so people fear to move at night to go to the hospital and people can attack you on the way" *[FGD, Men under 35].*

The health workers, the healthcare managers all admitted that this was a major problem. They acknowledged the circumstances and they recognized people's fears as understandable, pointing out that this was the price society paid on a daily basis for the chronic insecurity and unrest.

"And for people to access services there must be security, people should have peace of mind that if I walk five kilometers, I will go and come back without any problem. So one of the factors is .. if I go there and I feel threatened (on the way to getting to the facility), it will affect the utilization." [NGO Representative].

The findings above reveal that a variety of social fears also shape decisions around seeking maternal health care. In the discussion section, these fears, and the social processes driving them, are discussed in view of the theoretical insights on 'social fears'.

Dignity expectations not being fulfilled

In the study community, as in all communities in South Sudan, pregnancy is a matter of personal pride for women. It is something to be celebrated and dignified by the man's family. As the following quotes from an FGD among men illustrate, it is expected that a pregnant woman is treated nicely and is seen to be so too in society, particularly when she ventures out of the house and into public spaces.

"When you (a pregnant woman) get up to go to the health center, the culture and traditions are like ... the shoes on your feet and the clothes ... when you want to leave your house, you need to take a shirt and wear (good clothes)." [FGD, Men over 35].

Being able to dress nicely, and to be presentable in public spaces like the clinic, was very important to women. It was important to the extent that if they did not have soap to bathe and did not have a clean dress to wear, they would rather not go to the clinic – inspite of knowing well the importance of the antenatal, natal or postnatal visits.

"When they get pregnant, they want their husbands to buy them new dresses, new shoes, to braid their hair ... and to give her money ... then after ... that is when you leave home and go (out into public places, like the health centre)." [Woman under 35, Not in Union].

Women whose husbands were either away, or who had been abandoned by their husband, or had nobody to provide for them, would rather not be seen in public in an unpresentable state. Appearing disheveled and uncared for would give people an impression that this was someone whose pregnancy was not being celebrated and dignified by the family. Women in such circumstances would rather forgo care, than open themselves to dignity violations. While reliable data are not available, many women in the study community, and in South Sudan at large are in such a situation.

The 'pregnancy' - for the man's family, and also the man's responsibility

In some ways linked to all of the above themes, and in many ways shaping women's care seeking decisions and actions, albeit at a cognitively different level, is the status and role of women in the local society, and how women see themselves within and interact with these social arrangements. We found that women's role in society is seen to primarily be about bearing children for the man's family. The entrenched social norm is that women must bear as many children as the man and his family members wish; this norm relates to the idea that children replace the dead, and they allow inheritance and the continuation of the man's family name. The following two FGD interactions illustrate the local social reality and how men and women relate to it. The first interaction below, in an FGD among young women, illustrates how women see and experience their situation and role in the man's family; it also highlights how not bearing children as demanded by the man and his family, incurs the risk of being abandoned by the man.

Participant 1: "If you are married and already living with your husband and do not have a child, the husband can leave you and tell you to go back to your family."

Participant 2: "His relatives will come and argue that why you are not getting pregnant ...the man's relatives will complain why is this woman brought and eating our food for free if she is not going to deliver children."

Participant 1: "The relatives will tell the husband to leave you and go and get another woman who can have children."

Participant 3: "Or the (man's) relatives themselves will go and get a wife for their son." [FGD, Women under 35].

The second interaction below, in an FGD among men, men nonchalantly discuss their inalienable claim on the woman's womb and her fertility potential. They refer to the woman as 'our' wife – it signifies not just the man's claim, but rather the family's, for they have bought her, and brought her into the family, with the purpose of bearing children for the family. The discussion shows how the man, and the man's family not just expect the woman to give them children, her not doing so, is considered sufficient grounds to abandon her and replace her.

Participant 1: "Because this is our wife, we married her with money. Of course, marrying a woman is like

business ... is like business. Meaning that if you start a business you must profit from it."

Participants 2,3,4 (In chorus): "Yes, Yes."

Participant 1: "And if you take a woman with money and she does not give you children, that is not good."

Participant 2: "Yes, the family ... if a woman is pregnant your family is happy."

Participant 3: "They will say that this woman is now giving birth replacing the person who had died ... the one inside now is in place of the person who had died. The family will be happy."

Participant 4: "Like ... this is my son here. He married a woman. His wife is bearing children. I will be happy. Some people meet me and say ... Oh Peter! Your son's wife delivered. I'll be happy... But if my son married a woman and she does not bear a child, eating the 'Asida' (food) for free, I will not be happy." [FGD, Men under 35].

Women's awareness of their status in the man's household, and their cognizance of the social reality that they had been brought (even, bought) into the man's household to bear children, appeared to result in an ambivalent attitude towards pregnancies generally, including towards their own pregnancy. This layered sociality also shaped women's approach towards using maternal health services. Women seemed to view the (unborn) child as the man's family's, and also seemed to view the process of using maternal health services as not being about their own health, but rather being about the health of the (unborn) child, and thus the responsibility of the man and his family, and not their own.

Facilitator: "Some women do not go to the hospital what makes them not to go?"

Participant: "Sometimes the man says he does not have money that was why she could not go for check-up. So, she decides not to go and if the baby dies it is a loss for her husband's family and not her family." [FGD, Women under 35].

That having been said, this approach to pregnancy and maternity care was not universal. Many women, even when their husband did not provide them with the money, still used antenatal and delivery services; they did so through raising money from other sources. In such situations some women also resorted to using the services offered by traditional birth attendants who charged less, were open to being paid in kind, and to being paid in instalments.

Discussion

Consistent with Wilunda et al. [11] and Lawry et al's [12] studies from South Sudan [11, 12], and the global health services literature [18, 19], our study also found that women do not use the services, if they don't feel the need, if services are inaccessible (geographically and financially), if they perceive services to be of poor quality, and if they do not have confidence in the competence of providers. Instead of repeating what Wilunda et al. [11] and Lawry et al. [12] have reported in detail, in this paper we choose to focus upon an important, and often insufficiently reported dimension of access – 'social accessibility' [16]. In the following discussion section, we draw upon our insights about the context of South Sudan, theoretical insights, and empirical findings from literature, to discuss our findings about women's views on pregnancy, women's dignity expectations, and social fears around the act of seeking care. In doing so, we also extend the conceptual understanding of what constitutes accessibility of health services, to include the notion of 'social accessibility'; we make a case for inclusion of this understanding when studying access to health services and when intervening to improve access to services.

We begin with a discussion on what we consider a meta construct shaping women's thinking about pregnancy, and their approach to dealing with it. This background sets the stage to further discuss our findings within two broad and linked theoretical frames: social fears, and social dignity and its violations. Throughout the process, implications are drawn for public health policy and practice in South Sudan, and where appropriate, beyond; in the process, we add to and nuance this body of knowledge on multiple fronts. In doing so, the importance of 'location specific investigations' recommended by De Francisco et al. [6] and others [8], is reiterated.

Carrying a child for someone else

Women's ambivalent, sometimes even uncaring attitudes towards pregnancies, including their own pregnancy, need to be understood better. Oyewumi's work [20] on family structure and social relations in many African societies, provides a useful frame to understand this ambivalence; according to Oyewumi, in many African societies, the family unit is a "consanguinally-based family system built around a core of brothers and sisters-blood relations, wherein the spouses are considered outsiders and therefore not part of the family" [21]. This is unlike the Western family structure of a conjugally-based family built around a couple. In many communities of South Sudan, including in WBeG, the family unit is a consanguinally-based unit, and the woman remains an outsider whose primary role is to bear children for the man's family. This family structure and the social norms that accompany it, in some ways explains why many women viewed the child they were carrying as someone else's and for someone else, and its care was thus also seen by them as being someone else's responsibility – the someone else being the husband and his family. We argue that these social relational arrangements shape how women view and relate to their own pregnancy, and also what they are willing to do or not do, about it. These social-relational arrangements thus constrained women's use of maternal health and SRH services. Pregnant women seemed to also somehow use these social arrangements as a rationale to justify their actions or inactions, which they well knew as being not good for the health of the unborn.

Social fears

'Fears' of different kinds emerged as a key concern shaping the non-use of maternal health services. Findings show that the broader theme of 'social fears', is constituted by and subsumes sub-themes which reflect a wide range of social processes: unequal power relations between providers and patients, professional control over the patient-provider interaction and the linked sense of undermined agency, and the broader insecurity in region and country. The latter being a fear, but also perhaps an enabler of other fears; insecurity tends to undermine use of services through, among others, pushing up opportunity costs of accessing services. These sub-themes not just represent different facets of social fear experienced by women when interacting with or contemplating the use of maternal health services, they also help explain how the fear experience is mediated in a number of specific social contexts, and shapes women's decisions to use maternal health services.

Drawing on Tudor [22], we argue that the many fears articulated by women are perhaps best understood as 'social fears', where they relate to and are shaped by the attributes of the social worlds individuals inhabit. Social fears may be explicit or tacit, big or small, but they pervade all aspects of our lives and are a key feature of many social situations and interactions; Tudor argues that these fears featuring within social situations "have complex ramifications for the ways in which we live our lives" [22]. If one's environment, and social interactions repeatedly signal that a certain kind of activity or interaction is unpleasant, painful or dangerous, and could lead to trouble, and if these signals are experienced by others in one's environment, then this provides the conditions for fear to emerge for that particular activity or social interaction. Such fears, once established, have a powerful effect on the actions of individuals. Women who harbor fears, however big or small these fears might be, are unlikely to easily use the maternal health services on offer; furthermore, if sufficient number of women harbor such fears, it influences the thinking of others around them. Evidence shows that experts' and professionals' control over many areas of human activity, like healthcare, can promote fear also beyond the worries related to the direct consequences of specific actions and interventions – including, as in this case, rude/abusive behaviour [23, 24]. It can partly also explain why many women turn to and prefer traditional birth attendants.

Discussing the care experience of study participants within a relational context can help better understand the point regarding care providers. In South Sudan, including in Wau, the relations between the locals who stayed behind during the war, and the returnees who had fled to the erstwhile Sudan during the war, are tense. The returnees have brought valuable knowledge and skills back with them - a large proportion of health care providers are returnees. However, many returnees, because they have been away for decades, do not identify sufficiently with the locals, and tend to be judgmental of the locals. While on one hand the locals welcome and appreciate the returnees, they are keenly aware of the subliminal othering effected by the returnees. This, together with the underlying feelings of resentment amongst those who stayed, towards those who went away, makes the interaction between the locals and the returnee providers, complex, and presents a fertile ground for manifestation of fears. That said, the social dynamics between the returnees and locals was not the focus of our study; further investigation is needed to understand it and its possible public health implications.

Social dignity and dignity violations

Women's decisions to step out to seek care are the results of a complex trade-off they make or are willing to make between potential threats to their dignity in social spaces, their views on ownership and responsibility for the unborn, and their fears regarding the care encounter. Many of the fears expressed by women are perhaps better understood in terms of them being afraid of their dignity being violated in the various interactions entailed, and the spaces traversed, in the act of seeking care. We draw upon the notion of social dignity [25, 26], the social and cognitive processes around its maintenance and its violations, to better understand our major findings. Social dignity as a concept refers to the idea that in every social interaction, the dignity of one or more participant or bystanders, can potentially be upheld, promoted, threatened or violated. What entails social dignity, and perceptions of when it is upheld, threatened or violated, is socially constructed – it depends on the norms and traditions of a particular community or society. The socially constructed nature of

social dignity means that people in every society have tacit knowledge of how to assess it, when to expect its violation, and when to expect its upholdment. For a social interaction to become a dignity violation does not necessarily require explicit action or words being said, it can simply be an act of interpretation by the one whose dignity is at risk, or by others involved in the interaction, including the bystanders.

Consistent with the global literature on dignity and healthcare services [23, 25, 27, 28], women in our study reported being afraid of how they might be treated by healthcare workers in their care encounters. The mechanism underlying this fear of being abused, being reprimanded, being shamed, or being belittled during the care encounter, was fear of their social dignity being violated. This concern with social dignity, and its risk of being violated was however not restricted to the care encounter alone; women accorded great importance to, and were concerned about how they were seen in public spaces, be it on the way to the health facility, or in the health facility premises. These spaces were arenas for social interactions where community members, primarily women, asserted their social standing in relation to others. Those pregnant women who could not dress up, and look nice and be seen as being well taken care of, often preferred to stay at home and not seek care, to protect themselves from the judging eyes of other women and society at large, thereby guarding their social dignity. Not having the means to meet the social expectations, socially enforced or imagined, was a reality for most women in the study community. If a woman is in a position of vulnerability, she is more likely to interpret even a relatively minor social slight as violation of her social dignity [25, 26], and as discussed earlier, if the woman happens to see the process of making herself vulnerable to such a violation as not being in her benefit or her responsibility, she will avoid even initiating the process of seeking care. Jacobson [26] argues that in difficult circumstances, some, particularly those who are most disadvantaged and vulnerable, may be so worn down by the constant micro insults and violations of their social dignity, that they may isolate themselves and avoid social interactions as much as possible – this manifests as "a reluctance to seek help or access resources, passivity or 'learned helplessness'". Many women in our study community, and in many parts of South Sudan, are in such a position.

Limitations

The study has some limitations. There was a possibility that people would only give socially desirable answers with the view to not antagonize health workers. These constraints were anticipated, and steps were taken to loosen these constraints. Data collection with community members was done by researchers who hailed from the local community, were independent, and were in no way related to the NGOs delivering services. They also knew the local culture well, and took due care to ensure frank and open interactions. Visits were made to the study sites before the actual data collection to meet the villagers and the elders – to explain the nature of the study, to seek the village's agreement for our presence, and to reassure them that confidentiality will be maintained. We observed that participants were eager to participate and happy that they were being heard. Throughout data collection, the interactions with participants were frank and candid; it makes us confident about our study findings.

Conclusions

Barriers related to geographical accessibility, affordability, and perceptions (need and quality of care) hinder women from using maternal health services, and these barriers need to be addressed. Through this paper we show that it is equally important to also explicitly consider, and address barriers related to social accessibility – our findings highlight how social fears and fears of dignity violations may hold women back from using maternal health services. We argue and conclude that interventions to improve accessibility of maternal health services should have features that protect women from dignity violations in the care encounters, and should make and shape health facilities into spaces for dignity promotion, for one and all.

Making health facilities into spaces for dignity promotion requires the explicit embedment of dignity considerations in all aspects of service organisation, across provider-patient encounter settings, and across the health facility as a social space. Specifically, and drawing on Jacobson [29], among other things, this could entail the development of a local diagnostic tool which allows service users and practitioners to jointly reflect on "their own positions of vulnerability and antipathy, and on the nature of the gestures, interpretations, and responses that constitute dignity violation in their own settings, using this exercise to change the dignity dimensions of their interactions", and of the spaces in which these encounters occur. Doing so will not only draw women to health facilities, it can also contribute to broader social cohesion and social development by signalling social equality regardless of ethnicity, social and economic status.

Dignity violations in the healthcare encounter and in the health facility space are but reproductions and manifestations of the structural inequalities prevalent in a society. These structural problems require structural solutions at the societal level. While these solutions are beyond the purview of health workers,

public health programs and health workers can contribute to triggering social change by both, changing things in the health facility and creating exemplar islands of possibility, and also by actively making common cause with those who are working on promoting social justice, rule of law, and tackling gender and social inequalities in the society.

Summary

Women will use available maternal health services, if they feel the need for the services, if the services are geographically and financially accessible, and if they perceive the services to be of good quality. This study, adds that while these conditions are necessary, they may not be sufficient for women to step out of their homes to use services.

This study argues that the act of seeking care is a social act which entails many social interactions, in a variety of social spaces eg. the neighborhood to be traversed, the waiting area of the health facility, and the care encounter setting. And that, in the many potential social interactions that occur while traversing these spaces, depending on the local social norms, the woman's dignity may potentially be upheld, promoted, threatened or violated.

This study contends that women's decisions to use available services are shaped by a complex trade-off making process, between, on one hand, their beliefs about the importance of using services, and on the other, their fears about their dignity being violated during the interactions entailed in the act of seeking care.

This study concludes that policy makers should pay explicit attention to the embedment of social accessibility related considerations in all aspects of health services organisation, across provider-patient encounter settings, and across the health facility as a social space.

Abbreviations

FGD: Focus group discussion; MoH: Ministry of Health; SHARP: South Sudan health action and research project; SRH: Sexual and reproductive health; SSI: Semi structured interview; WBeG: Western Bahr el Ghazal State

Acknowledgements

Contributions of the Ministry of Foreign Affairs of the Government of The Netherlands, and of all SHARP project implementing partners, are duly acknowledged.

Funding

This study is part of the SHARP (South Sudan Health Action and Research Project) project funded by the Ministry of Foreign Affairs of the Government of The Netherlands.

Authors' contributions

SK is the Principal Investigator. SK, MK, MR collected and analysed the data. SK drafted the manuscript. MK, MR, MD, JB reviewed the draft manuscript and gave inputs. SK finalized the manuscript. All authors have read and approved the final manuscript.

Competing interests

All authors declare that they have no competing interests.

Author details

[1]KIT Royal Tropical Institute, Mauritskade 63, Amsterdam 1092 AD, The Netherlands. [2]Nossal Institute for Global Health, Melbourne School of Population and Global Health, University of Melbourne, Level 5, 333 Exhibition Street, Melbourne, VIC 3010, Australia. [3]Independent Consultant, Wau, Western Bahr el Ghazal, South Sudan. [4]School of Public and Environmental Health, University of Bahr el Ghazal, Wau, Western Bahr el Ghazal, South Sudan. [5]Athena Institute for Research on Innovation and Communication in Health and Life Sciences, Faculty of Earth and Life Sciences, VU University Amsterdam, Amsterdam, The Netherlands.

References

1. WHO. Trends in maternal mortality: 1990 To 2015: estimates by WHO, UNICEF, UNFPA, World Bank Group and the United Nations Population Division. 2015.
2. Ministry of Health. Republic of South Sudan. Health Sector Development Plan 2012–2016. 2012.
3. Roberts B, Guy S, Sondorp E, Lee-Jones L. A basic package of health services for post-conflict countries: Implications for sexual and reproductive health services. Reprod Health Matters. 2008;16(31):57–64.
4. World Bank. World development report 2011. Overview: Conflict, security, and development. The World Bank. 2011.
5. Haar RJ, Rubenstein LS. Health in post conflict and fragile states. Washington, DC: United States Institute of Peace; 2012.
6. de Francisco A, Dixon-Mueller R, d'Arcangues C. Research issues in sexual and reproductive health for low- and middle-income countries. In: Global forum for Health Research and world health Organization; 2007.
7. United Nations General Assembly. Right To Health: International covenant on Economic, Social and Cultural Rights. January. 1976.
8. Mugo N, Zwi A, Botfield JR, Steiner C. Maternal and child health in South Sudan: priorities for the Post-2015 agenda. Sage Open 2015; https://doi.org/10.1177/2158244015581190.
9. Mugo N, Agho KE, Zwi AB, Dibley MJ. Factors associated with different types of birth attendants for home deliveries: an analysis of the cross-sectional 2010 South Sudan household survey. Glob Health Action. 2016; https://doi.org/10.3402/gha.v9.29693.
10. Mugo N, Dibley MJ, Agho KE. Prevalence and risk factors for non-use of antenatal care visits: analysis of the 2010 South Sudan household survey. BMC Pregnancy Childbirth. 2015;15:68.
11. Wilunda C, Scanagatta C, Putoto G, Takahashi R, Montalbetti F, Segafredo G, API B. Barriers to institutional childbirth in Rumbek North County, South Sudan: a qualitative study. PLoS One. 2016; https://doi.org/10.1371/journal.pone.0168083.
12. Lawry L, Canteli C, Rabenzanahary T, Pramana W. A mixed methods assessment of barriers to maternal, newborn and child health in Gogrial west, South Sudan. Reprod Health. 2017;14:12.
13. Campbell OMR, Graham WJ. Strategies for reducing maternal mortality: getting on with what works. Lancet. 2006;368:1284–99.
14. Kane S, Kok M, Rial M, Matere A, Dieleman M, Broerse JEW. Social norms and family planning decisions in South Sudan. BMC Public Health. 2016; https://doi.org/10.1186/s12889-016-3839-6.
15. Kane S, Rial M, Matere A, Dieleman M, Broerse JEW, Kok M. Gender relations and women's reproductive health in South Sudan. Glob Health Action. 2016; https://doi.org/10.3402/gha.v9.33047@zgha20.2016.9.issue-s4.
16. Powell M. On the outside looking in: medical geography, medical geographers and access to health care. Health and Place. 1995;1(1):41–50.
17. Braun V, Clarke V. Using thematic analysis in psychology. Qual Res Psychol. 2006;3(2):77–101.
18. Say L, Raine R. A systematic review of inequalities in the use of maternal health care in developing countries: examining the scale of the problem and the importance of context. Bull World Health Organ. 2007;85(10):812–9.
19. Gabrysch S, Campbell OM. Still too far to walk: literature review of the determinants of delivery service use. Pregnancy Child Birth. 2009;9:34–10.
20. Oyewumi O. Gender Epistemologies in Africa: the gendering of African traditions, spaces, social identities and institutions. Basingstoke: Palgrave Macmillan; 2011. ISBN: 978–0–230–62345–3.
21. Oyewumi O. Conceptualizing gender: the Eurocentric foundations of feminist concepts and the challenge of African epistemologies. In: Anfred S, Bakare-Yusuf B, Kisiangani EW, Lewis D, Oyewumi O, Steady FC (Eds) 'African Gender Scholarship: Concepts, Methods and Paradigms'. Council for the Development of Social Science Research in Africa, 2004. Dakar, Senegal. ISBN: 2-86978-138-5.
22. Tudor A. A (macro) sociology of rear? Sociol Rev. 2003;51:238–56.
23. Bohren MA, Vogel JP, Hunter EC, Lutsiv O, Makh SK, Souza JP, et al. The Mistreatment of Women during Childbirth in Health Facilities Globally: A Mixed-Methods Systematic Review. PLoS. Med. 2015; https://doi.org/10.1371/journal.pmed.1001847.
24. Chi PC, Bulage P, Urdal H, Sundby J. A qualitative study exploring the determinants of maternal health service uptake in post-conflict Burundi and Northern Uganda. BMC Pregnancy Childbirth. 2015;15:18.
25. Jacobson N. Dignity and health: a review. Soc Sci Med. 2007;64:292–302.
26. Jacobson N. A taxonomy of dignity: a grounded theory study. BMC Int Health Human Rights. 2009;9:3.
27. Freedman LP, Kruk ME. Disrespect and Abuse of women in childbirth: challenging the global quality and accountability agendas. Lancet. 2015; 384:e42–4.
28. Miller S, Abalos E, Chamillard M, et al. Beyond too little, too late and too much, too soon: a pathway towards evidence-based, respectful maternity care worldwide. Lancet. 2016; https://doi.org/10.1016/S0140-6736(16)31472-6.
29. Jacobson N. Dignity violations in health care. Qual Health Res. 2009; 19(11):1536–47.

16

Attitudes of sperm, egg and embryo donors and recipients towards genetic information and screening of donors

David J. Amor[1,2,3*] ⓘ, Annabelle Kerr[1,2], Nandini Somanathan[1,2], Alison McEwen[4], Marianne Tome[3], Jan Hodgson[1,2] and Sharon Lewis[1,2]

Abstract

Background: Gamete and embryo donors undergo genetic screening procedures in order to maximise the health of donor-conceived offspring. In the era of genomic medicine, expanded genetic screening may be offered to donors for the purpose of avoiding transmission of harmful genetic mutations. The objective of this study was to explore the attitudes of donors and recipients toward the expanded genetic screening of donors.

Methods: Qualitative interview study with thematic analysis, undertaken in a tertiary fertility centre. Semi-structured in-depth qualitative interviews were conducted with eleven recipients and nine donors from three different cohorts (sperm, egg and embryo donors/recipients).

Results: Donors and recipients acknowledged the importance of genetic information and were comfortable with the existing level of genetic screening of donors. Recipients recognised some potential benefits of expanded genetic screening of donors; however both recipients and donors were apprehensive about extended genomic technologies, with concerns about how this information would be used and the ethics of genetic selectivity.

Conclusion: Participants in donor programs support some level of genetic screening of donors, but are wary of expanding genetic screening beyond current levels.

Keywords: Donor sperm, Donor conception, Assisted reproduction, Genetic screening

Plain English summary

A relatively small proportion of pregnancies are achieved with the assistance of sperm donors, egg donors or embryo donors. In most assisted reproductive clinics, donors or sperm, eggs or embryos undergo some genetic screening procedures in order to maximise the health of donor-conceived offspring. Recent advances in genetic testing technologies mean that it is now possible to perform more extensive genetic screening of donors than previously was possible.

In this study we conducted in depth interviews with sperm, egg and embryo donors, and with recipients of donor sperm, eggs or embryos, to explore their attitudes towards the collection and use of genetic information in the donor process, and towards the possibility of conducting more extensive genetic screening of donors. Donors and recipients all acknowledged the importance of genetic information and were comfortable with the existing level of genetic screening of donors. Recipients recognised some potential benefits of performing more extensive genetic screening of donors; however both recipients and donors were apprehensive about extended genomic technologies, with concerns about how this information would be used and the ethics of genetic selectivity. The study concludes that participants in donor programs support some level of genetic screening of donors, but are wary of expanding genetic screening beyond current levels.

* Correspondence: david.amor@mcri.edu.au
[1]Murdoch Children's Research Institute, Royal Children's Hospital, Parkville, Australia
[2]Department of Paediatrics, The University of Melbourne, Parkville, Australia
Full list of author information is available at the end of the article

Background

Individuals who donate gametes (eggs or sperm) and couples who donate embryos undergo genetic screening procedures that are designed to maximise the health and welfare of donor conceived children [1]. Practices vary between clinics, but typically include two main components: medical and family history of the donor and genetic screening tests. The medical and family history of the donor is designed to exclude the presence of major mendelian disorders, chromosome rearrangements and multifactorial disorders that have a significant genetic component [2, 3]. Genetic tests undertaken in donors may include karyotyping and genetic screening for the carrier status of specific conditions such as cystic fibrosis, spinal muscular atrophy, haemoglobinopathies, Tay--Sachs disease and Fragile X syndrome [2, 4, 5].

Despite implementation of these practices, it is inevitable that serious inherited conditions will, on occasion, occur in donor-conceived children or in individuals who have been donors in the past. Reporting of such instances has prompted calls for more extensive genetic screening of donors [6–8], and advances in genetic testing technology have now provided the opportunity for more expanded genetic screening of gamete and embryo donors [9–11]. To date, most attention has been directed towards expanded carrier screening for autosomal recessive disorders [2, 12, 13], although new genetic testing technologies could potentially be used to screen for undiagnosed autosomal dominant disorders and even for susceptibility to some multifactorial diseases [14].

There is little information about the attitudes of gamete and embryo donors and recipients towards donor genetic screening. A recent on-line survey of women who had used donor sperm found support for the implementation of more comprehensive genetic screening of donors [15]; however there are also concerns amongst health professionals about the effectiveness of expanded genetic screening protocols and the need to treat donors as 'interested stakeholders, not merely as providers of genetic material' [2]. In this research we aimed to explore the experiences and attitudes of gamete and embryo donors and recipients towards current donor genetic screening practices and towards potential future expanded donor genetic screening.

Methods

Study setting - Melbourne IVF donor program

This research was conducted in the setting of the donor program of Melbourne IVF, a large IVF provider based in Victoria, Australia. In Victoria, the donation of reproductive tissues must be altruistic, and it is illegal for donors to profit from their donation. In addition, a donor-conceived person is entitled to access identifying information about their donor. The Melbourne IVF donor program provides a service whereby people can donate, or be recipients of, gametes (eggs or sperm) and embryos. Donated embryos are from couples and individuals who have undergone IVF treatment and have completed their families. Donor program criteria stipulate that at the time of donation, sperm donors must be aged between 25 and 46 years and egg donors must be aged between 25 and 40 years. Embryos can be donated if the egg donor was aged less than 42 years at the time of embryo creation. All donors must be Australian citizens. Recipients of donor sperm must be aged less than 46 years and recipients of donor eggs or embryos must be aged less than 51 years.

At Melbourne IVF, donors complete a Genetic Health Questionnaire that collects information about personal and family history of conditions with a suspected genetic contribution. In addition to the genetic health questionnaire, donors undergo genetic screening to identify genetic abnormalities that could be transmitted to children that are conceived with their gametes or embryos. Screening comprises a standard karyotype (looking for structural rearrangements) and testing for three common single gene disorders: thalassemia, spinal muscular atrophy and cystic fibrosis. Female donors are also tested for Fragile X syndrome.

Participants

Two groups of participants were invited to participate in this study.

Recipients comprised recipients of gametes (sperm or eggs) and recipients of donor embryos who:

- had used received IVF treatment at Melbourne IVF using donor gametes or embryos between 2012 and 2014
- were not currently pregnant or undergoing IVF treatment
- had not used a genetically related person as a donor
- could speak English.

Demographic data about recipients, including whether or not a child had been born as a result of the donation, were not collected in order to preserve confidentiality.

Donors comprised donors of gametes (sperm or eggs) and embryo donors who:

- had donated between 2012 and 2014
- had not donated to a genetic relative
- could speak English.

Demographic data about donors, including whether or not a child had been born as a result of their donation, were not collected in order to preserve confidentiality.

Eligible individuals were contacted by phone and asked if they would like to receive information about the study; an invitation pack was sent to those who indicated interest. If no response was received from participants after two weeks, a reminder was sent. Once a consent form was received by the study team, the participants were contacted to arrange a convenient time to participate in the study. The most recently seen patients were contacted first and recruitment continued until thematic saturation had been reached.

Methodology

A qualitative methodological approach was employed in this research in order to enable exploration of the experiences of gamete donors and recipients in relation to genetic screening.

Interviews

A semi structured interview schedule was developed to address the specific research aims for each group (Table 1). It included an exploration of the background to being a donor or recipient, experiences of the health questionnaires, perceptions of important information transfer and participant attitudes to genetic information and genetic testing. Open ended questions were used to allow participants to take the discussion in any direction while maintaining focus of the topic under investigation. Interviews were conducted either face to face or by phone during a six month period in 2015. Interviews of donors were conducted by author NS and interviews of recipients were conducted by author AK. All interviews were digitally recorded.

Analysis

Digital recordings were transcribed verbatim using ExpressScribe Software (NCH Software, Inc., Greenwood Village CO, USA). Transcripts were de-identified and pseudonyms assigned. Transcripts were imported into NVivo Software (QSR International PTY Ltd., Melbourne, Australia) and analysed using thematic analysis. This involved a rigorous process of coding to identify differences and similarities in order to develop themes from within data [16]. A constant comparative approach was used - coding began immediately and continued throughout recruitment so that themes identified early in the process could be further explored with participants in later interviews [17]. The initial stages of coding were performed by NS and AK. The coding and categorizing of data were confirmed through co-coding by SL and AM.

Ethics committee approval

This study was approved by the Human Research Ethics Committee of Melbourne IVF, Victoria, Australia, reference number 39/15-MIVF.

Table 1 Interview Schedule used for donors and recipients

Domain	Areas to address	
	Donors	Recipients
Introduction	– Why the participant became a gamete or embryo donor	– Why the participant(s) required a gamete or embryo donor
Expectations about information	– Expectations of donor program – What information donors thought they would provide to potential recipients	– Expectations of recipient program – What information the recipients thought would be provided about potential donors
Experience of program regarding genetic information (obtained from the donor Genetic Health Questionnaire)	– Thoughts after seeing questionnaires – Unexpected information required – Donors experience with the questionnaires – How the donors thought the information would be used by recipients	– Thoughts after seeing completed questionnaires – Unexpected information given – More/less information than previously thought – How recipients used the donor information
Importance of genetic information	– What information donors thought would be most important to recipients – Medical – Genetic – Personal attributes	– What information was the most important to recipients and why – Medical – Genetic – Personal attributes – Did this remain consistent throughout the recipient process
Attitudes towards genetic information	– Thoughts on need for genetic information about donor – Options of further genetic screening – Personal and family implications	– Thoughts on need for genetic information about potential donors – Options for further genetic screening
Any other information required	– Any other information donors feel could have been provided to recipients	– Any other information recipients feel could have been provided about potential donors

Results
Response
Recipients
Thirty gamete/embryo recipients were identified from the MIVF database. Twenty-five gamete/embryo recipients were contacted by phone and 23 agreed to be sent an information pack. Nine recipients returned the consent forms and were interviewed, giving a participation rate of 39%. The recipient participants included three sperm recipients, three egg recipients and three embryo recipients. Two recipients were interviewed with their partner, resulting in a total of 11 participants.

Donors
Thirty gamete/embryo donors were identified from the Melbourne IVF database. All were contacted and agreed to be sent an information pack. Eleven donors returned consent forms and nine were available to be interviewed, giving a participant rate of 30%. The donor participants comprised three sperm donors, three egg donors and three (female) embryo donors. Participant demographics are shown in Table 2.

Recipient themes
Recipient themes are summarised in Fig. 1 and fall into two main categories.

Table 2 Demographics of participants

Participants (pseudonyms)	Donation	Relationship status
Recipients		
Cathy	Sperm	Different sex
Leonie and Cassie	Sperm	Same sex
Katrina	Sperm	Different sex
Anne	Egg	Different sex
Charlotte	Egg	Different sex
Lucy	Egg	Different sex
Jane	Embryo	Single
Kate	Embryo	Different sex
Dianna and Luke	Embryo	Different sex
Donors		
Anthony	Sperm	
Ethan	Sperm	
Euan	Sperm	
Paige	Egg	
Charlotte	Egg	
Becky	Egg	
Paula	Embryo	
Naomi	Embryo	
Lorna	Embryo	

A) *Existing genetic information and screening*

Recipients felt that donor genetic information was important and helpful information to receive during the donor program.

"Oh yeah, definitely, if you didn't know that then it is this world wide of unknown of what might happen in your child's future it's definitely something important that you need to know that" -Cathy, sperm recipient.

An egg recipient explained that the genetic information normalised the need to discuss the information with their known egg donor.

"The donor program is wonderful because it normalises that you need to look for that so it could feel quite intrusive like you are willing to give me a gift and now I'm going to give you the third degree and what's your health like"-Anne, egg recipient.

Sperm recipients explained that it helped in the selection of their donor.

"Yeah, it definitely impacted I think from what we saw on the form, it sort of helped us narrow it down to another couple of donors"-Leonie, sperm recipient.

While genetic information was important, for many recipients it did not play as significant a role as non-genetic information when selecting a donor.

"I guess whilst all the genetic information was kind of necessary the other side [non genetic information] was far more important"-Cassie, sperm recipient.

Recipients mentioned their hope that medical advances would mean that in the future many genetic conditions would be treatable.

"I was reasonably comfortable to take that risk and I think also 20 or 30 years down the track hopefully something would have come up"-Jane, embryo recipient.

Recipients explained that if they or their partner had a family history of a genetic condition, it wouldn't stop them from having a family.

"When you meet someone ...you don't sort of ask all the genetic information"-Leonie, sperm recipient.

Four recipients used donors who had a significant genetic or family history, and felt the information was helpful but did not influence their choice of donor.

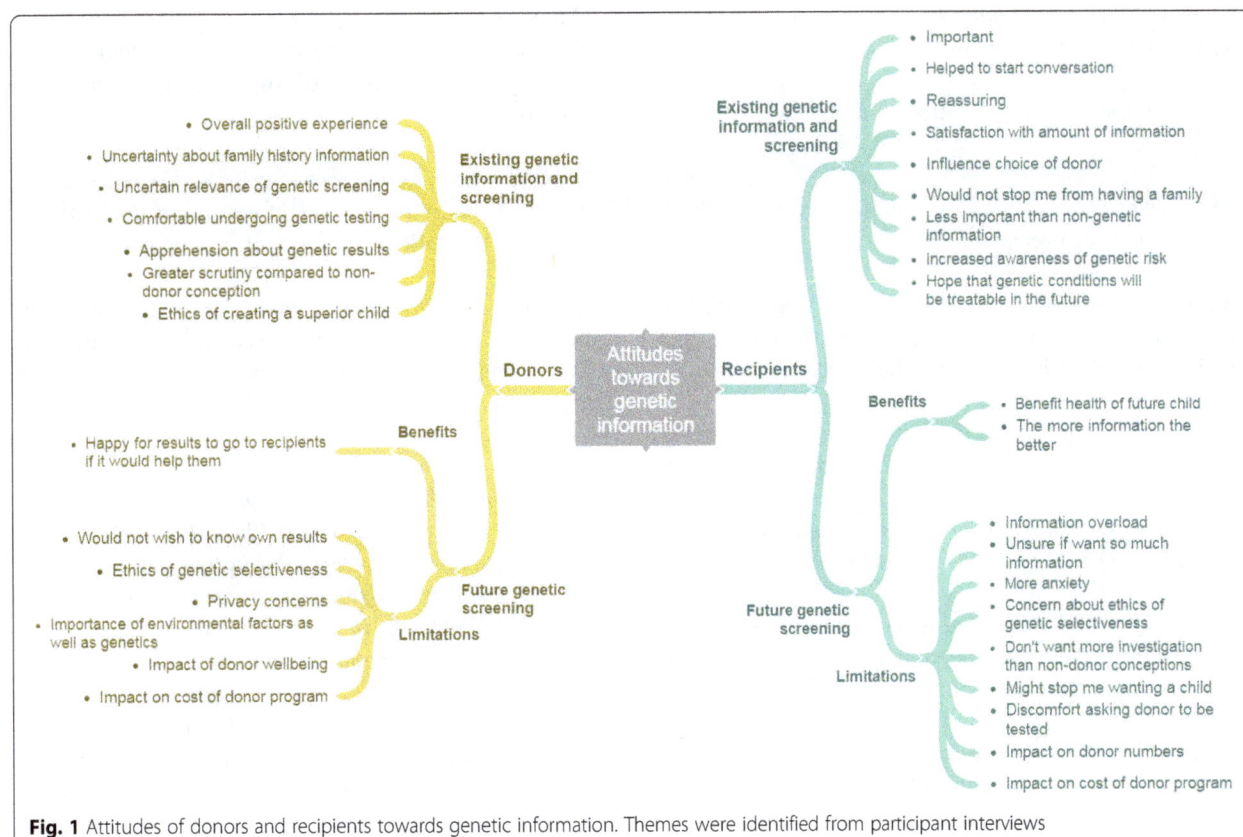

Fig. 1 Attitudes of donors and recipients towards genetic information. Themes were identified from participant interviews

"There was a letter saying that there is an increased chance that she could develop hearing loss, but we went with it because we thought well you know these days they do a lot with hearing"-Cathy, sperm recipient.

Recipients acknowledged that no donor was likely to be free of any genetic risk, and were satisfied with the amount of donor genetic information they received.

"The chances of getting someone with a perfectly clean medical history is just negligible we are all going to die from something whether it be a stroke, cancer, heart disease, so let's face it, when you put it on paper and it looks scary but that is the reality for all of us"-Jane, embryo recipient.

"For me I was happy with the knowledge that I had"-Anne, egg recipient.

The feeling of being reassured by the genetic screening process was a common theme among recipients.

"I actually found that to be very, very, very reassuring"-Cassie, sperm recipient.

Recipients mentioned that the genetic information provided an awareness of the risks for their future children.

"It reassured me because it meant that the medical team had looked at it and reviewed it and had given me their opinions and percentages so I could make an informed decision"-Charlotte, egg recipient.

Embryo recipients expressed how they had not previously thought about genetic information but they were glad they had received it.

"You know what was really good? Even though I hadn't thought of those things, I'm glad the questionnaire was there"-Lucy, egg recipient.

B) *Future genetic screening*

Recipients discussed future genetic testing technologies that might be used in the donor program and expressed that more information would be better in their situation.

"But yeah I certainly think the more information the better"-Jane, embryo recipient.

However the risk for too much information was also highlighted.

"You don't want to have information overload I think"-Lucy, egg recipient.

Recipients from all cohorts expressed their interest in having the option of more genetic information and found it difficult to determine if it would be wanted or not.

"It is a really hard one to know whether we would really have wanted more information"-Kate, embryo recipient.

"So it's not as important to me, but I think the option should be there"-Charlotte, egg recipient.

Recipients stated that more genetic information could benefit many aspects of the donor program. One was the wellbeing of the donor-conceived child.

"If you had more information it would be positive not only from the selection point of view but from a management point of view in the future"-Jane, embryo recipient.

Recipients went on to discuss potential adverse consequences from the introduction of new genetic technologies into the donor program. Ethical concerns were raised about choosing donors based on their genetic information, which they interpreted as a form genetic selectivity, or the creation of "designer" babies.

"It would have given me pause for thought just because it kind of...it sounds very much like it's starting to create designer babies"-Charlotte, egg recipient.

Recipients also felt that natural conceptions did not involve this amount of genetic investigation so questioned why donor conceived pregnancies should.

"You know it is what it is, you know, so it is the risk you take even if you are having your own children you don't know what is going to come"-Kate, embryo recipient.

Recipients also viewed extra donor genetic investigation as potentially unhelpful.

"I think that if we looked into it too much it might stop me from wanting a child"-Katrina, sperm recipient.

The potential of expanded genetic screening to cause anxiety was recognised by recipients, particularly when discussing the possibilities of knowing about uncertain genetic risks.

"For me if it was uncertain I would rather not know... and then it's not in the back of your head and you don't worry about it"-Cathy, sperm recipient.

Egg and embryo recipients were concerned about the impact that expanded genetic screening would have on donor numbers, with the majority claiming that they would much rather have more donors than more information.

"I don't think there is anything wrong with the information we have now so if I had the choice of more chance of a donor and less information or more information and less chance of a donor I would probably go with the information that I have now which is the current information and an increased number of donors"-Lucy, egg recipient.

Egg recipients were particularly concerned about the donors' wellbeing and thoughts on further screening.

"And then making a donor go through genetic screening because then...say by the way you have made the offer but I want you to go get screened"-Charlotte, egg recipient.

Egg recipients also felt that further genetic screening would be something they would find difficult to ask the donors to undergo.

"I'm not genetically screening myself, why would I do that to someone else?"-Charlotte, egg recipient.

Donor themes

Donor themes are summarised in Fig. 1 and fall into two main categories.

A) *Existing genetic information and screening*

The donors understood how important their medical and genetic information was for recipients and found the experience of providing this information to be a positive one. Donors mentioned the difficulty of having to find out their own family history, especially as some of the donors had not told their family members of their choice to donate. There were many factors identified within the genetic screening process and the providing of genetic information and these are outlined below.

Donors felt comfortable answering the medical questions. A few of the donors needed further testing due to a genetic condition being identified in the family history. These donors questioned the relevance of this process, partly because the genetic condition was in a distant family member.

"I was surprised that I then had to provide a lot more information about that, when...it was in relation to a family member and not in relation to me" -Euan, sperm donor.

Donors described their difficulty providing family history information. Donors had to ask other family members to help provide genetic histories, and some found the process very interesting, in terms of gathering all the information together.

"I found it good and I found it hard and sometimes you don't take notice of what happens in your grandparents or you know what I mean"-Paige, egg donor.

While all donors had to find out more about their family histories, many struggled to know what to write down on the Genetic Health Questionnaire, and were unsure if certain health conditions identified in their families were genetic or not.

"And it makes you think about things you do hear, whether they are genetic, and you feel, should I write this down, or shouldn't I..."-Naomi, embryo donor.

When asked about the importance of testing, there was a mixed response. Donors did not always see the relevance of genetic screening, but recognised that screening was important, especially if it could prevent the passing on of a serious genetic disease.

"Personally I don't see the relevance in it"-Becky, egg donor.

"Well, I don't have an issue with it. It's safer to know if you have an issue and to not donate, than to accidently pass on a genetic disease"-Charlotte, egg donor.

Although donors did not consistently recognise the importance of genetic screening tests, all were comfortable undergoing the tests. Donors mentioned their apprehension about finding out the results of their tests, even though they knew of no genetic condition in the family. They felt this was a normal anxious response to having a medical test.

"There is always that thing of ah discovering stuff you don't know about...that can be both good and bad at the same time"-Anthony, sperm donor.

The donors spoke about the level of scrutiny involved in genetic screening, and drew the comparison with natural conception: they noted that a couple conceiving naturally would not need to undergo genetic screening. Donors also expressed opinions about the ethics of genetic screening and whether this type of screening was creating a child that could be superior to a naturally conceived child.

"I mean I felt like they were trying to create a super human or something... It is a little off putting, that children, that people are selecting their children"-Euan, sperm donor.

B) *Future genetic screening*

Donors spoke about the future of genetic screening within donor programs. The participants expressed concerns about the ethics of expanded genetic screening in a donor program and whether this might lead to genetic selectivity. One participant compared this type of genetic screening to the movie 'Gattaca'. Participants raised the concept of the relative roles of genetic and environmental factors in child health, and thought that environmental factors play a greater role than genetics in a child's development.

"If it was me and the child was in my house, I would be providing the growing situation and buying the books, so I can influence what that person says more than their sperm donor"-Ethan, sperm donor.

The level of scrutiny in genetic screening lead many participants to voice their thoughts about the ethics of genetic selectivity and referred to children resulting as "designer babies". Participants felt that a high level of screening would promote the idea of the perfect child, and felt uncomfortable with the idea of selectivity, which they associated with a higher level of screening.

"...and the scary thing is then we can choose...choose what sort of babies we are going to have and that's scary to me"-Becky, egg donor.

"Um, it would have given me pause for thought just because it kind of...it sounds very much like it's starting to create designer babies"-Charlotte, egg donor.

Most donors, if required to go through this level of screening, would not want to know their results. The participants felt that the knowledge gained from these results would adversely affect their life and personal choices, especially if a detrimental disease was discovered. However, while the participants did not want to know their result, they were happy for the results to be given to recipients if it would help them choose a donor. Participants spoke about specific genetic diseases that have incomplete penetrance. These participants felt that knowing such a result would give them a lifelong fear and would leave them struggling to plan a future. However one participant also worried about the laboratory scientists knowing her information and what that would mean for her privacy.

"When you find out that your children have predispositions to illnesses and maybe if you don't know it could be...I don't know if it's good to know that much..."-Naomi, embryo donor.

"I don't think I would want those results personally but I don't mind if other people have those results or that it's tested for"-Ethan, sperm donor.

"But, then the scientists are going to know this information about me"-Becky, egg donor.

Participants questioned whether society was "crossing a line" by trying to create perfect human beings. Morally they felt this type of screening was wrong and would create inequality, especially for those who were conceived naturally. There was a general feeling that technology has advanced very quickly but the science is still lacking and more thought should be given as to whether these testing procedures could do more harm than good.

"There would be things that you would need to draw the line somewhere, things that are controllable and things that aren't controllable, to not create a society which is too bound by perfecting itself"-Charlotte, egg donor.

Donors were also concerned that an increased level of genetic screening would affect whether individuals would choose to donate. These participants thought they would still donate if expanded screening was introduced; however many of these participants would not want to know their own results. Participants worried about the impact this level of screening would have on their lives and thought that more thought should be given into whether this level of screening is ethical or beneficial.

"I think less people would [want to donate]. I mean... um...we all have a little something in our closet that we don't want to share with others"-Becky, egg donor.

Discussion

This qualitative study explored attitudes towards the genetic screening of gamete (sperm or egg) and embryo donors, from the dual perspectives of the donors and the recipients, providing valuable information that will assist in the design and implementation of donor programs in the context of the availability of expanded genetic screening. All donors and recipients had personal experience of the donor screening process at Melbourne IVF, which comprised a Genetic Health Questionnaire and limited genetic testing.

In relation to the Genetic Health Questionnaire, all donors and recipients understood the importance of the information contained in the questionnaire. However some donors had difficulty filling out the questionnaire because they were uncertain about aspects of their family history, and about whether or not certain medical conditions in their family history were genetic in origin. While the questionnaire is a cost effective way of gathering family history information, our results suggest that the process could lead to misinformation, and a face-to-face interview may be more effective. Recipients appreciated and valued the information provided by donors in the Genetic Health Questionnaire, but also felt that when selecting a donor, this information was less important than non-health related information, such as physical attributes, values and beliefs, and character descriptors. Most recipients did not feel that they would reject a donor based on family medical history information alone. Although previous studies have not addressed attitudes towards genetic information, our results are comparable to a previous Australian study which showed that health information was ranked as the most important type of donor information by sperm and egg recipients and by egg donors; sperm donors ranked health information as the second most important form of donor information, behind donor physical characteristics [18].

Donors and recipients supported the existing level of genetic testing in the donor program, which comprises karyotype and carrier screening for thalassemia, spinal muscular atrophy, cystic fibrosis and Fragile X syndrome. Some donors questioned the relevance of these tests but nonetheless were happy to be tested. However when asked about the opportunity for expanded genetic testing of donors, donors and recipients had reservations and questioned the desirability of expanded genetic screening. A specific concern expressed by donors and recipients alike was that choosing donors based on the results of expanded genetic screening might represent an undesirable move towards genetic selectivity, which they likened to having a "designer baby". In addition, donors and recipients expressed concern that increased genetic screening might deter donors from donating, resulting in a decline in donor numbers.

Donors also expressed concern about the psychological impact of them receiving this additional genetic information. Interestingly, some donors stated that although they would consent to expanded genetic screening being performed in them, they would not wish to be informed of the results. In practice, IVF clinics are unlikely to agree to such a request, as it would place both the clinic and the recipient in the position of holding undisclosed genetic information that might be important for the health of the donor. Recipients were concerned that expanded genetic screening of donors might cause increased anxiety to recipients, as well as increasing the financial cost of accessing the donor program. Although many recipients recognised potential benefits of having more genetic information about donors, such as an opportunity to maximise the health of their donor-conceived child, they were uncertain whether they would actually want this information themselves. In addition, participants highlighted the important contribution of environmental factors to child health, and did not view child health as being determined only by genetics.

No recipients were strongly in favour of receiving extended screening and genetic information about donors. Although attitudes towards extended carrier screening have not been studied in a donor population, reticence about the extended carrier screening has previously been observed amongst health professionals and patient representatives, with particular concerns centring on the ethical and psychological challenges of expanded carrier screening [9, 19, 20].

Genetic information was viewed differently by recipients of donor sperm compared to recipients of donor eggs/embryos. In particular, whilst genetic information was viewed by recipients of donor sperm as a factor in their selecting a sperm donor, recipients of donor eggs or embryos mostly saw genetic information as something to be passed on to their offspring. This was partly because recipients of donor eggs or embryos had less opportunity to choose between alternative donors, and because egg donors were known to their recipients. Egg recipients in particular reported not having considered the genetic history of the donor before they were provided with the genetic health questionnaires.

Overall, this research has highlighted that while donors and recipients are supportive of existing genetic screening of gamete and embryo donors, they have reservations about expanded genetic screening. This was particularly prominent amongst donors, but was also an issue for recipients who were concerned about the impact of expanded genetic screening on the cost and availability of accessing donors. These findings contrast to those of Sawyer et al. [15] who found support amongst recipients for expanded genetic screening of donors and a willingness from recipients to pay extra for this service. Notably, the study by Sawyer et al. was conducted as an on line survey, with 85% of respondents residing in the USA. Differences between the results of the two studies may be due to differences in study methodology, and between donor programs in USA and Australia. In Australia, the perspectives of donors and recipients are likely influenced by the fact that donation of reproductive tissues must be altruistic, and it is illegal for donors to profit from their donation. When interpreting this study, it is also important to note that the number of donors and recipients in each category (egg/sperm/embryo) is small and may not be representative of the donor community as a whole. In addition, the overall participation rate of 34% represents a potential source of bias.

Conclusion

Participants in our donor program support some level of genetic screening of donors, but have concerns about expanding genetic screening beyond current levels. The implementation of expanded genetic screening in donor programs may do more harm than good.

Acknowledgments
We thank Ms. Andrea Smales, Ms. Zoe Milgrom, and Ms. Melanie Nolan for their valuable assistance with recruitment. This research was undertaken in partial fulfilment of the Master of Genetic Counselling at The University of Melbourne. This work was supported by the Victorian Government's Operational Infrastructure Support Program.

Funding
This work was made possible through the Victorian State Government Operational Infrastructure Support and Australian Government NHMRC IRIISS. The authors report no competing interests.

Authors' contributions
DJA and SL formulated the study, interpreted the data and wrote the manuscript. AK and NS conducted the interviews, analysed and interpreted the data and co-wrote the manuscript. MT coordinated recruitment and co-wrote the manuscript, AM analysed and interpreted the data and co-wrote the manuscript; JH interpreted the data and co-wrote the manuscript. All authors read and approved the final manuscript.

Authors' information
Not applicable

Competing interests

The authors of this article have not competing interests to declare.

Author details

[1]Murdoch Children's Research Institute, Royal Children's Hospital, Parkville, Australia. [2]Department of Paediatrics, The University of Melbourne, Parkville, Australia. [3]Melbourne IVF, East Melbourne, Australia. [4]Graduate School of Health, University of Technology, Sydney, Australia.

References

1. Ethics Committee of the American Society for Reproductive M. Interests, obligations, and rights of the donor in gamete donation. Fertil Steril. 2009; 91(1):22–7.

2. Dondorp W, De Wert G, Pennings G, Shenfield F, Devroey P, Tarlatzis B, Barri P, Diedrich K, Eichenlaub-Ritter U, Tuttelmann F, et al. ESHRE task force on ethics and law 21: genetic screening of gamete donors: ethical issues. Hum Reprod. 2014;29(7):1353–9.

3. Isley L, Falk RE, Shamonki J, Sims CA, Callum P. Management of the risks for inherited disease in donor-conceived offspring. Fertil Steril. 2016;106(6):1479–84.

4. Landaburu I, Gonzalvo MC, Clavero A, Ramirez JP, Yoldi A, Mozas J, Zamora S, Martinez L, Castilla JA. Genetic testing of sperm donors for cystic fibrosis and spinal muscular atrophy: evaluation of clinical utility. Eur J Obstet Gynecol Reprod Biol. 2013;170(1):183–7.

5. Sims CA, Callum P, Ray M, Iger J, Falk RE. Genetic testing of sperm donors: survey of current practices. Fertil Steril. 2010;94(1):126–9.

6. Callum P, Urbina MT, Falk RE, Alvarez-Diaz JA, Benjamin I, Sims CA. Spinal muscular atrophy (SMA) after conception using gametes from anonymous donors: recommendations for the future. Fertil Steril. 2010; 93(3):1006. e1001-1002

7. Daar JF, Brzyski RG. Genetic screening of sperm and oocyte donors: ethical and policy implications. JAMA. 2009;302(15):1702–4.

8. Maron BJ, Lesser JR, Schiller NB, Harris KM, Brown C, Rehm HL. Implications of hypertrophic cardiomyopathy transmitted by sperm donation. JAMA. 2009;302(15):1681–4.

9. van der Hout S, Holtkamp KC, Henneman L, de Wert G, Dondorp WJ. Advantages of expanded universal carrier screening: what is at stake? Eur J Hum Genet. 2016;25(1):17–21.

10. Lazarin GA, Haque IS. Expanded carrier screening: a review of early implementation and literature. Semin Perinatol. 2016;40(1):29–34.

11. Edwards JG, Feldman G, Goldberg J, Gregg AR, Norton ME, Rose NC, Schneider A, Stoll K, Wapner R, Watson MS. Expanded carrier screening in reproductive medicine-points to consider: a joint statement of the American College of Medical Genetics and Genomics, American College of Obstetricians and Gynecologists, National Society of genetic counselors, Perinatal quality foundation, and Society for Maternal-Fetal Medicine. Obstet Gynecol. 2015;125(3):653–62.

12. Henneman L, Borry P, Chokoshvili D, Cornel MC, van El CG, Forzano F, Hall A, Howard HC, Janssens S, Kayserili H, et al. Responsible implementation of expanded carrier screening. Eur J Hum Genet. 2016;24(6):e1–e12.

13. Martin J, Asan, Yi Y, Alberola T, Rodriguez-Iglesias B, Jimenez-Almazan J, Li Q, Du HQ AP, Ruiz A, et al. Comprehensive carrier genetic test using next-generation deoxyribonucleic acid sequencing in infertile couples wishing to conceive through assisted reproductive technology. Fertil Steril. 2015;104(5):1286–93.

14. Dewey FE, Chen R, Cordero SP, Ormond KE, Caleshu C, Karczewski KJ, Whirl-Carrillo M, Wheeler MT, Dudley JT, Byrnes JK, et al. Phased whole-genome genetic risk in a family quartet using a major allele reference sequence. PLoS Genet. 2011;7(9):e1002280.

15. Sawyer N, Blyth E, Kramer W, Frith L. A survey of 1700 women who formed their families using donor spermatozoa. Reprod BioMed Online. 2013;27(4):436–47.

16. Corbin J, Strauss A. Basics of qualitative research (3rd ed.): techniques and procedures for developing grounded theory. Thousand Oaks: Sage; 2008.

17. Glaser BG. The constant comparative method of qualitative analysis. Soc Probl. 1965;12(4):436–45.

18. Rodino IS, Burton PJ, Sanders KA. Donor information considered important to donors, recipients and offspring: an Australian perspective. Reprod BioMed Online. 2011;22(3):303–11.

19. Cho D, McGowan ML, Metcalfe J, Sharp RR. Expanded carrier screening in reproductive healthcare: perspectives from genetics professionals. Hum Reprod. 2013;28(6):1725–30.

20. Holtkamp KC, Vos EM, Rigter T, Lakeman P, Henneman L, Cornel MC. Stakeholder perspectives on the implementation of genetic carrier screening in a changing landscape. BMC Health Serv Res. 2017;17(1):146.

17

Ebola virus disease outbreak in Guinea: what effects on prevention of mother-to-child transmission of HIV services?

Niouma Nestor Leno[1,2]*(iD), Alexandre Delamou[2,3,4], Youssouf Koita[5], Thierno Souleymane Diallo[6], Abdoulaye Kaba[1], Therese Delvaux[4], Wim Van Damme[4] and Marie Laga[4]

Abstract

Background: An unprecedented epidemic of Ebola virus disease (EVD) affected Guinea in 2014 and 2015. It weakened the already fragile Guinean health system. This study aimed to assess the effects of the outbreak on Prevention of Mother-to-Child Transmission of HIV (PMTCT) services in 2014.

Methods: We conducted a cross-sectional retrospective study. Data was collected from 60 public health centers (30 in the EVD affected areas and 30 in the unaffected areas). The comparison of PMTCT indicators between the period before Ebola (2013) and during Ebola (2014) was done using the t-test for the means and the Chi-square test for the proportions.

Results: This study showed a substantial and significant reduction in the mean number of antenatal care visits (ANC) in the affected localities, 1617 ± 53 in 2013 versus 1065 ± 29 in 2014, $p = 0.0004$. This would represent 41% drop in health facilities' performance. On the other hand, in the unaffected localities, the fall was not significant. The same observations were made about the number of HIV tests performed for pregnant women and the number of HIV positive pregnant women initiating ARVs. The study also noted an increase in the proportion of women tested HIV+ but who did not receive ARVs (12% in 2013 versus 44% in 2014) and HIV+ pregnant women who delivered at home (18% in 2014 versus 7% in 2013).

Conclusion: This study showed that PMTCT services, which are one of the key services to improve maternal and child health, were affected in Guinea during this Ebola outbreak in 2014 compared to 2013.

Keywords: Ebola, Effects, PMTCT, Health system, Guinea

Plain English Summary

Why was this study conducted?

This study aimed to assess the effects of the outbreak on PMTCT services in Guinée, in 2014.

How was the study conducted?

We assessed changes in PMTCT indicators during the first year (2014) of the epidemic. We have included 60 public health centers, including 30 in affected areas and 30 in unaffected areas. The data collected covers the period from January 1, 2013 to December 31, 2014. The ANC and PMTCT registers were used for this collection. For each of the two areas, we compared the 2013 values to the 2014 values to estimate the changes that occurred as effect of the outbreak.

What was found in this study?

In 2014, the number of pregnant women attending ANC visits fell by 41% in the EVD affected localities, compared to only 7% in the unaffected localities.

All PMTCT indicators fell sharply during the 2014 epidemic compared with 2013. This decline was statistically more pronounced in Ebola-affected areas than in non-affected areas.

* Correspondence: nnleno81@gmail.com
[1]Bureau de Stratégie et de Développement du Ministère de la Santé, Conakry, Guinea
[2]Chair de Santé Publique de l'Université Gamal Abdel Nasser de Conakry, Conakry, Guinea
Full list of author information is available at the end of the article

What have we learned?

The weak capacity of the health system to respond to emergencies while continuing the provision of routine services and the mistrust between health care workers and communities contributed to low utilization of health services during this epidemic. It's important to continue strengthening the Guinean health system to make it more resilient to mitigate the long-term effects of the epidemic and prepare it for future health crises. To this end, special emphasis should be placed on human resources for health.

Article summary
Strengths

- The comparison of indicators before and during the epidemic, as well as in Ebola-affected and unaffected areas, allow for a better estimate of the effect of the epidemic on PMTCT services;
- The study included PMTCT centers that did not have interruptions in supply (and therefore services) on a monthly basis of 5 or more days in 2013 to account for biases related to the unavailability of supplies.

Limitation

- The use of routine data could include under-reporting bias because of the lack of regular monitoring of management tools.
- The population coverage could not be calculated because denominator data were no available. This is because the estimate of the "Spectrum" software used in Guinea could not provide disaggregated target values by region, district, or heath facilities;
- Lack of information on how the pregnant women perceived the EDV epidemic situation and on the outcome of exposed children lost to follow-up.
- Retrospective data collection (design used in this study) could be one of the limitations of this study due to biases related to the management of data sources (e.g. registry) and the problem of reporting (under or overreporting).

Background
Introduction

An unprecedented epidemic of the Ebola virus disease (EVD) affected mainly three countries in West Africa, including Guinea, Sierra Leone and Liberia in 2014 and 2015. As of 17 January 2016, the cumulative number of cases in these three countries was 28,638, of which 11,316 died [1], representing a 39.51% lethality. This epidemic remains the largest in the world in terms of the number of cases, deaths and geographical distribution since the causative virus was isolated in 1970 [2].

In Guinea, the EVD outbreak experienced three major waves of transmission in 2014. The first two were located in Conakry and some prefectures of the forest region and the third was the phase of intense transmission at national level [3].

As of December 29, 2015, 3804 Ebola cases were reported in Guinea. Of these, there were 2536 deaths, a fatality rate of 66.6% [4]. In addition, it should be noted that more than 70% of country's total Ebola cases occurred in 2014. Also, the highest number of human-to-human transmissions of the Ebola virus occurred in 2014 compared to 2015 [5]. 148 Ebola cases were confirmed among Health Care Workers as of 28 December 2014, with a fatality rate of 58.78% [5].

These alarming statistics suggest that the Ebola epidemic had probably significant indirect effects beyond the mortalities and morbidities it caused in the social and development sectors of affected communities between 2014 and 2015 [3]. The scale of the epidemic further affected the fragile health systems in the three most affected countries (Guinea, Liberia and Sierra Leone), in a way that vital and limited resources had to be reallocated to cope with the crisis, reducing the ability of countries to manage health problems [2, 6]. One aspect of the health system that could be hardly hit was the provision of basic health care services [3].

Plucinski et al., in their study conducted in 2014 noted a steady decrease of 11% in the use of health services for malaria at the operational level in Guinea during the Ebola period (2014) compared to the year before the outbreak (2013). They also noted a 15% decrease in the number of malaria cases reported in these structures [3].

It should also be noted that given the high maternal and infant mortality ratio that existed well before Ebola [7, 8], disruption of health services could be particularly damaging to maternal and child health services. A study conducted by Camara et al. [9] in 2016 showed a 51% decrease in the use of family planning services during the Ebola period in Macenta health district (Guinea) compared to the period before Ebola. The same study reported a significant 41% decrease in the number of women visiting health facilities for antenatal care [9]. Because PMTCT services are integrated into the minimum package of primary health care in Guinea, it would be expected that these services would be similarly affected by the outbreak.

Prevention of vertical HIV transmission is one of the strategies to eradicate HIV worldwide by 2030 [10, 11]; and one of the priorities of Guinea's national AIDS strategy [12]. Many activities under this strategy occur in health care settings. Therefore, any reduction in the use of these services [13, 14], due to the EVD outbreak, could negatively impact the achievement of national targets for reducing vertical transmission of HIV and de facto reducing maternal mortality and child care in Guinea.

The purpose of this study was to describe and analyze the effects of the EVD outbreak in 2014 on PMTCT service provision in Guinea.

Country general context

Guinea is located in West Africa with a population estimated at 11.7 million inhabitants in 2014, of whom 52% are women [15] and more than half (65%) of this population lives in rural areas. The country is one of the poorest countries in the world with 55.2% of the population living in poverty [7]. The health status of the population remains worrying, with high rates of maternal and infant mortality and high prevalence of certain diseases such as malaria, and adding to these are emerging and re-emerging diseases such as Ebola (2013–2015). Maternal mortality ratio increased from 980 to 724 per 100,000 live births between 2005 and 2012 [7].

In the interim report of 2016 multiple indicators clusters survey (MICS 2016) found a maternal mortality rate of 550 per 100,000 live births in Guinea, suggesting that Guinea remains among the countries with high maternal mortality rate in Africa [8]. In addition, the health status of children under 5 remains a concern. Children in this age group are among the most affected by malaria, which is the leading cause of morbidity and mortality in Guinea [7, 8]. In this age group (children under 5 years), the mortality rate before the first birthday is 88 per 1000 live births [8]. This situation could be explained by the weakness of Guinea's traditional health care system, which is based on primary health care [16]. The system currently faces many challenges, including a low coverage of human resources for health (0.5 health personnel per 1000 inhabitants in 2016 for a norm of 2.3 per 1000 inhabitants), low immunization status in children (only 26% of children aged 12–23 months are fully immunized) and a concurrent high out of pocket payment for health expenditure (62% in 2014) [16].

HIV and PMTCT care in Guinea

In Guinea, the HIV epidemic is of generalized type with an estimated national prevalence of 1.7% among people aged 15 to 49 years in 2012 [7]. According to recent estimates from UNAIDS, about 120,000 people were living with HIV in Guinea in 2014 4600 people died as a result of this disease [17].

The HIV prevalence is higher among women (2.1%) than men (1.2%) of the same age group (15–49 years) [7]. This disparity is more pronounced among pregnant women aged 15–49, whose HIV prevalence was 2.5% in 2008 and 3.56% in 2015 [18, 19]. According to estimates of the national AIDS control program, in 2014, 14% of new infections occurred among children, with 64% of

them relating to vertical transmission (mother-child) [12]. The country's PMTCT program was initiated in 2003 with seven pilot sites, including five in Conakry and two in Forécariah. A Scaling-up Plan was developed in 2008. A National Plan to Eliminate Mother-to-Child Transmission of HIV (e-PMTCT) was also developed in 2012 [20]. The current treatment regimen, in the context of PMTCT, is based on triple therapy known as "Option B+", as recommended by the World Health Organization [21, 22]. It is initiated immediately after the diagnosis of HIV infection and continues for the rest of the mother's life. Strategies identified by the national AIDS program to achieve the goals of eliminating mother-to-child transmission of HIV in Guinea by 2017 include lifelong administration of antiretroviral to HIV-positive pregnant women (Option B+), decentralization of PMTCT services to peripheral health facilities, use of community health workers to engage target populations at PMTCT sites, active search for those lost to follow-up, and use of blotting papers to collect and transport blood samples for the virological diagnosis of HIV [12]. These activities take place in health centers providing ANC services. The geographical coverage of public facilities that have integrated PMTCT activities remains low (65% of the existing 453 facilities in 2016) [23]. In 2013, there were already significant PMTCT gaps to be addressed in Guinea before the EVD outbreak occurs in 2014. The epidemic might have therefore aggravated these already existing gaps.

Methods
Study's type

This was a retrospective cross-sectional evaluative study using routine data from public health facilities.

Study population

The study targeted three categories of users of maternal and child health services including pregnant women, HIV-positive pregnant women and children born to HIV-positive mothers enrolled in public health centers providing prenatal and PMTCT services from 1 January 2013 to 31 December 2014.

We chosed 2014 as the year of comparison because the epidemic was not yet widespread in the country compared to 2015 and thus, could allow good comparison of different geographical areas.

The study included a representative sample of health facilities from across the country. Due to the wide disparity in the reporting of EVD cases, we divided the country into two strata. Stratum 1 consisted of the five most EVD affected health districts in 2014 and included Guéckédou, Macenta, Nzérékoré, Coyah and Conakry. Stratum 2 consisted of five randomly selected health districts among the districts not affected by the EVD in

2014. It included the health districts of Labe, Mamou, Boké, Kankan and Siguiri. This stratification was done to allow for comparisons, not only between the periods before (2013) and during (2014) the EVD outbreak in the same area, but also among the EVD affected and non-affected localities. Within each of the two strata, a random selection of 30 health centers offering both antenatal care and PMTCT services was carried out [24].

The selection of the study sites was conducted in steps. Step 1 included the establishment of the exhaustive list of health centre's offering both ANC and PMTCT services by stratum. Step 2 included the identification of ANC/PMTCT sites that did not experience PMTCT services disruption for more than 5 days per month in 2013. Step 3 included the random selection of 30 ANC/ PMTCT sites in each of the two strata, using the list established in step 2.

Computer random generated numbers were used for the different selections. When a selected site did not meet the selection criteria, it was replaced by the one immediately following in the sampling frame, and so on.

Data collection
Antenatal care (ANC) and Prevention of Mother-to-Child Transmission of HIV (PMTCT) registers of the included public health facilities constituted the source for data collection.

A pre-elaborated survey questionnaire was used for data collection. The data collectors were selected from the national STI/HIV/AIDS prevention and management program (Programme National de Prise en Charge Sanitaire et Prévention des infections Sexuellement Transmissible et le Virus de l'Immunodéficience Humaine, (PNPCSP/IST/VIH) and the National AIDS Control Committee (Comité National de Lutte contre le Sida, CNLS) in Guinea.

They were selected based on their experience and knowledge of interventions to prevent mother-to-child transmission. Data collection was collected retrospectively. The approach was motivated by the low completeness of the statistical reports submitted to the national health information system and the results of previous evaluations showing discrepancies between data reported by health facilities and the actual data captured from facility registers [25]. The study focused on the PMTCT cascade. To this end, the following data was collected: 1) the number of pregnant women receiving ANC, representing pregnant women who made their first ANC visit for the current pregnancy and who were registered in the CPN registers; 2) the number of pregnant women tested for HIV which includes pregnant women who made their first ANC visit and received counselling about HIV testing, were screened for HIV and were registered in PMTCT registers; 3) the number of HIV+

pregnant women, representing women seen for their first ANC visit who were tested HIV positive and were registered in the PMTCT registers; 4) the number of HIV-positive pregnant women on ARVs, including HIV-positive pregnant women who initiated ARV treatment in PMTCT services and who were registered in PMTCT registers; 5) the number of exposed children on ARVs, representing infants born to HIV-positive mothers receiving antiretroviral prophylaxis for PMTCT; 6) the number of HIV+ pregnant women who gave birth at home, representing HIV-positive pregnant women registered in health facilities for PMTCT monitoring but who gave birth outside a health facility.

Data analysis
Data was analyzed using the EPI Info 3.5.4 software (CDC Atlanta, USA). The data of this study focused on the overall performance of health centers offering prevention of mother-to-child transmission services. After entering all the data into an excel database, we performed a quality check as follows: (i) a complete check of all the values of the study variables in the database to check for missing values and outliers and make necessary corrections and, (ii) quality check of a sample of the data collection cards to make comparisons between the database and paper copies.

The comparison covered two periods: period 1 from January 1 to December 31, 2013 (Pre-Ebola period) and period 2 from January 1 to December 31, 2014 (the first year of the Ebola epidemic in Guinea).

We used mean and standard deviations (SD) to examine the differences between absolute values. The t-test was used for normal distributions and the Wilcoxon test for asymmetric distributions. The absolute difference in performance between 2014 and 2013 was calculated for each stratum. We used the Chi-square test ($\chi2$) to compare proportions. The difference was considered statistically significant for values of $p < 0.05$.

Three main proportions were calculated including (i) the proportion of HIV-positive pregnant women on ARVs, obtained by dividing the number of HIV-positive pregnant women who initiated ARV treatment during our study period by the number of all pregnant women tested HIV-positive during our study period; (ii) the proportion of exposed children on ARVs, obtained by dividing the number of children born to HIV-positive mothers who received ARV prophylaxis by the number of pregnant women tested positive during our study period; and (iii) the proportion of HIV-infected pregnant women giving birth at home, obtained by dividing the number of HIV-positive pregnant women who gave birth at home by the number of pregnant women tested positive during the study period.

These proportions are based solely on the performance of the sites and not on the coverage of the population. This is because of the lack of available data that could provide disaggregated target values by region, district, or care structure. The estimate of the "Spectrum" software used in Guinea only gives nationwide estimates and projections.

Results

A total of 60 public health centers offering both ANC and PMTCT services were included in the analysis.

Among facilities located in EVD affected areas, there was a significant reduction in the mean number of pregnant women attending ANC visits, 1617 ± 53 in 2013 compared to 1065 ± 29 in 2014 ($p = 0.0004$. In non EVD affected localities, however, the decrease was not statistically significant (from 1817 ± 331 in 2013 to 1689 ± 280 in 2014 with, $p = 0.5696$ (Table 1). The same findings were made for the number of pregnant women tested for HIV, the number of HIV-positive pregnant women on ARVs and the number of exposed children who received prophylactic ARVs (Table 1).

Figure 1a presents the monthly trend of PMTCT activities in EVD affected localities in 2014. It appears that the monthly number of pregnant women attending ANC visits was more or less stable in 2013 with a peak in July. However, in 2014, the trend was modified. The fall began between February and March, peaking between July and September 2014 with a slight increase between October and December 2014 (Fig. 1a). In contrast, in unaffected localities, the monthly trends of the mean number of ANCs visits in 2013 and 2014 are almost similar (Fig. 1b).

Differences in the performance of health facilities between 2013 and 2014 in terms of PMTCT services are presented in Table 2. In 2014, the number of pregnant women attending ANC visits fell by 41% in the EVD affected localities, compared to only 7% in the unaffected localities. The fall in the number of HIV+ pregnant women who received ARVs was 55% in the EVD affected area compared to only 8% in the unaffected area. Similar trends were observed for two other indicators including

the number of pregnant women tested for HIV (with a 53% drop) and the number of exposed children receiving prophylactic ARVs (with a 69% drop) (Table 2). (In EVD affected areas, the changes were greater during the third quarter of 2014 compared to the same period in 2013. Regarding the number of HIV-infected pregnant women on ARVs, the fall did not change between the different quarters of 2014, except for the first quarter (Table 2).

Figure 2a compares the proportion of pregnant women tested positive for HIV who did not receive ARVs in order to reduce the risk of mother-to-child transmission of HIV, but also to improve their own health status. This proportion increased during the first year of the Ebola outbreak in the EVD affected areas, from 12% in 2013 to 44% in 2014, $p < 0.05$. However, in the unaffected areas, there were no statistically significant changes (12% in 2013 compared to 13% in 2014, $p = 0.427$) (Fig. 2b). Figure 3 shows that the proportion of HIV+ pregnant women who gave birth at home increased significantly during the EVD outbreak (7% in 2013 versus 18% in 2014) in the affected areas, $P < 0.0001$.

Discussion

Our study shows that in Guinea, the use of PMTCT services significantly decreased during the EVD outbreak (2014) compared to the period before the EVD (2013). In addition, our results show that the decrease in the use of PMTCT services was significantly more pronounced in the EVD affected areas compared to the areas not affected by the EVD in 2014.

Our results corroborate those reported by Delamou et al., in a study on the effects of the EVD on maternal and child health services in the forest region of Guinea [26]. The authors noted a significant reduction in the number of ANC visits and institutional deliveries during the epidemic compared to the pre-epidemic period. Similarly, they reported a significant drop in the number of immunized children and expressed concerns about the post-epidemic trends that were still below figures of the pre-epidemic period. Despite the methodological differences between our two studies (completeness of data in their

Table 1 PMTCT indicators comparison by year and by Ebola areas, 2014, Guinea

INDICATORS	Ebola areas affected means±SD			Ebola unaffected areas means±SD		
	2013	2014	P-value	2013	2014	P-value
Pregnant women receiving ANC	1617 ± 53	1065 ± 29	0.0004	1817 ± 331	1689 ± 280	0.5696
Pregnant women tested for HIV	1460 ± 266	717 ± 140	0.0000	1622 ± 247	1379 ± 212	0.1556
Pregnant women HIV+	44 ± 13	31 ± 9	0.1292	27 ± 7	27 ± 6	0.9723
HIV-positive pregnant women on ARVs	28 ± 6	13 ± 3	0.0000*	24 ± 7	22 ± 5	0.6513
Exposed children receiving prophylactic ARVs	22 ± 5	6 ± 1	0.0000*	17 ± 5	16 ± 3	0.6020

*=no - parametric test
Number of sites: 30 in the Ebola zone and 30 in the non-Ebola zone

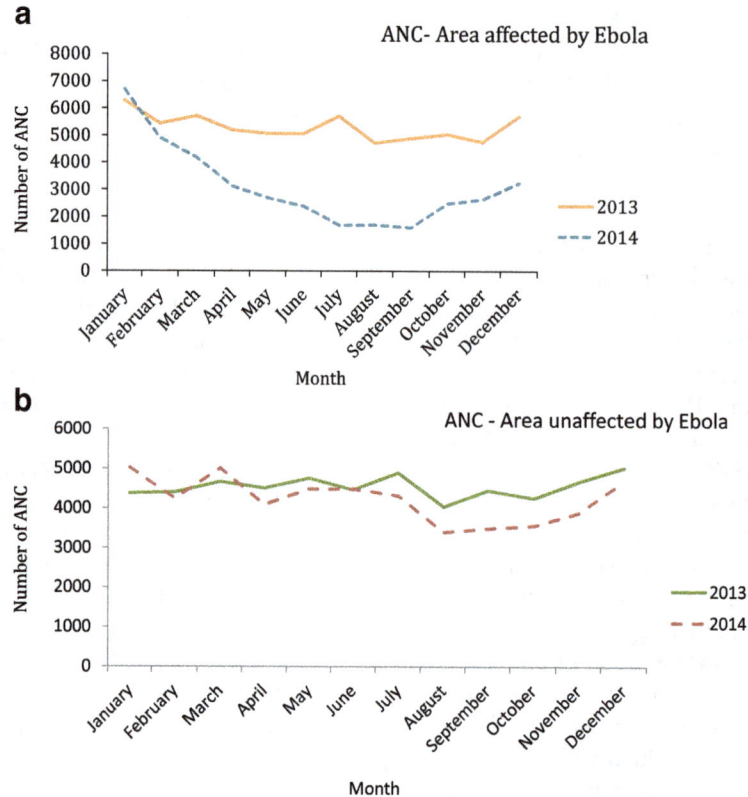

Fig. 1 a Comparison of the monthly change in the number of antenatal visits between 2013 and 2014 in 30 PMTCT facilities in EVD affected areas in 2014, Guinea. **b** Comparison of the monthly change in the number of antenatal visits between 2013 and 2014 in 30 PMTCT facilities in non EVD affected areas in 2014, Guinea

study and purposive sampling in ours), we reached the same conclusions. At the same time, this could also mean that PMTCT services would not probably regain the levels they had before the epidemic. Our results are also similar to the findings of a review of 22 studies conducted in 2016 by Ribacke et al., which reported a decrease in the number of ANC visits by 27% during the last six months of 2014 at national level in Sierra Leone and by 50% in Moyamba health district [13].

The significant drop in the number of ANC visits, pregnant women tested for HIV, and the number of HIV-positive pregnant women receiving antiretroviral

therapy may be due to a several factors. The first is the fear of communities to contract EVD in health facilities where many health workers were already infected [24]. This fear resulted from mistrust between health service providers and the community ([26]. This was the consequence of rumors around Ebola. One of the rumors circulating said that there was acomplicity between the political authorities and the International Non-Governmental Organizations (NGOs) to invent this epidemic in order to attract external funding and make financial profits. The second factor, a direct consequence of contaminations (lack of knowledge of the transmission modes and low protection of health workers) and deaths

Table 2 Changing in indicators by quarter and by the EVD status of the study areas, Guinea

	Area affected by Ebola					Area not - affected by Ebola				
	Q1	Q2	Q3	Q4	Global	Q1	Q2	Q3	Q4	Global
Pregnant women receiving ANC	−9%	−47%	− 67%	−46%	−41%	6%	−5%	−16%	−13%	−7%
Pregnant women tested for HIV	−8%	−69%	− 77%	−62%	− 53%	11%	− 14%	−31%	−25%	− 15%
Pregnant women HIV+	−15%	−19%	−29%	−52%	−28%	23%	16%	−18%	− 19%	−1%
HIV-positive pregnant women on ARVs	−14%	− 71%	−68%	−77%	−55%	22%	0%	−27%	−23%	−8%
Exposed children receiving prophylactic ARVs	−28%	−86%	− 86%	−89%	−69%	25%	−16%	−26%	−15%	−9%

Q Quarter, *Q1* January to March, *Q2* April to June, *Q3* July to September, *Q4* October to December

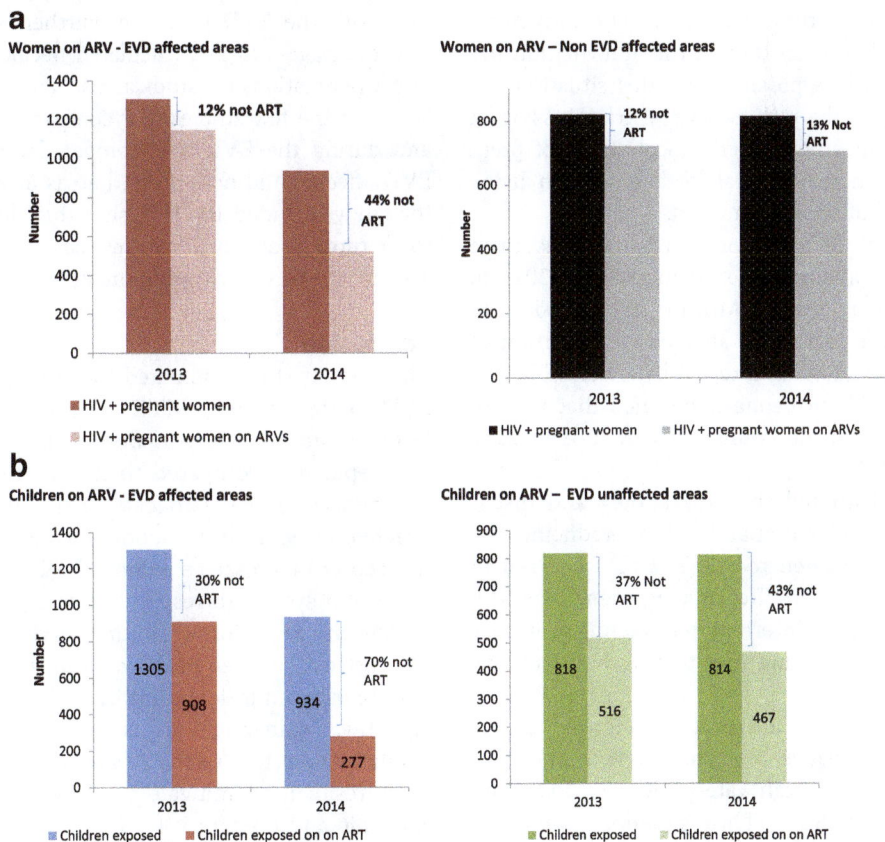

Fig. 2 a Comparison of the proportion of HIV-positive pregnant women who initiated ARVs between 2013 and 2014, stratified by EVD status of the study areas, Guinea. **b** Comparison of the proportion of HIV-positive pregnant women who were put on ARVs between 2013 and 2014, stratified by the EVD status of the study areas, Guinea

recorded among health personnel, would be the desertion of health facilities by the staff [27]. As a result, the supply and quality of health services might have been reduced. The third factor is the temporary closure of some health facilities during the peak of the epidemic [3]. The fourth factor is about the reorientation of a large number of health workers and available resources to EVD response activities (epidemiological surveillance, contact tracing, awareness raising) deemed less risky and more financially profitable.

The reduction in the number of ANC visits might have resulted in reduced demand for HIV testing among pregnant women in health centers. In fact, some women,

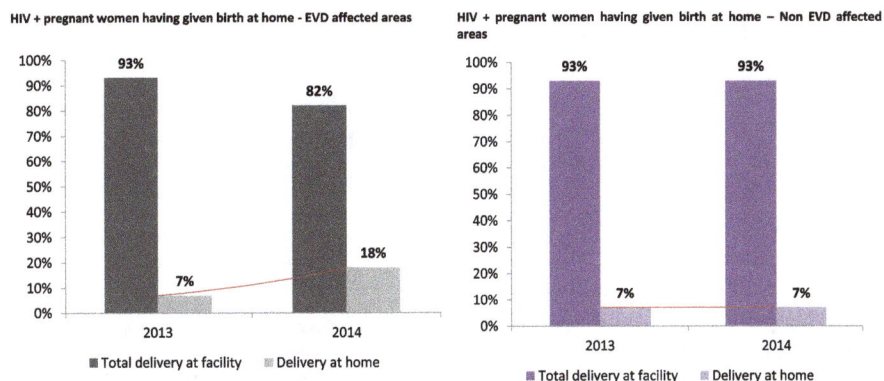

Fig. 3 Comparison of the proportion of HIV-infected pregnant women who gave birth at home (outside a health facility) between 2013 and 2014, stratified by the EVD status of the study areas, Guinea

even those who attended ANC, have been able to refuse HIV testing because of rumors about EVD transmission by blood and needles. Even though this information has not been collected, it is possible that this situation has led to an increase in the rate of vertical transmission of HIV due to ignorance of the serological status of pregnant women and increased viral load in women living with HIV, known but poorly managed.

Leuenberger et al. [26] also observed a 46% decrease in the number of patients screened for HIV in 2014 in the Medical Center of the African Phil Mission in Macenta (one of the most EVD affected district in forest Guinea in 2014). In addition, a report by UNICEF on the impact of EVD in Sierra Leone mentioned that the use of PMTCT services in the country fell by 23% in 2014 compared to 2013 [28].

EVD has also disrupted the HIV supply and distribution system at the national level by reducing the access of pregnant women to ARVs. EVD occurred in a context where HIV product management was still centralized and where international technical assistance may have been lacking due to travel restrictions and border closures [13].

Our study also showed a significant increase in the proportion of HIV-positive pregnant women who gave birth at home and the high rate of loss to follow-up among exposed children. This situation could be explained by two factors. First, even after having followed the ANC visit, women would fear to be contaminated by the EVD during deliveries in health facilities that were stigmatized for Ebola. Second, the reorientation of many community mediators, usually in charge of follow-up, to the EVD response activities might have negatively affected PMTCT services outcomes. A high number of HIV patients lost to follow-up (18.4% at six months) was reported in the study by Leuenberger in Macenta district [29]. Similar figures were reported in the systematic review by Ribacke et al., which showed a significant increase ($p < 0.001$) in the number of HIV patients lost to follow-up at 3 months, between June and October 2014 in Liberia [13].This could have led to an increased risk of mother-to-child transmission of HIV (MTCT) due to increased numbers of unsafe home deliveries, jeopardizing the investments of countries and their partners in the reduction of maternal and infant mortality that were in place before the EVD.

Our study had some limitations, in particular the lack of information on the perception of pregnant women and the future of exposed children lost to follow-up. In addition, only sites offering both ANC and PMTCT services were included in the study. This does not provide information about those offering only ANC. In addition, the collection of routine data could include under-reporting bias because of the lack of regular monitoring

of management tools as health care workers were occupied with the EVD response. Furthermore, the population coverage was not calculated because of the lack of target populations for study areas. Nevertheless, our study is one of the few studies that compared indicators before and during the EVD and compared indicators between EVD affected and non-affected areas in 2014. In addition, the study included PMTCT sites that did not experience stock rupture of more than five days a month in 2013 to account for biases related to unavailability of supplies.

Conclusion

The present study estimated the collateral effects of the EVD outbreak on PMTCT services in Guinea. All PMTCT indicators experienced a drastic fall during the 2014 epidemic compared to 2013. This fall was more pronounced in EVD-affected areas compared to non-affected ones. Lost to follow-up and home deliveries (unsecured) increased significantly. The weak capacity of the health system to respond to emergencies while continuing the provision of routine services (resilience) and the mistrust between health care workers and communities contributed to low utilization of health services during this epidemic. It is important to continue strengthening the Guinean health system to make it more resilient to mitigate the long-term effects of the epidemic and prepare it for future health crises. To this end, special emphasis should be placed on human resources health.

Abbreviations

ANC: Antenatal Care; ARVs: Antiretroviral; e-PMTCT: Eliminate Mother-to-Child Transmission of HIV; EVD: Ebola Virus Disease; HIV: Human Immunodeficiency Virus; IST: Infection Sexuellement Transmissible; Option B+: Antiretroviral therapy for all pregnant women tested positive for any immune status for life; PMTCT: Prevention of Mother-to-Child Transmission of HIV; PNCSP: Programme National de Prise en Charge Sanitaire et de Prévention des IST/VIH/Sida; SECNLS: Secrétariat Exécutif du Comité National de Lutte contre le Sida; Sida: Syndrome de l'Immunodéficience Acquise; UNICEF: United Nations Children's Fund; VIH: Virus de l'Immunodéficience Humaine

Acknowledgments

Our thanks go to the actors of the national STI/HIV/AIDS prevention and management program who worked hard during this epidemic and who facilitated the collection of the data used in this paper. We also thank the researchers from the Department of Public Health of the Institute of Tropical Medicine (ITM) of Antwerp, Belgium for their technical support in the design, data analysis and writing of this paper.

Funding

This study was conducted as part of the implementation of the Monitoring and Evaluation and Research activities of the national AIDS control program in Guinea. The supervision of HIV delivery services that enabled the collection of data from this study was funded by the National Development Budget (BND) of Guinea and the Global Fund to Fight AIDS Tuberculosis and Malaria on behalf of the new funding model's grant 2013–2017. This grant is co-managed by two Principal Recipients: the National AIDS Control Committee (CNLS) of Guinea and the NGO "Population Service International" (PSI). PNPCSP funds, one of the sub-recipients of this grant, were used for the implementation of data collection. The opinions expressed herein do not necessarily reflect those of the NCSPP, the Global Fund or CNLS.

Authors' contributions

LNN, LM initiated the study and developed the study protocol. All authors approved the study protocol. KY, TSD and NNL collected data. NNL, AD, TD and LM performed the analysis and wrote the manuscript. All authors commented on the manuscript project, then read and approved the final manuscript.

Competing interests

The authors declare that they have no competing interests.

Author details

[1]Bureau de Stratégie et de Développement du Ministère de la Santé, Conakry, Guinea. [2]Chair de Santé Publique de l'Université Gamal Abdel Nasser de Conakry, Conakry, Guinea. [3]Centre National de Formation et de Recherche en Santé Rurale de Maferinyah, Forécariah, Guinea. [4]Department of Public Health, Institute of Tropical Medicine, Antwerpen, Belgium. [5]Programme National de Prise en Charge Sanitaire et de Prévention des IST/VIH/Sida (PNPCSP) du Ministère de la Santé, Conakry, Guinea. [6]Secrétariat Exécutif du Comité National de Lutte contre le Sida (SECNLS), Conakry, Guinea.

References

1. Organisation Mondiale de la Sante. Rapport de situation sur la flambée de maladie à virus Ebola. 2016;(869). http://apps.who.int/iris/bitstream/handle/10665/204272/ebolasitrep_20Jan2016_fre.pdf?sequence=1.

2. Kieny M-P. Ebola and health systems: now is the time for change [internet]: Media center, WHO. Available from: http://who.int/mediacentre/commentaries/health-systems-ebola/en/

3. Plucinski MM, Guilavogui T, Sidikiba S, Diakité N, Diakité S, Dioubaté M, et al. Effect of the Ebola-virus-disease epidemic on malaria case management in Guinea, 2014: a cross-sectional survey of health facilities. Lancet Infect Dis. 2015;15(9):1017–23.

4. OMS. Rapport de situation sur la flambée de Maladie à virus Ebola au 29 décembre 2015. 2016.

5. Organisation Mondiale de la Sante. Feuille de route pour la riposte au virus Ebola, Rapport de situation au 31 décembre 2014; 2015. p. 1–20.

6. Save the Children. Épidémie Ebola: D'abord une crise Sanitaire; 2014. p. 2–5.

7. Institut National des Statistiques de Guinée du Ministère du Plan. Enquête Démographique et de Santé et à Indicateurs Multiples, Guinée 2012. Claverton: elINS & Macro. p. 2012.

8. Ministere du Plan et de la Coopération internationale/Institut de Statistique. Guinée_Rapport final des résultats cles. Enquête par grappes à indicateurs multiples 2016. 2017.

9. Camara BS, Delamou A, Diro E, Béavogui AH, El Ayadi AM, Sidibé S, et al. Effect of the 2014/2015 Ebola outbreak on reproductive health services in a rural district of Guinea: an ecological study. Trans R Soc Trop Med Hyg 2017;111(1):22–29.

10. UNAIDS. Accélérer la riposte. Mettre fin à l'épidémie de Sida d'ici à 2030; 2014. p. 19–20.

11. Ambia J, Mandala J. A systematic review of interventions to improve prevention of mother-to-child HIV transmission service delivery and promote retention. J Int AIDS Soc. 2016;19(1):1–11.

12. Comite National de Lutte contre le Sida de Guinée. Cadre Stratégique National de lutte Contre les IST/VIH/sida pour la periode 2013-2017de Guinée. 2013.

13. Brolin Ribacke KJ, Saulnier DD, Eriksson A, von Schreeb J. Effects of the West Africa ebola virus disease on health-care utilization - a systematic review. Front Public Health. 2016;4:222.

14. Parpia AS, Ndeffo-mbah ML, Wenzel NS, Galvani AP. Effects of Response to 2014–2015 Ebola Outbreak on Deaths from Malaria, HIV / AIDS, and Tuberculosis, West Africa. Emerg Infect Dis. 2016;22(3):433–41.

15. Institut National des Statistiques de Guinée du Ministère du Plan. Enquête Légère pour l'Evaluation de la Pauvreté en Guinée. 2002.

16. Ministère de la Santé G. Plan National de Développement Sanitaire 2015-2024. p. 2015.

17. UNAIDS. Zimbabwe HIV and AIDS estimates [Internet]. 2015. Available from: http://www.unaids.org/en/regionscountries/countries/guinea/

18. Secrétariat Exécutif du Comité National de Lutte contre le Sida-Guinée. Enquête Nationale de Surveillance sentinelle du VIH chez les Femmes enceintes en Guinée. Appui financier du Fonds mondial. 2015.

19. Ministere de la Sante et l'Hygiene Publique. Enquête Nationale de Surveillance sentinelle du VIH chez les Femmes enceintes en Guinée. Appui technique de GIZ et SE/CNLS. 2008.

20. PNPCSP/MS-Guinée. Plan National d'élimination de la transmission du VIH de la mère à l'enfant en Guinée (eTME). 2012.

21. WHO (World Health Organization). Summary: Consolidated guidelines on the use of ARV drugs for treating and preventing HIV infection - Key features and recommendations 2013; 2013. p. 16.

22. World Health Organisation. Consolidated guidelines on the use of antiretroviral drugs for treating and preventing HIV infection: recommendations for a public health approach - 2nd ed. WHO Guidel. 2016;(June):480.

23. SECNLS/PNPSCP/PSI. Cartographie nationale des services VIH (PEC, PTME, CDV) et des sites de fréquentation des populations clés (HSH et PS) en Guinée. RAPPORT FINAL. 2017.

24. Institut de Médecine tropicale d'Anvers (IMT). Belgique Epidemiologie et statistique de base; 2014. p. 1–158.

25. AMP-Agence de Médecine Préventive de Paris. Evaluation de la gestion et de la qualité des données du Programme Elargi de Vaccination (PEV) de la Guinée. 2014.

26. Alexandre D. Effect of Ebola virus disease on maternal and child health services in Guinea : A retrospective observational cohort study Eff ect of Ebola virus disease on maternal and child health services in Guinea : a retrospective observational cohort study. Lancet. The author(s). Published by Elsevier ltd. This is an Open Access article under the CC BY-NC-ND license; 2017;(February).

27. Ribacke KJB, Duinen AJ Van, Nordenstedt H, Molnes R, Froseth TW, Darj E, et al. The impact of the West Africa Ebola outbreak on obstetric health care in Sierra 2016;1–12.

28. Unicef. Sierra Leone Health Facility Survey 2014: Assessing the impact of the EVD outbreak on health Systems in Sierra Leone. Freetown: UNICEF. p. 2015. https://www.unicef.org/emergencies/ebola/files/SL_Health_Facility_Survey_2014Dec3.pdf.

29. Leuenberger D, Hebelamou J, Strahm S, De Rekeneire N, Balestre E, Wandeler G, Dabis F, IeDEA West Africa study group. Impact of the Ebola epidemic on general and HIV care in Macenta, Forest Guinea, 2014. AIDS. 2015;29(14):1883-7.

18

Factors affecting modern contraceptive use among fecund young women in Bangladesh: does couples' joint participation in household decision making matter?

Ahmed Zohirul Islam⬤

Abstract

Objectives: The purpose of the study was to explore the association between couples' joint participation in household decision making and modern contraceptive use (MCU) among fecund (physically able to bear child) young women in Bangladesh.

Methods: This study utilized a cross-sectional data ($n = 3507$) extracted from the Bangladesh Demographic and Health Survey (BDHS) 2011. Differences in the utilization of modern contraceptives (MC) by socio-demographic characteristics were assessed by χ^2 analyses. Binary logistic regression was used to identify the associated factors of usingMC, and the odds ratio with a 95% CI was computed to assess the strength of association. Multicollinearity was also checked by examining the standard errors in the fitted model.

Results: Desire for a child after two years go by and no child at all contributed the most to increasing MCU followed by receiving family planning (FP) methods from FP workers. Couples' joint decision making power on women's health care, child's health care and visiting family members or relatives emerged as the third most influential factor that might be associated with MCU.

Conclusions: Since spousal joint decision making increases the likelihood of using MC, government should include strategic interventions in FP programs to elevate women's status through creating educational and employment opportunities and encouraging more visible involvement in household decision making.

Keywords: Decision making power, women's empowerment, Young women, Modern contraceptives, Family planning, BDHS

Plain English summary

This study aimed to explore the association between couples' joint participation in household decision making and modern contraceptive use (MCU) among young women in Bangladesh. Present study utilized a cross-sectional data extracted from the Bangladesh Demographic and Health Survey 2011. A total of 3507 currently married women below 25 years old from total surveyed 17,842 women aged 15–49 years were selected for analyses.

The highest increase of the likelihood of using modern contraceptives (MC) was found among young women who desired a child after two years go by or no child at all, followed by those who were given family planning (FP) methods by FP workers. Remarkably, couples' joint participation in decision making on women's health care, child's health care and visiting family members or relatives emerged as the third most influential factor that might increase the likelihood of usingMC.

Correspondence: zohirul.18@gmail.com
Department of Population Science and Human Resource Development, University of Rajshahi, Rajshahi 6205, Bangladesh

In conclusion, government should include strategic interventions in FP programs to lift up women's status through creating educational and employment opportunities and encouraging more visible involvement in household decision making.

Introduction

Family planning (FP) is one of the major issues in many developing countries where poor maternal and child health care services are practiced [1, 2] . Studies show that contraceptive use averts 272,040 maternal deaths by reducing the chance of pregnancy and the associated complications (exposure reduction), lowering the risk of having an unsafe abortion (vulnerability reduction), delaying first pregnancy in young women who might have premature pelvic development, and reducing hazards of frailty from high parity and closely spaced pregnancies [3] and prevents almost 230 million births every year worldwide [4]. Statistics showed that an increase of 15 to 17% of using contraceptives reduces population growth by one birth for one woman [5]. However, 62% Bangladeshi women aged 15–49 years use some method of contraception, and 54% use modern methods [6]. Literature shows that women's lack of power restricts their ability to make decisions about FP practice [7, 8]. Although women's empowerment is a key to using contraceptives [9], most partners give inferior positions to women in all aspects of decision-making in developing countries [9–11]. Besides, little is known about how participation in household decision-making is associated with the utilization of modern contraceptives (MC) among young women in Bangladesh.

The population of the world became 7336 million in 2015 where South Asia contributed 1834 million people. Bangladesh, the third most populous country in South Asia comprises of 160.4 million people [12], where half of the population is aged below 25 years [13]. As this large cohort of young people enter the reproductive life span, the growth and size of the population of Bangladesh over the next few decades will largely depend on their reproductive behaviour. A considerable number of young adults get married every year. Fulfillment of their contraceptive demand is crucial to the ongoing FP programmes. Therefore, this study focuses on assessing the modern contraceptive use (MCU) status of women under 25 years old.

There is a body of literature that suggests some socio economic and demographic factors, such as residence [14], education [15, 16], age [16], economic status [17], employment status [18], religion [19, 20], parity [21], access to media [15, 19], autonomy [22, 23], desire for children [23], marital status [14] and partner communication [19], have been associated with the use ofMC. In addition, other studies revealed that women's power and autonomy is favorably related to better reproductive health and use of contraceptives [24–27]. These studies commonly provide evidence for one compelling proposition that women who exhibit substantial autonomy in the household have greater ability to control their body and achieve desired fertility. Decisions about adopting FP such as using contraceptives for either spacing or liming childbirth are often strongly shaped by spousal relationships [28]. Hence, this study attempted to address the question of whether couples' joint participation in household decision making or women's independent household decision making is more influential inMCU. Furthermore, since infecund women are physically unable to bear child and pregnant women are not currently in need of using contraceptives, including these women may bias the results. Therefore, this study aimed to address this gap in knowledge by exploring the association between couples' joint participation in household decision making and use of MC among currently married, fecund (physically able to bear child) and non-pregnant (who were not pregnant during the survey) young women in Bangladesh.

Methods

Data sources

This study used a representative set of cross-sectional data extracted from the Bangladesh Demographic and Health Survey (BDHS) 2011. The survey was conducted under the authority of the National Institute of Population Research and Training (NIPORT) of the Ministry of Health and Family Welfare, Bangladesh. Under this survey, Bangladesh was divided into seven administrative regions called divisions such as Barisal, Chittagong, Dhaka, Khulna, Rajshahi, Rangpore and Sylhet. Each division was subdivided into districts, and each district into *upazilas*. Each rural area in an *upazila* was divided into union parishads (UP) and *mouzas* within a UP. An urban area in the *upazila* was divided into *wards*, and into *mohallas* within a ward [29].

According to the official report of BDHS 2011 [29], a total of 47 people were trained to conduct household listing, to delineate Enumeration Areas (EAs), and to administer Community Questionnaires. They were also got training for the use of global positioning system (GPS) units, to obtain locational coordinates for each selected EA. The training hold out for seven days from May 11–21, 2011. A household listing operation was carried out in all selected EAs from May 22 to October 5, 2011 in four phases, each about three weeks in length. Training for the main survey was lasted for four weeks from June 6 to July 5, 2011. A total of 173 fieldworkers were recruited based on their educational level, prior experience with surveys, maturity, and willingness to spend up to six months on the project. Fieldwork for the 2011 BDHS was conducted by 16 interviewing teams, each consisting of one supervisor, one field editor, five female interviewers, two male interviewers, and one logistics staff member. The collection of data was accomplished in five phases, starting on July 8, 2011 and ending on December 27, 2011.

A nationally representative household based sample was created through a stratified, multistage cluster sampling strategy of which 600 primary sampling units were constructed (207 in urban areas and 393 in rural areas). The primary sampling units were derived from a sampling frame created for the 2011 Population and Housing Census, provided by Bangladesh Bureau of Statistics (BBS). Detailed information on survey design and sampling procedures has been reported elsewhere [29]. A total of 17,842 ever married women aged 15–49 were interviewed in the survey. After applying the definition of young people adopted by the United Nations [30], a total of 3507 currently married non-pregnant fecund women younger than 25 years, who were in actual need of using contraceptives, were selected for analyses (Fig. 1).

Response variable

The outcome variable of this study wasMCU, which is binary in nature (use or non-use). During the survey, sexually active women were asked if they were currently using any method to delay or avoid getting pregnant.

Those that reported using any method to delay or avoid getting pregnant were further asked to indicate what they were doing or the method they were using. MC, such as pills, condoms, Intra-Uterine Devices (IUD), injections and implants/norplants, refer to safe and effective methods to prevent pregnancy [29]. A binary variable is then created and categorized as using any type of MC and versus no use.

Statistical analyses

This study begins with descriptive exploration of both dependent and independent variables. Differences in MCU by socio-demographic characteristics were assessed by χ^2 analyses, with significance for all analyses set at $P < 0.05$. Since the response variable of this study had two categories, the binary logistic regression model was fitted to assess the net effect of selected socio-demographic variables. Because stepwise logistic regression analysis is a technique for selecting influential variables in multiple regression models [31], this study used this technique of analysis (backward LR method). All the variables significant in bivariate analyses were simultaneously included in the stepwise logistic regression model, and finally, the most influential predictors

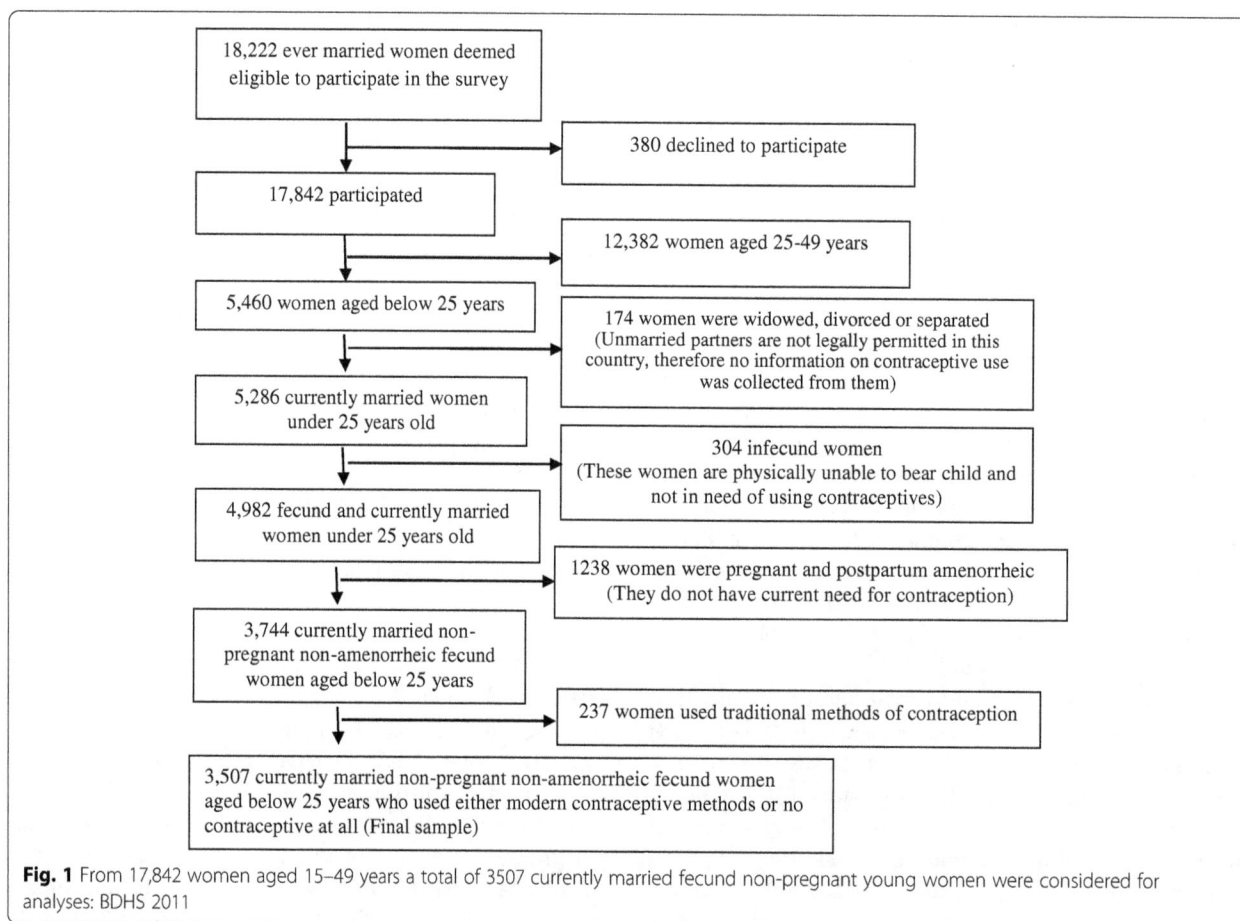

Fig. 1 From 17,842 women aged 15–49 years a total of 3507 currently married fecund non-pregnant young women were considered for analyses: BDHS 2011

for MCU were explored. Multicollinearity in the logistic regression analyses in this study was checked by examining the standard errors for the regression coefficients. A standard error larger than 2.0 indicates numerical problems, such as multicollinearity among the independent variables [32]. All of the independent variables in the fitted model had a standard error < 0.75 that indicate absence of multicollinearity in the study. Missing values are omitted from the analysis. Data were analyzed using SPSS Release 21.0 (SPSS Inc., Chicago, IL).

Results

Modern contraceptive use status and socio-demographic profiles

Table 1 describes the percentage distribution of using MC according to socio-demographic characteristics of 3507 currently married women younger than 25 years. Modern contraceptive prevalence was 69% among fecund women aged below 25 years. This study elucidates that 18% of women who wanted a child after two years go by were at risk of having mistimed pregnancies, 15% of women who wanted no child at all were at risk of encountering unwanted pregnancies in their young ages and 47% of women who were undecided about having child were at risk of getting unplanned pregnancies due to not using contraceptives.

This study also revealed several socio-demographic factors that might be associated with MCU at a bivariate level of analysis, using the chi-square test and hence, provided p-values for the differences of the groups within each explanatory variable according to the percentages of using versus not using MC (Table 1). MCU was found highest among fecund women aged 23–24 years, those who were non-Muslim, who got married before age of 15 years, who had two or more living children, those whose husbands were professional non-manual workers, who lived in Barisal division, who resided in the urban areas and who jointly took decision with their husbands regarding their own health care, child health care, large household purchases and visiting to family members or relatives.

Factors affecting modern contraceptive use of young women

Stepwise logistic regression analyses were performed to identify the most influential factors that might affect the likelihood of using MC. Table 2 shows that the highest increase of the likelihood of using MC was found among young women who desired a child after two years go by or no child at all, followed by those who were given FP methods by FP workers, who took decision together with their husbands about women's own healthcare, child's healthcare, and visiting family members or relatives, who had increasing number of living children, whose husbands were professional workers, and who were

non-Muslim. This study also indicated that the greatest decrease of the likelihood of using MC was observed among women who lived in Sylhet or Chittagong region, followed by women who did not know about their husbands' desires for the number of children and who lived in the rural areas of the country.

We observed that women who desired a child after two years go by were more likely to use MC [OR(95% CI): 14.004 (10.841–18.091), p < 0.001] and who wanted no child at all were also more likely to use MC [OR(95% CI): 10.854 (7.517–15.674), p < 0.001] than who desired a child within two years go by. Besides, women who were undecided about having a child were 3.477 times and who wanted another child but unsure about timing were 5.949 times likely to use MC compared to those who wanted another child within two years go by. Women who were given FP methods by the FP workers were 5.047 [(95% CI): (2.151–11.840), p = < 0.001] times likely to use MC than their counterparts who only talked with the FP workers.

The likelihood of using MC was increased when husband and wife jointly participate in decision making on respondent's own health care [OR (95% CI): 2.761 (1.925–3.960), p < 0.001], on child health care [OR (95% CI): 2.616 (1.808–3.786), p < 0.001], and on visiting family members or relatives [OR (95% CI): 1.830 (1.176–2.849), p = 0.007] than their counterparts who decided alone about these issues. It was also observed that if decisions about health care of women, child health care and visiting family members or relatives were taken by husband alone then the likelihood of using MC was increased by 2.698 times, 2.164 times and 1.559 times respectively compared to the women who took decision alone about these matters.

We also observed that number of living children played a significant role in contraceptive use since the likelihood of using MC was increased [OR (95% CI): 1.951 (1.516–2.511), p < 0.001] with increasing the number of children. The likelihood of using MC increased [OR (95% CI): 1.701 (1.354–2.138), p < 0.001] among women whose husbands were professional (non-manual) workers compared to their counterparts whose husbands were manual workers. Non-Muslim women were more likely to use MC than their Muslim counterparts.

Women residing in Sylhet, Chittagong, Dhaka, and Rangpur division were 0.231, 0.259, 0.479, and 0.589 times likely to use modern contraceptives than who lived in Barisal division, respectively. Women who resided in the rural areas were less likely to use [OR (95% CI): 0.617 (0.502–0.759), p < 0.001] modern contraceptives than who lived in the urban areas. The likelihood of using modern contraceptives was decreased among women who did not know about their husbands' desires for having children than those women who desired equal

Table 1 Percentage distribution of modern contraceptive use by socio-demographic characteristics of women: BDHS 2011 ($n = 3507$)

Characteristics	Modern contraceptive use (%)		p-value
	No	Yes	
Age (years)			< 0.001
15–19	37.3	62.7	
20–22	28.9	71.1	
23–24	26.6	73.4	
Husband's age (years)			0.072
15–25	33.7	66.3	
26–30	31.3	68.7	
31–77	29.0	71.0	
Age at marriage (years)			< 0.001
< 15	26.2	73.8	
15–17	31.8	68.2	
18–24	39.6	60.4	
Educational level			0.466
Illiterate	35.4	64.6	
Primary	30.5	69.5	
Secondary	31.1	68.9	
Higher	32.6	67.4	
Religion			0.011
Muslim	32.0	68.0	
Non-Muslim	25.1	74.9	
Place of residence			0.003
Urban	28.2	71.8	
Rural	33.1	66.9	
Region			< 0.001
Barisal	20.9	79.1	
Chittagong	42.8	57.2	
Dhaka	35.2	64.8	
Khulna	25.0	75.0	
Rajshahi	25.2	74.8	
Rangpur	24.3	75.7	
Sylhet	47.7	52.3	
Wealth index			0.109
Poorest	29.1	70.9	
Poorer	28.1	71.9	
Middle	32.8	67.2	
Richer	33.7	66.3	
Richest	32.2	67.8	
Husband's occupation			< 0.001
Manual	33.8	66.2	

Table 1 Percentage distribution of modern contraceptive use by socio-demographic characteristics of women: BDHS 2011 ($n = 3507$) (Continued)

	Modern contraceptive use (%)		p-value
	No	Yes	
Non-manual	24.5	75.5	
Did not work	38.1	61.9	
Visited by FP worker in past 6 months			< 0.001
Talked	24.3	75.7	
Gave family planning method	4.9	95.1	
Talked and gave method	4.8	95.2	
No	34.1	65.9	
Number of living children			< 0.001
0	61.1	38.9	
1	24.1	75.9	
2	15.5	84.5	
3–5	19.2	80.8	
Desire for more children			< 0.001
Wants within 2 years	76.6	23.4	
Wants after 2+ years	18.0	82.0	
Wants, unsure timing	48.1	51.9	
Undecided	47.0	53.0	
Wants no more	14.9	85.1	
Husband's desire for children			< 0.001
Both wanted same	30.4	69.6	
Husband wanted more	31.9	68.1	
Husband wanted fewer	26.6	73.4	
Did not know	66.1	33.9	
Person who usually decides on respondent's health care			< 0.001
Respondent alone	54.0	46.0	
Respondent and husband jointly	22.7	77.3	
Husband alone	28.0	72.0	
Someone else	54.3	45.7	
Other	68.8	31.3	
Person who usually decides on visits to family or relatives			< 0.001
Respondent alone	50.3	49.7	
Respondent and husband jointly	23.4	76.6	
Husband alone	27.9	72.1	
Someone else	49.6	50.4	
Other	57.1	42.9	
Person who usually decides on large household purchases			< 0.001
Respondent alone	52.3	47.7	
Respondent and husband jointly	24.3	75.7	

Table 1 Percentage distribution of modern contraceptive use by socio-demographic characteristics of women: BDHS 2011 (n = 3507) (Continued)

	Modern contraceptive use (%)		p-value
Husband alone	27.2	72.8	
Someone else	45.9	54.1	
Other	65.0	35.0	
Final say on: Child health care			< 0.001
Respondent alone	45.7	54.3	
Respondent & husband jointly	15.5	84.5	
Husband alone	20.0	80.0	
Someone else	45.8	54.2	
Other	60.8	39.2	
Total	31.4	68.6	

Note: Row percentages sum to 100%; p-values are based on chi-square tests

number of children with their husbands' desire. The likelihood of using MC was decreased with increasing age and increased with increasing age at marriage.

Discussion

This study assessed the relationship between household decision making and MCU and also identified the other factors contributed to the utilization of MC among currently married, fecund and non-pregnant women under 25 years old in Bangladesh using Demographic and Health Survey data of 2011.

Results showed that consensus in household decision making regarding women's own health care, visiting family members or relatives and child health care appeared as the third, fourth and sixth most influential contributing factor of MCU, respectively. The most significant factors contributed to using modern contraceptives were desire for children after two years, or want no child at all and receiving FP methods from FP workers. Other key factors that showed significant variability in using MC were number of living children, husbands engaged in professional non-manual jobs, regional variations and place of residence.

Present study demonstrated that women who were under collective decision-making with their husbands regarding their own health care, child health care and visiting family members or relatives were more likely to use MC than those who took decision alone about these matters. The likelihood of using MC decreased among young women who did not know about their husbands' desires for having children in comparison to women who shared the same feelings regarding parenthood as their husbands. Hence, this study clearly indicated that communication between husband and wife and eventually couples' joint participation in household decision

making emerged as one of the most influential factors that might be associated with MCU. Studies suggest that greater gender equality may encourage women's autonomy and may facilitate the uptake of contraception because of increased female participation in decision making [33]. Moreover, male participation in sharing the responsibility to practice and support family planning is identified as a vital strategy in increasing the contraceptive prevalence rate [34].

This study also revealed that women who desired another child after two years go by were more likely to use MC than those women who desired another child within two years go by. This finding is similar to previous study conducted in Bangladesh, Uganda and Pakistan [35–37]. Some of the reasons for this postponed childbearing as stated in other studies are: women's increased participation on the labour market, including their longer education [38–40] and career planning [38]. Furthermore, financial and practical circumstances during their studies may be difficult to combine with establishing a family, and a high educational level and a desire for career development and will increase the likelihood of delaying child birth in women [40–42]. Young women often express a need to avoid pregnancy because they may be too young to care for a baby, they may have to end or postpone their education [43].

Women who were given family planning methods by the FP workers were more likely to use MC than their counterparts who only talked with the FP workers. Consistently, other studies done in Bangladesh and Cambodia highlighted that outreach activities by FP workers and accessibility to FP related information to married women of reproductive age were significantly associated with use of modern contraceptives [19, 44, 45]. The likelihood of using MC was increased with increasing number of children. This finding is in line with the previous reports from Bangladesh, Tanzania and Pakistan [36, 37, 46].

This study described that women in Sylhet Chittagong, and Dhaka divisions were less likely to use MC than women living in Barisal division. Residing in the rural areas decreased the likelihood of using MC in comparison to their urban counterparts. Studies suggest that geographical variations in the utilization of contraceptives have been found to be influenced by a number of factors like cultural beliefs such as, value attached to child [47], the presence and quality of reproductive health care services [48], the physical characteristics of the area, and the presence of transport routes [49, 50].

Women whose husbands did professional jobs were more likely to use MC compared to women whose husbands were manual workers. This study supports findings from several other studies that showed that Muslim women were less likely to use MC than their

Table 2 Logistic regression model for modern contraceptive use

Predictors	Odds Ratio (95% CI)	p-value
Person who usually decides on respondent's health care		
Respondent alone *		< 0.001
Respondent and husband jointly	2.761 (1.925–3.960)	< 0.001
Husband alone	2.698 (1.875–3.885)	< 0.001
Someone else	1.186 (0.770–1.827)	0.439
Other	2.445 (0.577–10.368)	0.225
Final say on: Child health care		
Respondent alone *		< 0.001
Respondent & husband jointly	2.616 (1.808–3.786)	< 0.001
Husband alone	2.164 (1.430–3.277)	< 0.001
Someone else	1.156 (0.739–1.808)	0.526
Other	1.524 (0.982–2.364)	0.060
Person who usually decides on visiting family or relatives		
Respondent alone *		0.065
Respondent and husband jointly	1.830 (1.176–2.849)	0.007
Husband alone	1.559 (0.992–2.449)	0.054
Someone else	1.377 (0.851–2.229)	0.193
Other	0.876 (0.255–3.012)	0.833
Desire for more children		
Wants within 2 years *		< 0.001
Wants after 2+ years	14.004 (10.841–18.091)	< 0.001
Wants, unsure timing	5.949 (3.032–11.674)	< 0.001
Undecided	3.477 (1.902–6.358)	< 0.001
Wants no more	10.854 (7.517–15.674)	< 0.001
Visited by FP worker in past 6 months		
Talked *		< 0.001
Gave family planning method	5.047 (2.151–11.840)	< 0.001
Talked and gave method	4.479 (1.228–16.335)	0.023
No	0.781 (0.546–1.117)	0.176
Husband's occupation		
Manual *		< 0.001
Non-manual	1.701 (1.354–2.138)	< 0.001
Did not work	1.264 (0.711–2.248)	0.425
Husband's desire for children		
Both want same *		0.010
Husband wants more	0.761 (0.522–1.108)	0.154
Husband wants fewer	1.080 (0.734–1.589)	0.697
Did not know	0.462 (0.281–0.760)	0.002
Religion		
Muslim*		
Non-Muslim	1.628 (1.134–2.336)	0.008
Place of residence		
Urban *		

Table 2 Logistic regression model for modern contraceptive use (Continued)

Predictors	Odds Ratio (95% CI)	p-value
Rural	0.617 (0.502–0.759)	< 0.001
Region		
Barisal *		< 0.001
Chittagong	0.259 (0.179–0.375)	< 0.001
Dhaka	0.479 (0.333–0.690)	< 0.001
Khulna	0.790 (0.536–1.166)	0.235
Rajshahi	0.871 (0.585–1.298)	0.498
Rangpur	0.589 (0.396–0.877)	0.009
Sylhet	0.231 (0.150–0.358)	< 0.001
Age	0.932 (0.883–0.984)	0.011
Age at marriage	1.077 (1.018–1.140)	0.010
Number of living children	1.951 (1.516–2.511)	< 0.001
Constant	0.105	< 0.001

Note: * Reference category, CI is confidence interval

non-Muslim counterparts [19, 37]. The likelihood of using MC was decreased with increasing age and increased with increasing age at marriage among fecund women aged below 25 years. Therefore, establishment of youth-friendly service centers in convenient places and providing essential materials would encourage young people to use reproductive health services [45].

Limitations

This study must be considered with some limitations. There may be possibility of threats to internal validity. Firstly, major portions of the observations were dropped (approximately 79%) during data cleaning because this study considered only currently married, non-pregnant and fecund young women. Therefore, this study would suffer from the selection bias. Secondly, the possibility of under reporting cannot be ruled out since young women may be reluctant to reveal their contraceptive use status. Because, though the government and non-government organizations have a long history of investment in FP, contraceptive use is still a sensitive and often stigmatized subject in Bangladesh [37]. However, the personal interview method applied in this study is widely resorted to for this kind of research.

There may also be a possibility of threat to external validity. Although nationally representative data set was employed, this study cannot be generalized to all women in Bangladesh because it focused on only currently married and fecund young women. Finally, the questionnaire was filled out by the interviewers and their personal opinions might have biased the information. However, according to the BDHS report, interviewers were provided training for implementing the survey based on a training manual especially developed to enable the field staff to collect data in a friendly, secure, and ethical manner. In spite of these limitations, this study revealed important associations between couples' consensus in decision making and MCU, which have significant implications. Nevertheless, since a nationally representative dataset is used in this study, findings could be a true representation of the situation of this sub-group of women. Moreover, international comparisons of results are possible as DHS surveys take up similar instruments across the countries.

Conclusions

This study concludes that spousal joint participation in household decision making emerged to be a significant factor contributed to increasing the likelihood of MCU. Therefore, policy makers should focus on developing negotiation skills in young people by creating educational and employment opportunities. Government should include strategic interventions in FP programs to elevate women's status through encouraging more visible involvement in household decision making in order to increase MCU. Besides, desire for a child after two years go by or no child at all contributed the most to increasing the likelihood of MCU, followed by getting FP methods from FP workers. Therefore, this study also suggests that FP interventions should be tailored through wide spreading the activities of FP workers and introducing reproductive and sex education in schools to prepare the young for healthy and responsible living. Because remarkable portions of fecund young women want to either postpone or delay pregnancies but do not use contraceptives, this study suggests a qualitative study to investigate in depth why this sub-group of women does not use contraceptives. In last but not least, contraceptive discontinuation and switching of methods among young and older women would be our future research.

Abbreviations

BDHS: Bangladesh Demographic and Health Survey; CI: Confidence Interval; FP: Family planning; MC: Modern contraceptives; MCU: Modern contraceptive use; OR: Odds Ratio

Acknowledgements

I would like to acknowledge Dr. Md. Golam Mostofa, Professor, Department of Population Science and Human Resource Development, University of Rajshahi, Bangladesh for his valuable suggestions in carrying out this study. I also acknowledge the MEASURE DHS for providing the data set and all individuals and institutions in Bangladesh involved in the implementation of the BDHS 2011.

Competing interests

The author declares that he has no conflict of interests.

Authors' contributions

The author read and approved the final manuscript.

References

1. Yigzaw M, Zakus D, Tadesse Y, Desalegn M, Fantahun M. Paving the way for universal family planning coverage in Ethiopia: an analysis of wealth related inequality. Int J Equity Health. 2015;14(1):77.
2. Onarheim KH, Taddesse M, Norheim OF, Abdullah M, Miljeteig I. Towards universal health coverage for reproductive health services in Ethiopia: two policy recommendations. Int J Equity Health. 2015;14(1):86.
3. Ahmed S, Li Q, Liu L, Tsui AO. Maternal deaths averted by contraceptive use: an analysis of 172 countries. Lancet. 2012;380(9837):111–25.
4. Liu L, Becker S, Tsui A, Ahmed S. Three methods of estimating births averted nationally by contraception. Popul Stud. 2008;62(2):191–210.
5. Cleland J, Conde-Agudelo A, Peterson H, Ross J, Tsui A. Contraception and health. Lancet. 2012;380(9837):149–56.
6. National Institute of Population Research and Training (NIPORT). Bangladesh demographic and health survey 2014. Mitra and Associates, Dhaka, Bangladesh and ICF International, Calverton, Maryland, USA 2016.
7. Blanc AK. The effect of power in sexual relationships on sexual and reproductive health: an examination of the evidence. Stud Fam Plan. 2001;32(3):189–213.
8. Bawah AA, Akweongo P, Simmons R, Phillips JF. Women's fears and men's anxieties: the impact of family planning on gender relations in northern Ghana. Stud Fam Plan. 1999;30(1):54–66.
9. Do M, Kurimoto N. Women's empowerment and choice of contraceptive methods in selected African countries. Int Perspect Sex Reprod Health. 2012:23–33.
10. Bogale B, Wondafrash M, Tilahun T, Girma E. Married women's decision making power on modern contraceptive use in urban and rural southern Ethiopia. BMC Public Health. 2011;11(1):342.
11. Bourey C, Stephenson R, Bartel D, Rubardt M. Pile sorting innovations: exploring gender norms, power and equity in sub-Saharan Africa. Global public health. 2012;7(9):995–1008.
12. Population Reference Bureau. World population data sheet. In: Population reference bureau Washington; 2015.
13. Central Intelligence Agency. Country comparison to the world. In: The world Factbook; 2015.
14. Audu B, Yahya S, Geidam A, Abdussalam H, Takai I, Kyari O. Polygamy and the use of contraceptives. Int J Gynecol Obstet. 2008;101(1):88–92.
15. Ekani-Besala M, Carre N, Calvez T, Thonneau P. Prevalence and determinants of current contraceptive method use in a palm oil company in Cameroon. Contraception. 1998;58:29–34.
16. Oye-Adeniran BA, Adewole IF, Umoh AV, Oladokun A, Gbadegesin A, Ekanem EE. Community-based study of contraceptive behaviour in Nigeria. Afr J Reprod Health. 2006;10(2):90–104.
17. Gakidou E, Vayena E. Use of modern contraception by the poor is falling behind. PLoS Med. 2007;4(2):e31.
18. Islam A, Mondal N, Khatun L, Rahman M, Islam R. Prevalence and determinants of contraceptive use among employed and unemployed women in Bangladesh. International Journal of MCH and AIDS. 2016;5(2):92–102.
19. Rahman M, Islam A, Islam M. Rural-urban differentials of knowledge and practice of contraception in Bangladesh. Journal of Population and Social Studies. 2010;18(2):87–110.
20. Islam AZ, Mostofa MG, Islam MA. Factors affecting unmet need for contraception among currently married fecund young women in Bangladesh. Eur J Contracept Reprod Health Care. 2016:1–6.
21. Islam R, Islam AZ, Rahman M. Unmet need for family planning: experience from urban and rural areas in Bangladesh. Public Health Research. 2013;3(3):37–42.
22. Cleland J, Bernstein S, Ezeh A, Faundes A, Glasier A, Innis J. Family planning: the unfinished agenda. Lancet. 2006;368(9549):1810–27.
23. Nagase T, Kunii O, Wakai S, Khaleel A. Obstacles to modern contraceptive use among married women in southern urban Maldives. Contraception. 2003;68(2):125–34.
24. Govindasamy P, Malhotra A. Women's position and family planning in Egypt. Stud Fam Plan. 1996:328–40.
25. Rahman M. Women's autonomy and unintended pregnancy among currently pregnant women in Bangladesh. Matern Child Health J. 2012;16(6):1206–14.
26. Haque SE, Rahman M, Mostofa MG, Zahan MS. Reproductive health care utilization among young mothers in Bangladesh: does autonomy matter? Womens Health Issues. 2012;22(2):e171–80.
27. Hindin MJ. Women's autonomy, women's status and fertility-related behavior in Zimbabwe. Popul Res Policy Rev. 2000;19(3):255–82.
28. Allendorf K. Couples' reports of women's autonomy and health-care use in Nepal. Stud Fam Plan. 2007;38(1):35–46.
29. National Institute of Population Research and Training (NIPORT). Bangladesh demographic and health survey 2011. Mitra and Associates, Dhaka, Bangladesh and ICF International, Calverton, Maryland, USA 2013.

30. General Assembly Resolutions, A/RES/62/126 *United Nations* 2008.
31. Chatterjee S, Hadi AS. Simple linear regression. Regression Analysis by Example, Fourth Edition. 2006:21–51.
32. Chan Y. Biostatistics 202: logistic regression analysis. Singap Med J. 2004; 45(4):149–53.
33. Hakim A, Salway S, Mumtaz Z. Womens autonomy and uptake of contraception in Pakistan. Asia-Pac Popul J. 2003;18(1):63–82.
34. Manaf A, Manaf M. Male participation and sharing of responsibility in strengthening family planning activities in Malaysia Malaysian Journal of Public Health Medicine. 2010; 10(1):23–27.
35. Asiimwe JB, Ndugga P, Mushomi J, Ntozi JPM. Factors associated with modern contraceptive use among young and older women in Uganda; a comparative analysis. BMC Public Health. 2014;14(1):926.
36. Stephenson R, Hennink M. Barriers to family planning service use among the urban poor in Pakistan. Asia-Pac Popul J. 2004;19(2):5–26.
37. Islam AZ, Rahman M, Mostofa MG. Association between contraceptive use and socio-demographic factors of young fecund women in Bangladesh. Sexual & Reproductive Healthcare. 2017;
38. WHO, UNICEF, UNFPA,the World Bank. Trends in Maternal Mortality: 1990 to 2008. Estimates Developed by WHO, UNICEF, UNFPA and the World Bank. Geneva, Switzerland. 2010.
39. OsayiOsemwenkha S. Gender issues in contraceptive use among educated women in Edo state, Nigeria. *African health sciences*. 2004;4(1):40–9.
40. Mensch BS, Bruce J, Greene ME. The uncharted passage: girls adolescence in the developing world. New York: Population Council; 1998.
41. Haberland N, Chong E, Bracken H, Parker C. Early marriage and adolescent girls YouthLens on reproductive health and HIV. AIDS. 2005;15:99–119.
42. Chowdhury A, Phillips JF. Predicting contraceptive use in Bangladesh: a logistic regression analysis. J Biosoc Sci. 1989;21(02):161–8.
43. United Nations. Goal 5: improving maternal health. 2012.
44. Thou C. Factors influencing modern contraceptive use among currently married women in Cambodia: Mahidol University; 2008.
45. Islam AZ. Association between modern contraceptive use and socio-demographic factors among fecund young women in Bangladesh. Journal of Women's Health, Issues & Care. 2017;6(5)
46. Lwelamira J, Mnyamagola G, Msaki M. Knowledge, Attitude and Practice (KAP) towards modern contraceptives among married women of reproductive age in Mpwapwa District, Central Tanzania. *Current Research Journal of Social Sciences*. 2012;4(3):235–45.
47. Ntozi J. High fertility in rural Uganda. Kampala: Fountain publishers; 1995.
48. Tsui AO, Ochoa LH. The role of family planning programs as a fertility determinant. In: Ross JPJ, editor. Service proximity as a determinant of contraceptive behavior : evidence from cross-National Studies of survey data. London: Oxford University Press; 1992.
49. Nielsen KK, Nielsen SM, Butler R, Lazarus JV. Key barriers to the use of modern contraceptives among women in Albania: a qualitative study. Reproductive health matters. 2012;20(40):158–65.
50. Stephenson R, Baschieri A, Clements S, Hennink M, Madise N. Contextual influences on modern contraceptive use in sub-Saharan Africa. Am J Public Health. 2007;97(7):1233–40.

19

Antenatal tobacco use and iron deficiency anemia: integrating tobacco control into antenatal care

Ritesh Mistry[1][*], Andrew D. Jones[2], Mangesh S. Pednekar[3], Gauri Dhumal[3], Anjuli Dasika[1], Ujwala Kulkarni[2], Mangala Gomare[4] and Prakash C. Gupta[3]

Abstract

Background: In India, tobacco use during pregnancy is not routinely addressed during antenatal care. We measured the association between tobacco use and anemia in low-income pregnant women, and identified ways to integrate tobacco cessation into existing antenatal care at primary health centers.

Methods: We conducted an observational study using structured interviews with antenatal care clinic patients ($n = 100$) about tobacco use, anemia, and risk factors such as consumption of iron rich foods and food insecurity. We performed blood tests for serum cotinine, hemoglobin and ferritin. We conducted in-depth interviews with physicians ($n = 5$) and auxiliary nurse midwives ($n = 5$), and focus groups with community health workers ($n = 65$) to better understand tobacco and anemia control services offered during antenatal care.

Results: We found that 16% of patients used tobacco, 72% were anemic, 41% had iron deficiency anemia (IDA) and 29% were food insecure. Regression analysis showed that tobacco use (OR = 14.3; 95%CI = 2.6, 77.9) and consumption of green leafy vegetables (OR = 0.6; 95%CI = 0.4, 0.9) were independently associated with IDA, and tobacco use was not associated with consumption of iron-rich foods or household food insecurity. Clinics had a system for screening, treatment and follow-up care for anemic and iron-deficient antenatal patients, but not for tobacco use. Clinicians and community health workers were interested in integrating tobacco screening and cessation services with current maternal care services such as anemia control. Tobacco users wanted help to quit.

Conclusion: It would be worthwhile to assess the feasibility of integrating antenatal tobacco screening and cessation services with antenatal care services for anemia control, such as screening and guidance during clinic visits and cessation support during home visits.

Plain english summary

Tobacco use and anemia are harmful to pregnant women and their fetuses. In India, tobacco use during pregnancy is not addressed when woman receive antenatal care, while anemia and other nutritional problems, which are more common, make up key components of care. We studied the relationship between tobacco use and anemia to find opportunities to integrate tobacco cessation into antenatal care at governmental health centers in Mumbai, India. We interviewed patients and did

blood tests for tobacco use, anemia and iron-deficiency. We also interviewed providers and had focus group discussions with community health workers who worked at antenatal care clinics.

We found that 16% of patients used tobacco, 72% were anemic, 41% had iron deficiency anemia (IDA) and 29% were food insecure. Tobacco use dramatically increased the risk of IDA and consumption of green leafy vegetables lowered the risk. Tobacco users compared to non-users were just as likely to consume iron-rich foods and to be food secure. Clinics had a system for screening, treatment and follow-up care for anemic and iron-deficient patients, but no services were present for tobacco use. Clinicians and community health workers were interested in integrating tobacco screening and

* Correspondence: riteshm@umich.edu
[1]Department of Health Behavior and Health Education, University of Michigan School of Public Health, 1415 Washington Heights, SPH I, Room 3806, Ann Arbor, MI 48109-2029, USA
Full list of author information is available at the end of the article

cessation services with current maternal care services such as anemia control. Tobacco users wanted help to quit. It would be worthwhile to assess the feasibility of integrating antenatal tobacco screening and cessation services with antenatal care services for anemia control, such as screening and guidance during clinic visits and cessation support during home visits.

Background

The rate of tobacco use among adult women and pregnant women in India is about 10% with widely varying rates by region [1, 2]. Despite the harms associated with tobacco use, tobacco cessation services are not routine parts of reproductive health care, including antenatal care. In contrast, the prevalence of anemia in India is 65% [3], and anemia prevention and control are key components of antenatal care services [4]. The National Health Missions' (NHM) guidelines require every pregnant woman be tested for anemia and iron deficiency, and anemic women be given a free 90-day supply of iron folic acid (IFA) tablets. The NHM uses antenatal clinics and a cadre of community health workers (CHWs) called ASHA workers (Accredited Social Health Activist) to provide pregnant women relevant healthcare, education and support. In contrast, even though many women in India use tobacco even during pregnancy, there is no national scheme to address antenatal tobacco use, despite international recommendations [5].

Antenatal tobacco use and anemia appear to be correlated [6, 7], and are important risk factors for poor pregnancy outcomes [8–11]. Biochemically, tobacco use may affect iron metabolism [12], iron stores [13], inflammation [14], and hemoglobin levels [6]. Behaviorally, tobacco use may act as an appetite suppressant [15–17], and has been linked with lower food intake and household food insecurity [18–20], while tobacco abstinence may increase appetite [16, 21]. It is unclear how the relationships between tobacco use, anemia and iron status may be relevant to the delivery, uptake and efficacy of tobacco cessation services during pregnancy. We examined the links between tobacco use, anemia and iron deficiency anemia in the context of antenatal care in Mumbai, India to explore ways to integrate tobacco control services into routine antenatal care services.

In observational studies of clinical settings in India, tobacco use screening and motivational guidance to quit have been reported [22–24]. In a study of pregnant women, patients were screened [25] and users were monitored and counseled about the harms of tobacco use on the mother and fetus, but there was no effect on cessation rates. Also in a clinical setting, an observational study of tuberculosis patients used a brief application of 5-A's model (Ask, Advise, Assess, Assist

and Arrange) to help tobacco users to quit and showed promise [26].

From a community-based perspective, CHWs at antenatal clinics can help address antenatal tobacco use during home visits and community events. Their health promotion activities involve frequent contact with pregnant women at home, including coordination with antenatal care visits. When employed to address antenatal tobacco use, CHW strategies appear feasible in observational studies from India [25, 27] and elsewhere in the region [28]. One cluster randomized trail in low-income communities in India [29], used a brief (2 session) CHW delivered intervention and showed a small positive effect, a 2% improvement in cessation rates.

The current study, conducted at urban governmental Primary Health Centers (PHCs) aimed to: 1) measure the association between tobacco use and anemia; 2) assess the role of iron-rich food consumption and household food insecurity; 3) identify ways to integrate tobacco cessation services with existing antenatal care services. We hypothesized that tobacco use would be strongly associated with anemia and iron deficiency anemia and consumption of iron-rich foods and household food insecurity would be associated with tobacco use, anemia and IDA. We identified opportunities to address tobacco use as part of antenatal anemia care.

Methods
Design

This observational study was conducted in Mumbai, India at antenatal clinics in 5 PHCs. We recruited 100 pregnant women (20 per clinic) from waiting areas by approaching all patients. A research staff person recruited patients, screened for eligibility, and enrolled those who gave informed consent. Inclusion criteria were: receiving antenatal care at the PHCs; first or second trimester; no major pregnancy complications; and age 18–45. We also recruited 75 antenatal care providers from the five clinics (five doctors, five auxiliary nurse midwives (ANMs), and 65 CHWs). Current antenatal providers at the PHCs were eligible. Data were collected from April 2015 to April 2016.

Measures
Pregnancy questionnaire

We conducted 60-min face-to-face structured interviews in *Marathi* with pregnant women in private settings after antenatal care appointments.

Tobacco use

Tobacco use items were adapted from the Global Adult Tobacco Survey [30]. Current tobacco use was defined as past 30-day use of smoked / chewed / applied tobacco. Amount of tobacco use was measured as number of days and number of times per day in the last 30 days tobacco was smoked / chewed / applied. We measured reasons for using tobacco (helps with morning motions, satisfies craving, helps to relax, etc.); desire to quit and to receive cessation counseling; and antenatal cessation services received (screening, cessation guidance and referral).

Consumption of iron-rich foods
We administered a 31-item food frequency questionnaire to assess past 90-day consumption of iron-rich foods, vitamin A and folate as well as foods high in facilitators (e.g., ascorbic acid) and inhibitors (e.g., tannins) of iron absorption. The food list was adapted from a previously validated tool used in a similar context to our study population [31]. We measured weekly beef, lamb, chicken (meat/poultry) consumption by taking the median frequency value (0.35) for these items and grouping the sample into *no weekly consumption* (0), *less than median weekly consumption* (< 0.35) *or more than median weekly consumption* (≥ 0.35). A similar approach was used to categorize weekly consumption of fenugreek greens, spinach, black-eyed pea greens, and mustard greens (dark green leafy vegetables). The median value was 0.5 times a week. Because only one respondent reported no weekly consumption of green leafy vegetables, we combined that group with the "less than median weekly consumption" group.

Iron supplementation
Women were asked if they currently take an iron-folic acid tablet (Yes/No).

Household food insecurity
Household food insecurity (HFI) was measured using the Household Food Insecurity and Access Scale (HFIAS) [32], which includes nine Yes or No questions focused on three dimensions of household food access—anxiety about food access, food quality and food quantity—and a series of sub-questions to define the frequency of experiencing conditions linked to these three dimensions. We categorized HFI into four levels (i.e., food secure, mildly food insecure, moderately food insecure, and severely food insecure) based on standard protocols [32]. For the purpose of data analysis, we combined the moderately and severely food insecure categories because some cell sizes were small.

Socio-demographics covariates
We measured age, education (none, primary school, middle school, secondary school, college graduate, postgraduate), employment in the past 12 months, wealth index of household assets [33], religion (Hindu, Muslim or other) and parity (zero, one, two or more).

Blood tests
All blood tests were done as part of routine antenatal care clinic visits. Blood samples were stored and tested by labs used by the PHCs. In total, 9 mL of blood was drawn from each participant. Portable Hemocue photometers (Hemocue, Inc., Brea, CA) were used to assess hemoglobin (Hb). Serum cotinine and serum ferritin (SF) were assessed using Chemiluminescence Immunoassay and Chemiluminescent Microparticle, respectively. Cutoffs were as follows: tobacco use (cotinine ≥15 ng/mL), anemia (Hb < 110 g/L), iron deficiency (SF < 15 µg/L) and IDA (SF < 15 µg/L and Hb < 110 g/L).

Key informant interviews and focus groups
We conducted Key Informant Interviews (KIIs) with physicians and auxiliary nurse midwives (ANMs) and Focus Group Discussion (FGDs) with CHWs to determine the content of services provided during antenatal clinic and home visits. We asked to what extent anemia and tobacco use were evident among antenatal clinic patients; the content of anemia, IDA and nutrition-related services; how tobacco use is identified; what tobacco cessation services were provided; and how tobacco cessation could fit into the existing structure of care? We asked about the role of clinicians and CHWs in antenatal care including about anemia and tobacco use. We audiotaped all interviews and FGDs with prior permission of respondents.

Data analysis
Quantitative data analysis was conducted using Stata 12.1 [34]. First, we examined the distribution of study variables to characterize the sample with respect to socio-demographic factors and other measures. Secondly, because we examined both self-reported tobacco use and serum cotinine we measured the sensitivity and specificity of the self-reported use against the serum cotinine cut-off described above. Sensitivity was defined as the proportion of self-reporting tobacco users who had cotinine levels at or above the cut-off. Specificity was defined as the proportion of women not reporting tobacco use who had cotinine levels below the cut-off. Third, in order understand the role of iron-rich food consumption and food insecurity, we measured the bivariate association (chi-squared test or Fisher's exact tests when cell sizes were < 5) between tobacco use based on serum cotinine levels ($n = 16$, cotinine ≥15 ng/mL), anemia, IDA, IFA supplementation, consumption of iron-rich foods and HFI. Fourth, we used logistic regression to measure the association between IDA and tobacco use based on serum cotinine ($n = 16$, cotinine ≥15 ng/mL), controlling for IFA supplementation, consumption iron-rich foods, HFI and socio-demographic factors. We used the Stata's *cluster* subcommand to

account for nesting of pregnant women within clinic sites. Finally, we measured the Variance Inflation Factor (VIF) for each covariate to identify multicollinearity in our regression model [35].

We used a standard approach to conduct qualitative data analysis [36, 37]. In addition to the written notes taken during qualitative interviews and FGDs, the audio recordings were transcribed verbatim. The notes and transcripts were reviewed and discussed by members of the research team. We identified themes based on our discussions about the data. In our effort to accurately make sense of the qualitative data, we corroborated our interpretations throughout the data analysis process by checking with all members of the research team, including the field investigators.

Results

All antenatal care patients were married, mostly young, educated up to secondary school, and lived in low-income households (Table 1). The sample was 66% Hindu and 22% Muslim. There were high levels of anemia (72%), iron-deficiency (44%), and IDA (41%). No one reported past 30-day smoking tobacco use, but 13% reported past 30-day smokeless tobacco use. In contrast, 16% had cotinine levels indicating tobacco use. The sensitivity and specificity of self-reported tobacco use was 92.3% and 95.4%, respectively. *Mishri*, a form of dried and powdered tobacco rubbed on gums, was the most common form of tobacco used (54%). Every tobacco user reported using 20 or more days out of 30 days, and 69% used two to five times a day. The top reported reasons for using tobacco were: helps with morning motions (46%), satisfies a craving (46%), enjoy using (38%), and helps when upset or relaxes (23%). One (8%) woman said she used when feeling hungry. Ninety-two percent wanted to quit, and 77% wanted help to quit. Tobacco use was not well addressed during antenatal care visits; only two tobacco-using women were asked about tobacco use and advised to quit.

Tobacco user had higher rates of anemia ($p = .13$ and IDA ($p < .05$) than non-using pregnant women (per cotinine blood tests) (Table 2). There was no statistically significant difference in past 30-day intake of IFA supplementation among those who used (33%) and those who did not (24%) ($p > .05$). Green leafy vegetable consumption was less common in tobacco users (31%) than non-users (52%), but the difference was not statistically significant ($p = .12$). Nearly one-third of households were food insecure (29%), but HFI was not associated with tobacco use status or IDA. None of the tobacco users reported 'mild' food insecurity, while 12% of non-users did. Table 3 shows that IDA was strongly associated with tobacco use (OR = 14.3, 95% CI [2.6, 77.9]), and negatively associated with weekly meat (OR = 0.1, 95% CI [0.03, 0.6]) and green leafy vegetable consumption (OR = 0.

Table 1 Characteristics of pregnant participants ($n = 100$)

	number of participants
Age in years (mean = 25.5; SD = 0.5)	
18–19	7
20–29	72
30–39	18
40–41	1
Missing	2
Parity	
0	43
1	32
2 or more	25
Currently Married	100
Education	
None	6
Primary or middle school (grade 1–7)	22
Secondary school (grade 8–12)	62
College or more	10
Monthly household income	
Less than 10,000 INR	39
10,001–15,000 INR	43
More than 15,000 INR	15
Don't Know	3
Employed in the last 12 months	
Yes	28
No	71
Missing	1
Religion	
Hindu	66
Muslim	22
Other	12
Current smoking tobacco use (self-report)	0
Current smokeless tobacco use (self-report)	13
Current tobacco use (serum cotinine[a])	16
Anemia[b]	72
Iron deficiency[c]	44
Iron deficiency anemia[d]	41

[a] cotinine≥15 ng/dL
[b] hemoglobin< 110 g/L
[c] ferritin< 5 mg/L
[d] hemoglobin< 110 g/L & ferritin< 15 mg/L

6, 95% CI [0.4, 0.9]), and not associated with HFI. There was no indication of multicollinearity in our regression analysis (VIF mean = 1.47, range [1.17, 2.28]).

Key informant interviews with physicians and nurses

There was no systematic approach to address tobacco use during antenatal care at the PHCs. Services for

Table 2 Distribution of antenatal anemia, iron status and other nutritional factors by tobacco use and iron deficiency anemia ($n = 100$)

	Percent				Overall Sample ($n = 100$)
	Tobacco use[d]		Iron deficiency anemia[c]		
	User	Non-user	Yes	No	
Anemia[a]	[e]88	69	.	.	72
Iron deficiency[b]	**69	40	.	.	44
Iron deficiency anemia[c]	**69	36	.	.	41
Taking iron / folic acid supplements	33	24	23	27	25
Meat / Poultry Consumption					
None (0)	13	19	*27	12	18
Less than median	50	42	46	52	50
More than median	38	39	27	36	32
Green Leafy Vegetable Consumption					
Less than median	[f]69	48	46	54	65
More than median	31	52	54	46	34
Household Food Insecurity					
Food secure	75	70	71	71	71
Mildly food insecure	0	12	10	10	10
Moderate or severely food insecure	25	18	20	19	19
Overall Sample	16	84	41	59	100

[a] hemoglobin< 110 g/L
[b] ferritin< 15 mg/L
[c] hemoglobin< 110 g/L & ferritin< 15 mg/L
[d] cotinine≥15 ng/dL
[e] $p = 0.13$
[f] $p = 0.12$
* $p < 0.10$, ** $p < 0.05$
Note: Since only one person reported no weekly consumption of green leafy vegetable, she was grouped with the less than median category

anemia screening, treatment and supportive services were provided during clinic visits by nurses and doctors and home visits by CHWs. Clinics conducted anemia screenings at every visit and provided appropriate treatment, which included iron supplementation, guidance about nutrition, and other services as needed. Anemic patients were referred to a CHW program. Antenatal anemia was of high priority. Antenatal tobacco use was seen as a concern but not as common in the patient population. There were no systematic services in place for tobacco use screening and cessation. Providers advised known tobacco users to quit, but were not trained to provide cessation guidance and had nowhere to refer patients for cessation services, which were said to be offered at addiction centers. Providers wanted to learn about integrating tobacco use screening and cessation guidance into their routine practices. There was some concern about competing health priorities.

CHW focus groups
CHWs were provided with a list of pregnant mothers from the PHCs, including anemia status. Their main role was to provide supportive services for anemia control during home visits that include dietary guidance, provision of and guidance about taking IFA supplementation, and reminders for follow-up clinic visits. Anemia during pregnancy was seen as a major problem. CHWs were trained to identify signs of anemia, provide advice about taking IFA tablets and offer dietary advice to pregnant women about eating iron-rich foods. They also helped women address any logistical barriers to accessing antenatal care and delivery care.

There was variability in the perception that tobacco use was a problem. At an FGD in one clinic, CHWs reported that 40% of pregnant women used tobacco, while tobacco use was not perceived as a problem at an FGD in a different clinic. CHWs do not provide any tobacco control services. They had some knowledge about the harms of smoking tobacco use, but not specifically about harms during pregnancy. Smokeless tobacco use was not universally seen as harmful. Some CHWs noted that they used fear tactics to encourage users to quit. In addition, CHWs did not receive training to deliver cessation guidance and support, but wanted to be trained, particularly if they were paid to deliver services.

Table 3 Logistic regression of maternal iron deficiency anemia[a] (n = 98)

	OR	95% CI
Tobacco use[b]	**14.3	(2.6, 77.9)
Taking iron-folic acid supplements	0.6	(0.1, 4.0)
Meat Consumption		
None (0)	Referent	–
Less than median	**0.3	(0.1, 0.7)
More than median	**0.1	(0.03, 0.6)
Green Leafy Vegetable Consumption[c]		
None or less than median	Referent	–
More than Median	*0.6	(0.4, 0.9)
Household Food Insecurity		
Food secure	Referent	–
Mildly food insecure	2.3	(0.4, 11.5)
Moderate or severely food insecure	1.6	(0.7, 3.8)

[a] hemoglobin< 110 g/L & ferritin< 15 mg/L
[b] cotinine≥15 ng/dL
[c] There was only one individual in the "None" category, which was therefore combined with "Less than median" category
* p < 0.05
** p < 0.001
Note: Adjusted for age, education, employment, wealth index, religion and parity

Discussion

We hypothesized that tobacco-using pregnant women would have lower consumption of iron-rich foods (i.e. meats and green leafy vegetables) and higher household food insecurity, and therefore would be at increased risk of anemia and IDA. This hypothesis was not fully supported. The regression analysis suggested that there were independent associations between IDA and tobacco use as well as consumption of iron-rich foods (meats and green leafy vegetables), but not household food insecurity. The rate of anemia was higher in tobacco users than non-users but the difference was not statistically significant, though almost every tobacco-using pregnant women was anemic. In addition, tobacco-users compared to non-users tended to eat less than the median frequency of green leave vegetable consumption. There was no notable difference in meat consumption between users and non-users.

We also hypothesized that tobacco use would be more common among individuals from food insecure households, assuming that tobacco was used to increase satiety/lower appetite, and would therefore help cope with psychological effects of food insecurity. We found no evidence that HFI was associated with tobacco use or IDA. None of the tobacco users reported 'mild food insecurity', that is, anxiety about food access, while 12% of non-users did. In addition, only one (8%) participant reported that tobacco was used to address hunger, while 23% said they used when upset or for relaxation.

We found that almost nine out of ten tobacco users were anemic and that tobacco use was strongly, positively and independently associated with IDA. This has important implications for antenatal care visits. In low- and middle-income countries, antenatal care, particularly anemia control services, are missed opportunities for addressing antenatal tobacco use. Tobacco control services could parallel and be integrated with anemia control services, because nearly all tobacco users appear to be anemic and would therefore receive services for anemia. Providers in our study did not screen for tobacco use, but sometimes provide quit guidance if they notice use (e.g. stained teeth or gums). They said that tobacco use screening and cessation services at clinics and home visits would be useful and feasible, especially if they integrated with current practices. Given the link between tobacco use and iron deficiency anemia found in our current study and elsewhere [6, 12–14], when discussing harms of tobacco with patents antenatal care providers can inform anemic tobacco users that their use may worsen anemia.

The integration of antenatal tobacco cessation services could face many challenges. First, CHWs and clinicians are not currently trained to look for and address tobacco use in their patients. There is a need to increase awareness about the prevalence and risks associated with antenatal smokeless tobacco use (including the increased risk of anemia and IDA) as well as to increase the clinics capacity to provide evidence-based cessation guidance and support. Unfortunately, the literature about effective antenatal *smokeless* tobacco cessation strategies is sparse, particularly in India. Second, the antenatal care system appears burdened. Competing demands was an important concern raised by providers. Antenatal tobacco cessation services should not be resource intensive, and should be well integrated with current practices. Third, the rate of current IFA supplementation in anemic women is already low at 25%, while the rate of anemia and IDA is high. This indicates that the current approaches to address anemia and IDA need improvement, and may portend a relatively small impact on antenatal tobacco use, if parallel tobacco use screening and cessation services are added. Finally, in an environment of scarce resources, additional funds will be required, particularly for capacity building activities and labor costs.

Strengths and limitations

The key strength of this study is the use of multiple data sources (questionnaires administered to patients, biomarkers from blood tests, and qualitative information from providers) to make a careful assessment of tobacco use, anemia and iron deficiency in pregnant. Although we collected data from multiple sources, our sample size of pregnant women was not large, but it was sufficient to detect moderate effects. Smaller effects, such as those found for the association between food insecurity and tobacco use (odds ratios between 1.6 and 2.3), we not detected. The data were cross-sectional, and the observed relationships between indicate direction rather than magnitude of association or causation. The self-reported measures of tobacco use, dietary practices, IFA supplementation and HFI are prone to social desirability and recall bias. However, measures of this type are routinely used in public health surveillance systems. We used biomarkers to supplement the self-report measures. For example, our self-reported measure for tobacco use had very good but not perfect sensitivity and specificity when compared to our serum cotinine cut-off. Our cut-off was higher ($\geq$15 ng/ml) than recommended to identify smokeless tobacco use (> 5 ng/ml) [38, 39], which was the only form of tobacco used by the participants. Our budget limited our ability to use a more sensitive blood test for cotinine. It is likely that the true rate of tobacco use in our sample was higher than 16%.

Conclusions

We found that antenatal tobacco use was strongly associated with maternal anemia and iron status. There was less supportive evidence of the involvement of nutritional factors such as consumption of iron-rich foods and HFI. Tobacco-using pregnant women were highly interested in receiving cessation services. There were missed opportunities for addressing tobacco use as part of antenatal care. Although antenatal clinics did not have a formal strategy to address tobacco use, there was interest among providers to add routine tobacco control services, if they were integrated with current practices such as services which address anemia and iron deficiency.

Acknowledgments
This study could not have been completed without support from the Municipal Corporation of Greater Mumbai, and the participation of clinic staff, community health workers and patients. We thank them all, and the dedicated research staff at the Healis Sekhsaria Institute for Public Health and University of Michigan.

Funding
This work was supported by a seed grant from the University of Michigan Global Public Health (Co-PIs: R. Mistry and A. Jones). The contents of this paper do not represent the views of the funders.

Authors' contributions
RM and AJ conceived of the original study. MP provided critical inputs in the development of the study. RM drafted the paper, and all authors contributed to the implementation of the study, edited drafts of the paper, and agreed to the content of the submitted version. All authors read and approved the final manuscript.

Competing interests
The authors declare that they have no competing interests.

Author details
[1]Department of Health Behavior and Health Education, University of Michigan School of Public Health, 1415 Washington Heights, SPH I, Room 3806, Ann Arbor, MI 48109-2029, USA. [2]Department of Nutritional Sciences, University of Michigan, Ann Arbor, USA. [3]Healis Sekhsaria Institute for Public Health, Navi Mumbai, India. [4]Municipal Corporation of Greater Mumbai, Mumbai, India.

References
1. Mistry R, Dasika A. Antenatal tobacco use and secondhand smoke exposure in the home in India. Nicotine Tob Res. 2018;20:258–61.
2. Sinha DN, Suliankatchi RA, Amarchand R, Krishnan A. Prevalence and sociodemographic determinants of any tobacco use and dual use in six countries of the WHO south-East Asia region: findings from the demographic and health surveys. Nicotine Tob Res. 2016;18:750–6.
3. India Institute of Population Sciences and Macro International. National Family Health Survey 3, 2005–06: India. Vol. 1. Mumbai: India institute population Sciences; 2007.
4. Maternal Health Division. Guidelines for antenatal care and skilled attendance at birth. New Delhi: Governement of India; 2010.
5. World Health Organization. WHO recommendations for the prevention and management of tobacco use and second-hand smoke exposure in pregnancy. pp. 103. Geneva: World Health Organization; 2013. p. 103.
6. Subramoney S, Gupta PC. Anemia in pregnant women who use smokeless tobacco. Nicotine Tob Res. 2008;10:917–20.
7. Ganganahalli P, Pratinidhi A, Patil JA, Kakade SV. Smokeless tobacco use & anaemia among pregnant women in Karad taluk western Maharashtra: A cross sectional study. Ntl J of Community Med. 2015;6:622–5.
8. Ratsch A, Bogossian F. Smokeless tobacco use in pregnancy: an integrative review of the literature. Int J Public Health. 2014;59:599–608.
9. United States Department of Health and Human Services. The health consequences of smoking: a report of the surgeon general. Atlanta: US Department of Health and Human Services, Centers for Disease Control and Prevention, National Center for Chronic Disease Prevention and Health Promotion, Office on Smoking and Health; 2004. p. 62.
10. Klebanoff MA, Shiono PH, Selby JV, Trachtenberg AI, Graubard BI. Anemia and spontaneous preterm birth. Am J Obstet Gynecol. 1991;164:59–63.
11. Scholl TO, Hediger ML, Bendich A, Schall JI, Smith WK, Krueger PM. Use of multivitamin/mineral prenatal supplements: influence on the outcome of pregnancy. Am J Epidemiol. 1997;146:134–41.
12. Kocyigit A, Erel O, Gur S. Effects of tobacco smoking on plasma selenium, zinc, copper and iron concentrations and related antioxidative enzyme activities. Clin Biochem. 2001;34:629–33.
13. Northrop-Clewes CA, Thurnham DI. Monitoring micronutrients in cigarette smokers. Clin Chim Acta. 2007;377:14–38.
14. Chelchowska M, Ambroszkiewicz J, Gajewska J, Jablonska-Glab E, Maciejewski TM, Oltarzewski M. Hepcidin and iron metabolism in pregnancy: correlation with smoking and birth weight and length. Biol Trace Elem Res. 2016;173(1):14–20.
15. Blaha V, Yang ZJ, Meguid M, Chai JK, Zadak Z. Systemic nicotine administration suppresses food intake via reduced meal sizes in both male and female rats. Acta Med (Hradec Kralove). 1998;41:167–73.
16. Koopmann A, Bez J, Lemenager T, Hermann D, Dinter C, Reinhard I, Hoffmann H, Wiedemann K, Winterer G, Kiefer F. Effects of cigarette smoking on plasma concentration of the appetite-regulating peptide ghrelin. Ann Nutr Metab. 2015;66:155–61.
17. Miyata G, Meguid MM, Fetissov SO, Torelli GF, Kim HJ. Nicotine's effect on hypothalamic neurotransmitters and appetite regulation. Surgery. 1999;126:255–63.
18. Chaloupka FJ. Smoking, food insecurity, and tobacco control. Arch Pediatr Adolesc Med. 2008;162:1096–8.
19. Cutler-Triggs C, Fryer GE, Miyoshi TJ, Weitzman M. Increased rates and severity of child and adult food insecurity in households with adult smokers. Arch Pediatr Adolesc Med. 2008;162:1056–62.

20. Kim JE, Tsoh JY. Cigarette smoking among socioeconomically disadvantaged young adults in association with food insecurity and other factors. Prev Chronic Dis. 2016;13:E08.

21. Shiffman S, West R, Gilbert D. Recommendation for the assessment of tobacco craving and withdrawal in smoking cessation trials. Nicotine Tob Res. 2004;6:599–614.

22. Anczak JD, Claire E. Tobacco cessation in primary care: maximizing intervention strategies. Clin Med Res. 2003;1:201–16.

23. Panda R, Persai D, Venkatesan S, Ahluwalia JS. Physician and patient concordance of report of tobacco cessation intervention in primary care in India. BMC Public Health. 2015;15:456.

24. Pati S, Patnaik S, Swain S. 5A tobacco cessation strategy and physician's practice in Odisha, India: a cross-sectional study. Int J Prev Med. 2014;5:325–32.

25. Pratinidhi A, Gandham S, Shrotri A, Patil A, Pardeshi S. Use of 'mishri' a smokeless form of tobacco during pregnancy and its perinatal outcome. Indian J Community Med. 2010;35:14–8.

26. Kaur J, Sachdeva KS, Modi B, Jain DC, Chauhan LS, Dave P, Singh RJ, Wilson N. Promoting tobacco cessation by integrating'brief advice'in tuberculosis control programme. WHO South-East Asia J Public Health. 2013;2:28.

27. Nair S, Schensul JJ, Begum S, Pednekar MS. Use of smokeless tobacco by Indian women aged 18 – 40 years during pregnancy and reproductive years. PLoS One. 2015;10:1–18.

28. Shelley D, Tseng T, Pham H, Nguyen L, Keithly S, Stillman F, Nguyen N. Factors influencing tobacco use treatment patterns among vietnamese health care providers working in community health centers. BMC Public Health. 2014;14:14–68.

29. Sarkar BK, West R, Arora M, Ahluwalia JS, Reddy KS, Shahab L. Effectiveness of a brief community outreach tobacco cessation intervention in India: a cluster-randomised controlled trial (the BABEX trial). Thorax. 2017;72:167–73.

30. Ram F, Lahir S, Parasuraman S, Singh LL, Paswan B, Singh SK, Das KC. Global adult tobacco survey: India 2009-2010. Pp. 289. Mumbai: WHO and International Institute for Population Sciences; 2010. p. 289.

31. Bowen L, Bharathi AV, Kinra S, Destavola B, Ness A, Development ES. Evaluation of a semi-quantitative food frequency questionnaire for use in urban and rural India. Asia Pac J Clin Nutr. 2012;21:355–60.

32. Coates J, Swindale A, Bilinsky P. Household food insecurity access scale (HFIAS) for measurement of food access: Indicator guide (v3): Food and nutrition technical assistance project (FANTA). Washington DC.: Academy for Educational Development; 2007.

33. Rutstein SO, Johnson K. DHS comparitive reports 6: The DHS wealth index. Pp. 71. Calverton, Maryland USA: ORC Macro; 2004. p. 71.

34. StataCorp. 12.1 edition. College Station. StataCorp LLC: Texas; 2012.

35. Craney TA, Surles JG. Model-dependent variance inflation factor cutoff values. Qual Eng. 2002;14:391–403.

36. Miles MB, Huberman AM. Qualitative data analysis: an expanded sourcebook. Thousand Oaks: Sage; 1994.

37. Strauss A, Corbin J. Basics of qualitative research. Newbury Park: Sage; 1990.

38. Agaku IT, King BA. Validation of self-reported smokeless tobacco use by measurement of serum cotinine concentration among US adults. Am J Epidemiol. 2014;180:749–54.

39. Benowitz NL, Bernert JT, Caraballo RS, Holiday DB, Wang J. Optimal serum cotinine levels for distinguishing cigarette smokers and nonsmokers within different racial/ethnic groups in the United States between 1999 and 2004. Am J Epidemiol. 2009;169:236–48.

20

Weighted log-linear models for service delivery points in Ethiopia: a case of modern contraceptive users at health facilities

Demeke Lakew Workie[1*], Dereje Tesfaye Zike[1], Haile Mekonnen Fenta[1] and Mulusew Admasu Mekonnen[2]

Abstract

Background: Ethiopia is among countries with low contraceptive usage prevalence rate and resulted in high total fertility rate and unwanted pregnancy which intern affects the maternal and child health status. This study aimed to investigate the major factors that affect the number of modern contraceptive users at service delivery point in Ethiopia.

Methods: The Performance Monitoring and Accountability2020/Ethiopia data collected between March and April 2016 at round-4 from 461 eligible service delivery points were in this study. The weighted log-linear negative binomial model applied to analyze the service delivery point's data.

Results: Fifty percent of service delivery points in Ethiopia given service for 61 modern contraceptive users with the interquartile range of 0.62. The expected log number of modern contraceptive users at rural was 1. 05 (95% Wald CI: − 1.42 to − 0.68) lower than the expected log number of modern contraceptive users at urban. In addition, the expected log count of modern contraceptive users at others facility type was 0.58 lower than the expected log count of modern contraceptive users at the health center. The numbers of nurses/midwives were affecting the number of modern contraceptive users. Since, the incidence rate of modern contraceptive users increased by one due to an additional nurse in the delivery point.

Conclusion: Among different factors considered in this study, residence, region, facility type, the number of days per week family planning offered, the number of nurses/midwives and number of medical assistants were to be associated with the number of modern contraceptive users. Thus, the Government of Ethiopia would take immediate steps to address causes of the number of modern contraceptive users in Ethiopia.

Keywords: Negative binomial, Number of contraceptive users, Service delivery points, Weighted log-linear

Plain English summary

In Ethiopia, there is a high total fertility rate and unwanted pregnancy due to low contraceptive prevalence rate. This study aimed to investigate the major factors that affect the number of modern contraceptive users at service delivery point in Ethiopia. The weighted log-linear negative binomial model applied to analyze the Performance Monitoring and Accountability2020/ Ethiopia data.

The 461 eligible service delivery points were in this study. Fifty percent of service delivery points in Ethiopia given service for 61 modern contraceptive users with the interquartile range of 0.62. Among different factors considered in this study, residence, region, facility type, the number of days per week family planning offered, the number of nurses/midwives and number of medical assistants were found to be associated factors for the number of modern contraceptive users in Ethiopia.

In conclusion, the Government of Ethiopia both regional and federal would take immediate steps to address the causes of the number of modern contraceptive users in Ethiopia.

* Correspondence: demay_gu06@yahoo.com
[1]Statistics Department, Science College, Bahir Dar University, Bahir Dar, Ethiopia
Full list of author information is available at the end of the article

Background

Globally, each year, nearly 350,000 women die while another 50 million suffer illness and disability from complications of pregnancy and childbirth [1]. In developing countries, millions of sexually active women aged 15–49 want to avoid pregnancy and delay childbearing for at least 2 years or want to stop pregnancy and limit their family size but have an unmet need for family planning (FP) [2]. About 25% of women who would like to postpone their next birth by 2 years do not currently use a contraceptive method. This need could be met by improving contraceptive knowledge and the supply of reproductive health services so that women can better plan their families [3]. It has been reported that Ethiopia is one among six countries that contribute to about 50% of the maternal deaths along with India, Nigeria, Pakistan, Afghanistan and the Democratic Republic of Congo [1]. The total fertility rate of Ethiopia is 4.6 children per woman, contraceptive prevalence rate (CPR) is only 36% and an unmet need for family planning is 22% for married women [4], 24% of total women age 15–49 years [5] and 16.2% among all women aged 15–49 years [6]. If Ethiopia follows its current rate of growth, its population will double in the next 30 years, hitting 210 million by 2060. For fertilities to fall to those low levels, increases the use of modern contraceptive methods and family planning service delivery points play a significant contribution especially in less developed countries including Ethiopia. At present, contraceptive methods which are free of cost is provided in both governmental and NGO health facilities in Ethiopia at hospitals, clinics, health centers, and health posts [7]. But, Ethiopia is among countries with low contraceptive prevalence rate, with only 36% [4]. This resulted in high total fertility rate and unwanted pregnancy which intern affects the maternal and child health status [8].

Current use of modern contraceptive methods is one of the indicators most frequently used to assess the success of family planning programs. In Ethiopia, the variations of modern contraceptive use observed among regions, place of residence, marital status, wealth index and other factors [4, 5]. This situation indicated that the assumption of conditional independence of responses of individuals on the probability of contraceptive users who are living in the same area (cluster) given the covariates may not be longer valid. This indicates that current contraceptive use may be affected by unobserved regional and clustering effects at the different level of the factors [9]. The modern contraceptive prevalence rate in Ethiopia is varied from 1.4% in Somali to 50.1% in Addis Ababa across regions and 49.8% in Urban to 32.4 in rural via residence [4]. The success of any policy or family planning program intervention depends on a correct understanding of the socioeconomic, geographic, demographic, and behavioral factors which

may influence the family planning health facilities and modern contraceptive users. It is believed that population growth and family planning health facilities are closely related concepts. The principal findings and recommendations for strengthening the modern contraceptive users are availability and access to services, health facilities readiness, staffing training and improving the quality of care [10, 11]. Therefore, this study aimed to investigate the major factors that affect the modern contraceptive users at service delivery point in Ethiopia using weighted log-linear negative binomial model.

Methods

Data source, sampling design, and sample size

The PMA2020/Ethiopia-R4 data was collected by Addis Ababa University's School of Public Health at the College of Health Sciences (AAU/SPH/CHS), in collaboration with regional universities, the Federal Ministry of Health and the Central Statistics Agency under the aegis of the Bill & Melinda Gates Institute for Population and Reproductive Health at the Johns Hopkins Bloomberg School of Public Health. The PMA2020/ Ethiopia project was applied a two-stage stratified sample selection and stratification was achieved by separating each region into urban and rural areas. A sample of 461 eligible service delivery points (SDP) was considered for this study. The data collection was conducted between March and April 2016 by trained women who attained a high school diploma or higher level of education using smartphones. The study area and data collection procedures revealed in Fig. 1 [12].

Measurements

The response variable for this study was defined as the total number of visitors for modern contraceptive users at service delivery points during the last complete month preceding the survey. The predictor variables that included in this study were Region, residence (rural and urban), type of health facility (Health center and others (include: Health post, Hospital, Clinic and Pharmacy/drug shop/retail), advanced facility (Yes or No), facility supports by CHVs (Yes or No), the number of opening days per a week to offer family planning (5 days or below and above 5 days), total number of doctors, total number of nurses/midwives, total number of health officers and total number of pharmacists [13]. Data were entered into STATA-12 and analyzed using SAS-9.2.

Statistics analysis

A common model for count data is the Poisson model by assuming that the distribution has mean and variance equally [14]. Often, this does not hold true in real data, the sample variance is considerably larger than mean called over-dispersion and rarely smaller called under-

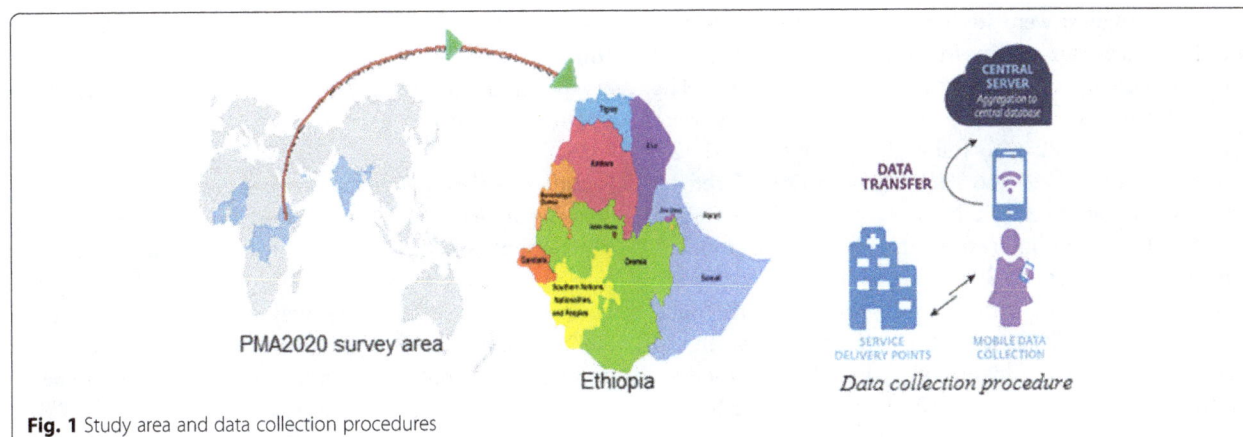

Fig. 1 Study area and data collection procedures

dispersion [15]. An over-dispersed model which assumes equidispersion can result in misleading inferences and conclusions, as over-dispersion can lead to the underestimation of parameter standard errors and falsely increase the significance of beta parameters [16, 17]. Hinde and Demetrio have published the issue of over-dispersion in both binary and count data whereas more recently, Hayat and Higgins have published a review of Poisson regression and over-dispersion [18, 19].

Contraceptive user's data which is an example of count data, often exhibit larger variance than would be expected from the Poisson assumption [20]. There are a number of strategies for accommodating over-dispersion. One of the approaches among a lot is a model in which μ was a random variable with a gamma distribution leading to a negative binomial distribution (NB) for the count data [20]. NB regression handles dispersion issues by modeling the dispersion parameter of the response variable. The relationship between variance and mean for NB distribution has the form of var. $(Y_i) = \mu_i + k\mu_i^2$, where k is a constant [18, 20, 21]. This is becausethe NB distribution accounts for further variance in count outcomes than the Poisson distribution through an additional shape parameter to the Poisson scale parameter [22]. In addition, classical methods of fitting statistical models canbe invalid in the presence of complex sampling designs involvingunequal weights, stratification or multi-stage sampling. To address this concern, there has been a considerable development of methods which do take account of complex designs [23–25]. One advantage of this approach is applicable to a very broad class of complex sampling schemes [26].

Along these lines, in this study researchers fitted a weighted log-linear negative binomial model for the number of modern contraceptive users from service delivery point as the data was over-dispersion due to cluster sampling.

The link function for negative binomial distribution is natural logarithm and then the model can be fitted as: $\log(\mu_i) = X\beta$, where μ_i be the expected number and variance of women who used the modern contraceptive method in i^{th} SDP, **X** is the predictors and β is the parameter of the model. As the data was over-dispersed due to cluster sampling the model leads to the negative binomial with mean and variance of women who used the modern contraceptive method in i^{th} SDP. Here the data was collected from a disproportionate number of population size across nine regions grouped into two residences (rural and urban). Thus in this study, the weighted log-linear model was used that proposed by Agresti [27]. The advantage of the weighted analysis is that it removes the bias due to the unequal population sizes. Then the weighted log-linear model link function can be fitted as: $\log(\mu_{ij} / W_{ij}) = X\beta$, where Wij be the total population size in i^{th} region and j^{th} residence, μ_{ij} be the expected number of women in i^{th} region and j^{th} residence at a given SDP, **X** is the predictors and β is the parameter of the model. This model has an equivalent representation as: $\log\mu_{ij} - \log W_{ij} = X\beta$, where -$\log W_{ij}$ is the adjustment term to the log link of the mean called an offset [27]. As the maximum likelihood estimate is biased, restricted maximum likelihood technique was used for parameter estimation [28].

Result
Descriptive statistics
Among the study service delivery points (SDP) 206 (44. 7%) modern contraceptive providers were health centers whereas 255 (52.3%) were collectively hospital, health post, health clinic, and pharmacy and retail outlet. Out of 10, service delivery points seven had no community health volunteer (CHV) supports, of which more than half 166 (52.2%) were located in the rural area. Among all family planning (FP) services provided at the study

SDPs, the smallest were sterilization 76 (2.7%) for female and 57 (2.0%) for male) followed by IUD 268(9.6%) whereas female condom and beads were null. The majority maternal services that offered by SDPs were antenatal care 406(28.3%) followed by delivery 391 (27. 3%). The majority 296 (66.8%) of SDPs were offered FP below 5 days per week (Table 1).

The outcome of interest is the number of modern contraceptive users at SDPs during the last complete month preceding the survey. As a summary of the data, Fig. 2 shows a frequency plot, overall users, in all regions. We observe a highly skewed number of modern contraceptive users, (mean = 105.51 and standard deviation = 195.12), with 1.1% zero values.

Table 2 revealed that the median, quartiles and interquartile range statistic for quantitative variables including the response one. Fifty percent of service delivery points in Ethiopia had given service for 61 modern contraceptive users with the interquartile range of 0.62. Fifty percent of service delivery points in the urban area had given service for 99 modern contraceptive users

whereas 50% SDPs in rural had given only to 45 modern contraceptive users. In addition, 50% of service delivery point in urban had 17 nurses whereas 50% SDPs in rural had only 9.

Factors associated with the number of modern contraceptive users at SDPs, Ethiopia

The weighted Poisson and a negative binomial regression model were fitted. The deviance values for weighted Poisson and negative binomial regression model were 56821.95 and 351.08 respectively. Thus, the negative binomial regression model estimates the dispersion coefficient as a value 1.52 with a 95% CI 1.30–1.73 signifying that it is more appropriate than the Poisson. Therefore, Table 3 below revealed the regression coefficients, standard errors, the Wald 95% confidence intervals for the coefficients, chi-square tests and p-values for each of the model variables based on the analysis of ML parameter estimates.

The variables residence, region, the number of days per week FP offered, type of facility, the total number of

Table 1 Frequency distribution for qualitative predictors

Variables			Residence area		Total
			Urban	Rural	
Type of facility	Hospital Center	Count (%)	99(48.1)	107(51.9)	206(44.7)
	Others[b]	Count (%)	121(47.5)	134(52.5)	255(55.3)
Advanced Facility	No	Count (%)	24(96.0)	1(4.00)	25(5.4)
	Yes	Count (%)	196(45)	240(55)	436(94.6)
CHV supports	No	Count (%)	152(47.8)	166(52.2)	318(69.0)
	Yes	Count (%)	44(38.9)	69(61.1)	113(24.5)
Types of FP Provide[a]	female sterilization	Count (%)	47 (61.8)	29(38.2)	76 (2.7)
	male sterilization	Count (%)	39 (68.4)	18(31.6)	57(2.0)
	implants	Count (%)	164(43.9)	210(65.1)	374(13.4)
	IUD	Count (%)	152(56.7)	116(43.3)	268(9.6)
	injectables	Count (%)	206(47.5)	228(52.5)	434(15.6)
	pills	Count (%)	211(48.2)	227(51.8)	438(15.7)
	progestin pills	Count (%)	181(52.5)	164(47.5)	345(12.4)
	male condoms	Count (%)	210(48.5)	223(51.5)	433(15.5)
	female condoms	Count (%)	8(80.0)	2(20.0)	10(0.4)
	EC	Count (%)	202(58.0)	146(42.0)	348(12.5)
	beads	Count (%)	1 (50.0)	1(50.0)	2(0.1)
Type of maternal Services Provide[a]	antenatal services	Count (%)	180 (44.3)	226(55.7)	406(28.3)
	delivery services	Count (%)	164(49.2)	169 (50.8)	333(23.2)
	postnatal services	Count (%)	173(44.2)	218(55.8)	391(27.3)
	post-abortion services	Count (%)	161(53.0)	143(47.0)	304(21.2)
Number of days per week FP offered	Below 5 days	Count (%)	133(44.9)	163(55.1)	296(66.8)
	Above 5 days	Count (%)	80(54.4)	67(45.6)	147(33.2)

Key: [a] multiple responses, CHVs (Community health volunteers), FP (Family planning), [b] includes Hospital / Polyclinic, Health post, Health clinic, Pharmacy and Retail outlet

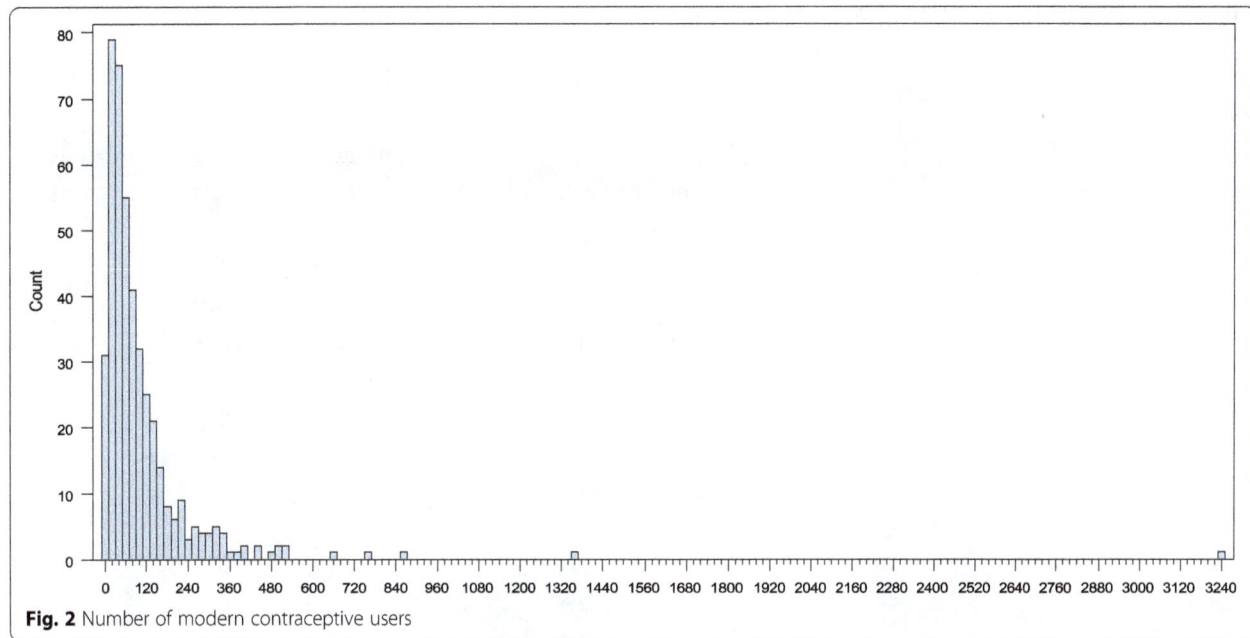

Fig. 2 Number of modern contraceptive users

nurses/midwives, the total number of pharmacists and the total number of medical assistants were statistically significant. Keeping the other variables constant, the expected log count for a rural modern contraceptive user is 1.05 lower than the expected log count for urban modern contraceptive users. The expected log count of modern contraceptive users at others facility type was 0.58 lower than the expected log count of modern contraceptive users at the health center. The numbers of nurses/midwives were positively affecting the number of modern contraceptive users. Thus, the incidence rate of modern contraceptive users increased by more than one (1.01) as one additional nurse in the given service delivery point (Table 3).

Discussion

Fifty percent of service delivery points in Ethiopia had given service for 61 modern contraceptive users with the interquartile range of 0.62. Considering the place of residence, urban modern contraceptive users were higher

than that of rural modern contraceptive users. The contributors to this positive association may be the better socioeconomic status of women in urban, easy access to family planning services, cultural disparity compared to rural areas, and the high level of women literacy in urban areas. This result is in line with the study conducted at Afghanistan [29].

At the regional level, the disparity was observed among regions.

The expected log number of modern contraceptive users at Gambella, Harari, SNNP, and Somali was lower than that of Addis Ababa. This result is similar with the study in Ethiopia from EDHS data by Tesfaye. He recommended as efficient distribution of health care facilities offering family planning services in urban and rural residents are required and designed for family planning services targeting on Somali region greatly increase the rate of the number of contraceptive use [30]. This is because geographical variations in the number of modern contraceptive use have been found to be

Table 2 Descriptive statistic for numerical predictors

Variables	Urban				Rural				Total			
	M	Q1	Q3	IQR	M	Q1	Q3	IQR	M	Q1	Q3	IQR
Number of Modern Contraceptive users	99	45	174	0.59	45	21	74	0.56	61	29	123	0.62
Total number of doctors	0	0	9	1.00	0	0	2	1.00	0	0	5	1.00
Total number of nurses/midwives	17	7	44	0.73	6	0	12	1.00	9	2	28	0.87
Total number of health officers	3	1	6	0.71	2	1	2	0.33	2	1	4	0.60
Total number of pharmacists	2	1	5	0.67	0	0	2	1.00	1	0	3	1.00
Total number of medical assistants	0	0	2	1.00	0	0	0	–	0	0	1	1.00
Total number of other medical staff	4	1	14	0.87	2	1	4	0.60	2	1	8	0.78

Key: M (median), Q1 (lower quartile), Q3 (upper quartile), IQR (inter quartile range)

Table 3 Analysis of maximum likelihood parameter estimates

Variable	DF	Estimate	Std Err	95% Wald CI		Chi-Square	Pro>ChiSq	Exp(Est)
				Lower	Upper			
Intercept	1	−3.64	0.60	−4.81	−2.47	37.28	0.00[c]	
Residence of SDP	1					29.79[b]	0.00[c]	
Rural	1	−1.05	0.19	−1.42	−0.68	31.19	0.00[c]	0.35
Urban[a]								
Region of SDP	10					99.43[b]	0.00[c]	
Afar	1	4.18	0.73	2.76	5.61	33.14	0.00[c]	65.65
Amhara	1	1.07	0.49	0.11	2.03	4.78	0.03[c]	2.91
Benishangul Gumz	1	0.23	0.65	−1.03	1.50	0.13	0.72	1.26
Dire Dawa	1	0.34	1.01	−1.63	2.31	0.12	0.73	1.41
Gambela	1	−1.64	0.97	−3.54	0.27	2.83	0.09	0.19
Harari	1	−0.02	0.84	−1.68	1.63	0.00	0.98	0.98
Oromiya	1	0.20	0.49	−0.76	1.15	0.16	0.69	1.22
S.N.N.P	1	−0.30	0.40	−1.09	0.49	0.56	0.45	0.74
Somali	1	−1.55	0.63	−2.78	−0.32	6.08	0.01[c]	0.21
Tigray	1	0.39	0.50	−0.59	1.36	0.60	0.4	1.47
Addis Ababa[a]								
# of days per week FP offered	1					30.86[b]	0.00[c]	
Five or below days	1	−1.33	0.26	−1.84	−0.82	26.33	0.00[c]	0.26
Above days[a]								
CHV Supporters	1					0.54[b]	0.46	
No	1	−0.20	0.28	−0.74	0.34	0.53	0.47	0.82
Yes[a]								
Type of facility	1					4.80[b]	0.03[c]	
Others	1	−0.58	0.26	−1.08	−0.08	5.13	0.02[c]	0.56
Health Center[a]								
Total # of doctors	1	−0.01	0.02	−0.04	0.03	0.32	0.57	0.99
Total # of nurses/midwives	1	0.01	0.00	0.00	0.01	4.21	0.04[c]	1.01
Total # of health officers	1	0.04	0.04	−0.04	0.11	0.87	0.35	1.04
Total # of pharmacists	1	−0.16	0.03	−0.22	−0.10	29.18	0.00[c]	0.85
Total # of medical assistants	1	−0.19	0.04	−0.27	−0.10	19.46	0.00[c]	0.83
Dispersion	1	1.52	0.11	1.30	1.73			

Key: *CI* (Confidence Interval), [a] (Reference category), [b] (Type 3 chi-square value), [c] (the relationship is significant at alpha value of 0.05 and or below), Exp(Est) (Exponentiating estimate)

influenced by community-level cultural beliefs like value attached to the child, the presence and quality of reproductive health services, shortage of midwives in most SDPs, remote geographical areas, and the presence of transport routes [29, 31–33]. Whereas the expected log number of modern contraceptive users from Afar, Amhara, Benishangul Gumiz, Oromia, Tigray, Dire Dawa was higher than that of Addis Ababa. This result contradicts with the result done by [4] stated as the modern contraceptive prevalence rate in Ethiopia is varied from 1.4% in Somali to 50.1% in Addis Ababa across regions. This contradicts might be mainly due to confounding

variables and slightly under estimation in regional towns. The main courses of under estimation may as regional women feeling shame to take contraceptive methods publically.

An increasing of nurse/midwives health officers, the expected log number of modern contraceptive users was increased by 0.01 and 0.04 respectively. Several studies have confirmed to the key role of nurses/midwives and health officers in providing guidance and effective counseling, resulting in an increased number of modern contraceptive users [34, 35]. Other studies have reported an increase in a couple–year protection following the engagement of midwives in family planning services in service delivery points [34, 35]. In Ethiopia, the involvement of health extension workers increased the contraceptive prevalence rate from 14 to 30% in 4 years [34, 35]. In Iran, increased community participation consequent to the involvement of midwives and other stakeholders resulted in the number of modern contraceptive users this intern a decline in total fertility rate. In addition, the incident rate of the modern contraceptive user for below 5 days per week FP offered is 0.35 times compared to above 5 days per week FP offered. This is the fact that increasing the access days to offer modern contraceptive methods leads to increases the number of modern contraceptive users at SDPs.

Conclusion

This study was aimed to investigate the major factors that affect the number of modern contraceptive users at service delivery point in Ethiopia. Among different factors considered in this study, residence, region, facility type, the number of days per week family planning offered, number of nurses/midwives and number of medical assistants were found to be significantly associated factors for the number of modern contraceptive users in Ethiopia. The influence of these factors can be used to develop the strategies of increasing the number of modern contraceptive users at service delivery points in Ethiopia. The median number of experts at the rural area is very few compared to the urban area in Ethiopia. This intern leads the median number of modern contraceptive users at rural service delivery points in Ethiopia is very few. Few numbers of modern contraceptive users at service delivery points in Ethiopia might potentially lead to high total fertility rate which intern affects the maternal and child health status. Finally, this affects negatively the 2030 ambitious goals for universal access to sexual and reproductive health services, including family planning. Thus, the regional and federal Government of Ethiopia would take immediate steps to address causes of the number of modern contraceptive users in Ethiopia, especially in rural areas.

Abbreviations

AAU: Addis Ababa University; AOR: Adjusted odds ratio; CHS: College of Health Sciences; CI: Confidence interval; COR: Crude odds ratio; EDHS: Ethiopia demographic health survey; ESA: Ethiopian statistical agency; FP: Family planning; GTP: Growth and transformation plan; LAM: Lactational amenorrhea method; OR: Odds ratio; PMA2020: Performance monitoring and accountability 2020; REs: Resident enumerators; SAS: Statistical analysis system; SPH: School of public health; SPSS: Statistical packages for social Sciences

Acknowledgments

The authors are indebted to Selamawit Desta, MSPH, MIA, Program Officer, PMA2020 give us permission access to the PMA2020/Ethiopia dataset.

Funding

The data collection funding was provided by the Bill & Melinda Gates Foundation. No additional funding was sought to complete this article.

Authors' contributions

MA supervised the data collection. DL analyzed the data and wrote the manuscript. MA, DT, and HM critically edited the manuscript. All authors read and approved the final manuscript.

Competing interests

The authors declare that they have no competing interests.

Author details

[1]Statistics Department, Science College, Bahir Dar University, Bahir Dar, Ethiopia. [2]PMA2020/Ethiopia project & John Snow Inc (JSI) SEUHP/Ethiopia projecthttp://www.pma2020.org/Ethiopia.

References

1. Hogan MC, et al. Maternal mortality for 181 countries, 1980–2008: a systematic analysis of progress towards millennium development goal 5. Lancet. 2010;375(9726):1609–23.
2. Darroch, J.E., S. Singh, and J. Nadeau, Contraception: an investment in lives, health and development. Issues in brief (Alan Guttmacher Institute), 2011(5): p. 1–4.
3. Guengant J, May J. Africa 2050: African demography Washington. In: DC: centennial Group for Emerging Market Forum; 2013.
4. EDHS, Ethiopia demographic and health survey 2016: key indicators report. The DHS Program ICF, 2016.
5. PMA2020 and AAU. Detailed Indicator report: Ethiopia, 2014, BILL AND MELINDA GATES INSTITUTE for POPULATION and REPRODUCTIVE HEALTH, PMA2020 project, School of Public Health – Addis Ababa University. Baltimore: PMA2020; 2014.
6. Workie DL, et al. A binary logistic regression model with complex sampling design of unmet need for family planning among all women aged (15-49) in Ethiopia. Afri Health Sci. 2017;17(3):637–46.
7. UN. World contraceptive use. New York: UN Department of Economic and Social Affairs, Population Division; 2011.
8. Berhane Y, Hailemariam D, Kloos H. Epidemiology and ecology of health and disease in Ethiopia. Addis Ababa: Shama books; 2006.
9. Tesfay Gidey Hailu. Determinants and cross-regional variations of contraceptive prevalence rate in Ethiopia: a multilevel modeling approach. J. Math. Stat. 2015;5(3):95–110. https://doi.org/10.5923/j.ajms. 20150503.01.
10. Miller K, et al. Clinic-based family planning and reproductive health Services in Africa: findings from situation analysis studies. New York: Population Council, Inc; 1998.
11. Lewis N, et al. AN ASSESSMENT OF CLINIC-BASED FAMILY PLANNING SERVICES IN KENYA. Nairobi: Division of Family Health; 1997.
12. PMA2020. Performance monitoring and accountability 2020. 2017 [cited 2017 Sep.].
13. [Ethiopia], C.S.A. Ethiopia mini demographic, and health survey 2014. Addis Ababa: Central Statistical Agency, CSA; 2014.
14. Molenberghs GVG. Models for discrete longitudinal data. New York: Library of Congress; 2005.
15. Iddi S, Molenberghs G. A combined overdispersed and marginalized multilevel model. Computational Statistics and Data Analysis. 2012;56:1944–51.
16. Faddy M, Smith D. Analysis of count data with covariate dependence in both mean and variance. J Appl Stat. 2011;38(12):2683–94.
17. Hilbe JM. Negative binomial regression. Cambridge: Cambridge University Press; 2011.
18. Hinde, J. and C.G. Demétrio, Overdispersion: models and estimation. Computational statistics & data analysis, 1998. 27(2): p. 151–170.
19. Hayat MJ, Higgins M. Understanding Poisson regression. J Nurs Educ. 2014; 53(4):207–15.
20. Greenwood M, Yule GU. An inquiry into the nature of frequency distributions representative of multiple happenings with particular reference to the occurrence of multiple attacks of disease or of repeated accidents. J R Stat Soc. 1920;83(2):255–79.

21. Joe H, Zhu R. Generalized Poisson distribution: the property of mixture of Poisson and comparison with negative binomial distribution. Biom J. 2005; 47(2):219–29.

22. Booth JG, et al. Negative binomial loglinear mixed models. Stat Model. 2003;3(3):179–91.

23. Skinner C, Vallet L-A. Fitting log-linear models to contingency tables from surveys with complex sampling designs: an investigation of the Clogg-Eliason approach. Sociol Methods Res. 2010;39(1):83–108.

24. Chambers RL, Skinner CJ. Analysis of survey data. University of Southampton UK: Wiley; 2003.

25. Lumley T. Analysis of complex survey samples. J Stat Softw. 2004;9(1):1–19.

26. Asparouhov T. Sampling weights in latent variable modeling. Struct Equ Model. 2005;12(3):411–34.

27. Agresti A. Wiley series in probability and statistics, Analysis of ordinal categorical data, second edition; 2002. p. 397–405.

28. Venables WN, Ripley BD. *Random and mixed effects*, in *Modern applied statistics with S*. New York: Springer; 2002. p. 271–300.

29. Osmani AK, et al. Factors influencing contraceptive use among women in Afghanistan: secondary analysis of Afghanistan health survey 2012. Nagoya J Med Sci. 2015;77(4):551.

30. Hailu TG. Determinants and cross-regional variations of contraceptive prevalence rate in Ethiopia: a multilevel modeling approach. American Journal of Mathematics and Statistics. 2015;5(3):95–110.

31. Asiimwe JB, et al. Factors associated with modern contraceptive use among young and older women in Uganda; a comparative analysis. BMC Public Health. 2014;14(1):926.

32. Kragelund Nielsen K, et al. Key barriers to the use of modern contraceptives among women in Albania: a qualitative study. Reprod. Health Matters. 2012; 20(40):158–65.

33. Stephenson R, et al. Contextual influences on modern contraceptive use in sub-Saharan Africa. Am J Public Health. 2007;97(7):1233–40.

34. Jabbari H, et al. Effectiveness of presence of physician and midwife in quantity and quality of family planning services in health care centers. J Family Community Med. 2014;21(1):1.

35. Alayande A, et al. Midwives as drivers of reproductive health commodity security in Kaduna state, Nigeria. Eur J Contracept Reprod Health Care. 2016; 21(3):207–12.

21

Understanding modern contraception uptake in one Ethiopian community

Erica Sedlander[1*], Jeffrey B. Bingenheimer[1], Mark C. Edberg[1], Rajiv N. Rimal[1], Hina Shaikh[1] and Wolfgang Munar[2]

Abstract

Background: In the last decade, the proportion of Ethiopian women using contraceptive methods has increased substantially (from 14% in 2005 to 35% in 2016 among married women). Numerous factors have contributed to the increased uptake. An important one is the implementation of the Health Extension Program, a government-led health service delivery strategy that has deployed more than 38,000 health extension workers (HEWs) throughout the country. Key mechanisms underlying the success of this program are not well understood. Using a case study approach, the goal of this study is to describe how key features of local contexts, community perceptions, and messaging by HEWs have contributed to the increased use of modern contraception in one community in Ethiopia.

Methods: We conducted focus groups and individual interviews with men, women, adolescents, and key informants, including (HEWs), in Oromia, Ethiopia. We used a random sampling protocol to recruit all participants except key informants, with whom purposive sampling was used to ensure participants were knowledgeable on family planning in the village. Interviews were audio recorded, translated, transcribed, and then analyzed using applied thematic analysis and NVivo v.11 qualitative research software.

Results: We identified four themes that may explain uptake of contraception: (1) HEWs are seen as trusted and valued community members who raised awareness about family planning; (2) the HEW messaging that contraception is useful to space pregnancies among married women was effective; (3) the message that spacing is healthy for mother and child was also effective; and (4) communicating to the entire community (including men, women, adolescents, and religious leaders), contributed to changing attitudes around contraception.

Conclusion: The four aspects of the Health Extension Program approach increased uptake of contraception in our sample. In contexts where community health workers are valued by the health systems and local communities they serve, this type of approach to widening modern contraception use could help increase uptake and address unmet need. Understanding these granular aspects of the program in one local context may help explain how use of contraception increased in the country as a whole.

Keywords: Family planning, Contraceptives, Health extension worker, Ethiopia, Sub Saharan Africa, Community based interventions

* Correspondence: esedlander@gwu.edu
[1]Department of Prevention and Community Health, The George Washington University, Milken Institute School of Public Health, 950 New Hampshire, Washington, DC, USA
Full list of author information is available at the end of the article

Plain English summary

In the last decade, the proportion of Ethiopian women using contraceptive methods has increased substantially (from 14% in 2005 to 35% in 2016 among married women). One of the reasons for this increase is the government-initiated health program that hired and trained over 38,000 female Health Extension Workers (HEWs). Although this program has shown a high level of success in increasing the use of family planning methods, little is known about how the program works on the ground. In this study, we wanted to understand how uptake of contraceptive methods occurred in one community in Ethiopia. To do so, we conducted interviews and focus groups in the Oromia region of Ethiopia. We found four main themes: (1) HEWs are seen as trusted and valued community members who raised awareness about family planning; (2) the message that contraception is useful to space pregnancies was effective; (3) the message that spacing is healthy for mother and child was also effective; and (4) communicating to the entire community (including men, women, adolescents, and religious leaders), contributed to changing attitudes around contraception. Understanding these specific components of the program in one local context may help explain how use of contraception increased in the country as a whole.

Background

Between 2005 and 2016, total fertility in Ethiopia dropped and contraceptive use increased significantly. According to Demographic Health Surveys (DHS), total fertility dropped from 5.4 in 2005 to 4.1 in 2014. Additionally, married women more than doubled their use of modern contraception from 14% in 2005 to 35% in 2016 [1, 2]. Knowledge of modern contraceptive methods among women is almost universal: It increased from 80.0% in 2005 to 97.1% by 2011 [3, 4]. Various factors have been proposed to explain this increase in contraceptive use, including growing political will, substantial external funding, non-governmental and public-private partnerships, and implementation of the Health Extension Program (HEP) to train health extension workers (HEWs) to work at community health posts [5].

Ethiopia's large, government-sponsored HEP, operationalized in 2004, brings health education and a range of primary care health services to rural areas. Some of the services include personal hygiene, water sanitation, disease prevention and control, maternal and child health, and family planning [5]. Across Ethiopia, some 38,000 HEWs work in over 1500 villages and serve as an intermediary between the community and the government-provided primary health services to expand health infrastructure and services [6]. In contrast to the prevailing practice in other low-income countries, HEWs in Ethiopia are salaried and receive one full year of intensive training based on a curriculum developed by a team of national and international experts [7, 8]. The recruitment criteria require that candidates be females who have at least a secondary school education; are 18 years or older and residents of the *kebele*, or village, where they will work (a community made up of about 500 households); and are committed to returning to their respective *kebele* after training is complete. The HEWs are recruited from within their own community to ensure delivery of locally needed care and to facilitate trust between the community and the HEWs [9].

The program adopts a diffusion model, which posits that community change occurs incrementally, by training early adopters first and then moving to the next group that may be ready to change [10]. One example of this is the Health Development Army (HDA), a component of the HEP introduced in 2012. Within the HDA, HEWs train "model families" – households that adopt specific healthy behaviors and receive 96 h of training. Model families are considered early adopters of desirable health practices and become leaders of a group of five families known as the "one to five network," who subsequently form a group of 25 to 30 households within a village [11].

Several studies have identified key elements for the effectiveness of the HEP platform, including the use of data to monitor performance, clearly defined roles among various program actors and stakeholders, and standardized support from the Minister of Health for HEWs [6, 11]. Specifically, the training and deployment of HEWs have been shown to reduce barriers, increase access, and help change fertility and family planning social norms in Ethiopia [12–14].

Although the success of the HEP has been lauded by many international organizations, to our knowledge, no study has examined the specific components within the family planning program administered by the HEWs that led to select achievements [15–17]. Several calls have been made to document the process of the Ethiopian HEWs as a successful service delivery model and to reduce the implementation gap for other health facilities and communities [5, 8]. While our initial focus of this study was more broadly focused on how uptake of contraception increased in one community, our data quickly revealed the substantial influence that the HEWs had on uptake. Therefore, our findings are primarily focused on their influence and specific aspects of the HEP program.

In this paper, adopting a case study approach, we describe *how* Ethiopia's public sector HEWs helped to increase modern contraception in one rural district. We focus on the following questions:

(1) Which behavior change outcomes were targeted by the HEWs?

(2) Which framing and key messages were communicated to the community?

(3) What approach was used by HEWs to engage the local community?

Methods

In July and August 2016, we conducted a case study of one community in Ethiopia. The goal of case study research is to understand the complexity of the behavior patterns of the catchment area or bounded system (in this case, the geographic community) [18]. To understand how modern contraceptive use increased in this community, we conducted five focus groups and 13 individual interviews with men, women, adolescents and key informants in one rural area in Oromia, Ethiopia ($n = 59$). (See Appendix #1 for number of total interviews and focus groups for each type of participant). Key informants included HEWs, teachers, and religious leaders. All interviews were conducted face-to-face in the local languages, Afan Oromo or Amharic, by native speakers trained in qualitative interviewing, using pretested and open-ended discussion guides that covered where and how women receive information about family planning and attitudes around use of family planning. To explore family planning norms in a less personal and threatening way within the focus groups, we used vignettes, short stories about hypothetical characters who live in a rural village in Oromia [19]. We chose qualitative methods to better understand the local approaches used to increase modern contraceptive uptake in one community and to understand how these approaches were carried out on the ground. We chose to two types of individual interviews to gather different information: key informant interviews focused on a broader profile of village-level patterns; and life-history interviews obtained in-depth narratives about experiences with childbearing, contraceptive use, and decision-making factors.

Setting

The Oromia region (population 279,639) is one of the nine ethnically based regional states of Ethiopia. Over 90% of its residents live in rural areas [20]. We chose Oromia because it exemplifies the dramatic increase in family planning use and drop in fertility. In 2005, the total fertility rate in Oromia was 6.2, and 12.9% of currently married women ages 15–49 reported use of family planning [4]. In 2014, the percentage of married women using family planning more than tripled, with 39.4% reporting use of family planning, and the total fertility rate dropped to 4.4, higher than the national average of 4.1 [2]. In Oromia, we collected data in one verdant, hilly and rural *gare* (a community made up of approximately 90 households). The gare is located in the Yebu District of Jimma Zone, Southwestern Ethiopia which is

approximately 200 miles southwest of Addis Ababa. We chose a rural gare because it is more representative of the predominantly rural Oromia region. Focus groups were conducted in the village primary school and interviews were conducted outside of homes or at the HEWs stations/health posts.

We used a random sampling procedure to select participants for focus group discussions and life history interviews. Research team members conducted a household enumeration activity in the *gare* (an area of approximately 90 households). Based on the number of individuals needed for focus group discussions and interviews, against a sampling frame that consisted of the entire gare, we used a proportional skip pattern that began with a randomly selected initial participant in order to identify households from which to select every succeeding participant for each category (e.g., mothers, adolescent girls). We used purposive, critical case sampling to select key informants based on their level of knowledge about family planning in the village. [21] For the purpose of this study, we define community as the *gare* from which we recruited participants.

Analysis

Interviews and focus group discussions were audio-recorded, transcribed, and translated to English by our research partners in Jimma Ethiopia. Transcripts were uploaded to NVivo v.11 qualitative software for analysis [22]. We analyzed transcripts using applied thematic analysis, an inductive set of procedures designed to identify and examine emerging themes from conceptual data [23]. Following the procedures outlined by Bradley, Curry and Devers (2007), we used both inductive and deductive coding [24]. Specific a priori codes were used to identify text related to attitudes and practices around family planning, and additional codes were then generated based on new themes that emerged. Two experienced qualitative researchers independently reviewed transcripts to develop an initial codebook and modified the codebook as themes emerged. One researcher coded all transcripts and another coded 20% to ensure consistency across coding. They met over the course of the analysis to discuss codes and reconcile discrepancies. Using NVivo v.11, we identified themes by comparing codes and content across sources, and by running specific word queries, associations between themes, and creating hierarchal visual displays of codes to identify linkages and patterns in the data. This study was approved by the Institutional Review Boards of Jimma University in Ethiopia and The George Washington University in the United States.

Results

Participants ranged in age from 14 to 55 years, the median and mean ages being 18 and 23, respectively. Most participants (68.5%) were female. All identified themselves as

Muslims and as members of the Oromo ethnic group. We identified four main themes that may help explain uptake of modern contraception in Oromia: (1) high acceptance of and impact on uptake of family planning services provided by HEWs in the community; (2) a focus on changing behaviors to increase spacing between births; (3) framing the spacing message as "healthy" for mother and baby but only targeting married women who have already given birth; and (4) delivering the message to everyone in the community, including men, women, adolescents, and religious leaders. Themes are further described below with quotes.

Theme 1: HEWs are seen as trusted and valued members of the community responsible for increasing use of family planning

We found that most participants valued the increased awareness and use of family planning methods, which they primarily attributed to the HEWs. Many participants mentioned that this was a fairly new and positive change within their community. According to one adolescent boys' focus group participant, "*Since the health extension workers have been teaching and giving advice throughout the meetings, mothers started to use contraceptives. Before five/ten years, people didn't have awareness about using these contraceptives.*"

The HEWs were also perceived as trusted community members. In the men's focus group, one participant said, "*Previously people consulted traditional midwifery which resulted in so many problems but now they [women] don't discuss the issue with their family or relatives. Rather they talk with the health workers. So they even discuss the secrets that they don't tell their husbands with the health extension workers.*"

Theme 2: HEWs focused on the use of contraception to "space births" among married women

Our data illustrate three main sub-themes within family planning behavior change. We describe these themes on a spectrum from least acceptable (substantial resistance) to the most acceptable (a relative openness) within the community. The themes are the following: (1) substantial resistance to the idea of delaying the initiation of childbearing after marriage; (2) some resistance to the idea of deliberately stopping childbearing or limiting; and (3) a relative openness to spacing births.

Substantial resistance to the idea of delaying the initiation of childbearing after marriage

Our data show that all newly married couples in our sample experience a great deal of internal and normative pressure to conceive soon after marriage. A mother in a focus group stated, "*After she gets married having children is necessary; so that, she does have the first child*

after getting married, and then she can stay some years to have the second child. But, she can't wait initially without children." A boy from a focus group supported this cultural norm, expressing, "*If she has planned to get marriage, what will follow is to have a child.*"

Some resistance to the idea of deliberately stopping childbearing or limiting

Clearly, delaying birth after marriage does not align with the community norms. A mother in a focus group reported that there is more openness to limiting total number of children, "*The mistake we did with lack of awareness at previous times is not available now and everyone knows to limit the number of children they have.*" However, according to a midwife, some religious push back still lingers in regards to limiting, "*In many households about this regulating the number of children is not common because of considering child as a gift from Allah....they don't want to limit.*"

A relative openness to spacing births

Conversely, once the first child is born, couples are more flexible in making decisions about family size and spacing. A mother's statement in a focus group illustrates the rigidity of giving birth immediately after marriage but the flexibility in regards to spacing, "*After she gets married having children is necessary; so that, she does have the first child after getting married, and then she can stay some years to have the second child.*" In this community, HEWs focused on increasing the practice of spacing after the first birth. All participants knew of and accepted family planning to space childbirth. As a result of HEWs efforts, in this community, spacing is not only perceived as an accepted practice, but it is also a highly regarded one. A mothers' focus group participant said, "*You know, it was great problem in the past when we didn't know. But, now we are spacing our births and most women are doing so in our community.*" Clearly, this strategy of targeting married women who have already given birth and primarily promoting one behavior, spacing, is effective within this community.

Theme 3: Messaging that "spacing is healthy for mother and baby" among married women resonated within the community

In regards to changing behavior to space births, HEWs communicated that spacing is a "healthy" practice for both mother and baby. One adolescent girl's statement during a focus group illustrates this common sentiment: "*Giving birth frequently without gaps affects the mothers physical health and their health in general. Spacing or limiting is important for children's development and for mothers as well.*"

Additionally, spacing for "five years" was cited by almost all participants who referenced a specific number of years to space; this may likely reflect the consistent message disseminated by the HEWs. A mother from an individual interview stated that the HEWs provide awareness to the whole community about contraception and the health benefits of spacing, "*Now I am left only with one year; I planned to give birth after five years. If the gap between children is narrow, it hurts both preceding child and the newborn.*"

Spacing and use of contraception for married women only

Although participants were not asked about use of contraception among adolescents specifically, throughout the interviews, all participants discussed use of contraception as commonplace among married women only. In the adolescent girls' focus groups, all participants stated that they were aware of contraception and discussed the benefits in reference to married women, not themselves. As one health extension worker said, "*Almost all adolescent boys in this village were educated and they have positive thoughts about the benefits of family planning.*" However, several participants stated that family planning education and services for adolescents were inadequate though a few felt that it was sufficient. One health extension worker reported that the HEP curriculum includes a module on adolescent reproductive health but that it is not emphasized.

"Reproductive health of adolescents is one of the health extension packages and it concerns awareness for the adolescents. But it is not practically dealt as it is put on the packages. There is initiation on some of the places on youth friendly services, but it is still not wide. This gap is created from the higher policy level."

We observed a discrepancy between awareness about family planning as reported by the adolescents in the focus groups and actual use among them. As one HEW said, "*They get some information at school and from health extension professionals working in the community, but; adolescents visit the health facility when they face problems rather than for consulting what to do to protect themselves.*"

Theme 4: A whole-community approach to HEWs engagement may have been critical for changing fertility norms and attitudes about the use of modern contraception

According to all participants who mentioned the target population, family planning education offered by the HEWs was made available to all members of the community, including men, women, adolescent boys and girls, and religious leaders. Including men in the dialogue may be particularly important because most participants stated that the husband is the "decision-maker" within a family. A participant in a mother's focus group said, "*It is husband's word that is given great place in using contraceptives. Husbands were not positive at initial period, but as time goes on, they see its advantage and they are encouraging us to take it. Now those health professionals are also giving advice to males as well.*" Building upon this, according to one HEW, they also help mediate differences between couples in the use of family planning, "*If, she faced challenge from her husband in using family planning, there will be negotiation with him by the help of health extension professionals.*"

In addition to the influence from the husbands and religious leaders, another HEW said that although some women make decisions without external influence, "*the majority of the families involve the mother-in-law in decisions around some of the issues in a family,*" including use of family planning. Given these multiple influencers, communicating to all members of the community, not solely to women as contraceptive users, may be a critical step for acceptance within the community.

Respondents also highlighted the role that HEWs play in influencing the perceptions of religious leaders about spacing, which is critical given that, according to one health extension worker, religious leaders have "*a lion share role in terms of influencing people to use family planning.*" According to another health extension worker, "*As time goes on, religious leaders were called at health facilities and they were given repeated training and awareness to convince them. After that, they never complained about using contraceptives to space birth at all. Fortunately, now a days religious leaders, husbands, women as well as community as a whole understand the advantage of birth spacing and feel happy about it.*"

Discussion

Our findings illuminate some key areas where HEWs effectively increased use of family planning within one Ethiopian community. The HEWs have helped make family planning a widely accepted practice to space births among married women who have previously given birth. Participants reported that spacing was "healthy" for mother and baby and that it improved their quality of life, thus reflecting positive valuation of HEWs and, in turn, increasing trust in them as individuals and in the services they provide. The HEWs educate not just women but men, teachers, and religious leaders about family planning. Our data suggest that changing norms related to the social acceptance of discussing family planning with husbands and religious leaders may be a critical step for reducing normative barriers to the adoption of modern contraception. Some participants also mentioned that practices related to family planning for adolescents have not been prioritized. We encountered conflicting accounts about whether or not adolescents receive adequate sexual health education. Adolescents were familiar with contraception, but they spoke about it solely in regards to married women, suggesting that there may be a general resistance to adolescents using it, perhaps because of a presumption that unmarried adolescents should not be sexually active.

Our finding that the HEP may have contributed to increasing the use of contraception is in line with the Health and Health Related Indicator report issued by the Ethiopia Federal Ministry of Health that shows the contraceptive acceptance rate increased significantly following the launch of the HEP, from 23% in 2004 to 61.7% in 2011 [25]. A 2011 evaluation of the HEP found that that family planning practices were rated highest among community members using services administered by HEWs, and the leading reason that they visited HEWs was for family planning [26]. Other studies have found that HEWs are trusted and valued members of the community, and that they are the primary communicators and educators about family planning [9, 12].

A 2015 review of community-based reproductive health interventions for young married couples in developing countries included eight studies from Malawi, India and Nepal. While the studies varied in their targeted behavioral outcomes, target population, and to whom they delivered key messages, the review found that the most successful interventions included counseling for the women themselves, husbands, family members, and the community as a whole [27]. Other studies have shown that including men in discussions around family planning is critical [28, 29]. Similarly, including religious leaders in the dialogue may shift community norms. A study in Rwanda found that religious leaders were named as the primary community members who changed perceptions about family planning [30]. In certain contexts, gaining approval from religious leaders may be key for shifting norms and practices, if such leaders are perceived as trusted and important influencers in the community.

Our findings that adolescent sexual health education and use of family planning need improvement are echoed in the literature. One study suggests that health workers in Ethiopia (primarily consisting of HEWs) may not have the required training to effectively communicate with adolescents [31]. The same study found that health workers have mixed attitudes about providing family planning services to unmarried adolescents; nearly one third had negative attitudes and almost half had unfavorable responses about providing reproductive health services to unmarried adolescents. According to the Family Planning 2020 website, at the 2012 London Family Planning Summit, the Ethiopian Minister of Health pledged to improve "the needs of adolescent girls" and "to expand youth

friendly services" [5, 32]. Clearly, there is a need but also a desire to improve services for adolescents.

Limitations

This work has several limitations. Participants were from one rural area in Ethiopia and are not representative of all Ethiopian perspectives. However, our focus groups included a diverse sample of participants and the majority of sub-Saharan Africa is rural, so our findings may be applicable to similar settings. Additionally, we only included one community. A comparison of different approaches to family planning from different communities using the HEP curriculum may yield helpful information. This is especially critical given that HEWs are selected from their own community and tailor their approach to locally appropriate content. Another limitation is that focus group-based study designs may produce selection biases; those who choose to participate in research may be a different population than those who do not. However, to reduce this threat to validity, we utilized a random sampling approach as described in the methods section.

Social desirability bias is another threat. Because information related to family planning and the HEWs are government services and employees, respectively, we tried to minimize this potential bias by reminding participants that discussions were anonymous, using vignettes within focus group guides for participants to be able to speak about someone hypothetical, and gathering data from a variety of participants and comparing responses. Although we purposefully conducted interviews and focus groups with a wide range of participants, we do not have a large number of data sources from each demographic group. Additionally, although we describe how participants learn about family planning and which messages they hear, we cannot account for all of the sources of information that may be influencing this community, which may include the internet or public health campaigns. Lastly, we did not specifically ask questions about family planning practices among unmarried women or adolescents.

Future research

While focusing on married women was successful in this community, future research should include adolescent and unmarried women's perceptions of family planning among themselves, not just married women. While there are adolescent sexual health modules within the initial HEW curriculum, prioritizing these sub-populations more or a continued education module for the HEWs after targeting married women may be a logical approach [23]. Additionally, this study highlights a single Ethiopian community, but a comparison of strategies across select villages would illustrate how other approaches may be similarly effective or ineffective. Furthermore, additional information on the HEP training and curriculum development may highlight a nationwide incremental strategy versus a local approach. Lastly, longitudinal qualitative data could examine how HEWs adapt their approaches (e.g., a change in the sub-population they target, the behavior and messaging) as the attitudes and behaviors around family planning shift within the community where they work.

Conclusion

To the extent that the HEWs have been effective in changing attitudes and behaviors related to family planning, their success may be attributable in part to a strategy of incremental change. It appears that the HEP focuses on less controversial approaches to increasing family planning uptake (e.g., contraception among married women *after* their first child to space births). Even if the education remains focused around spacing for married women only, the HEWs in this community in Oromia include men and religious leaders in the discussion, who comprise a seemingly less traditional group to bring into conversations about contraception use. Although religious leaders, adolescents, and unmarried women are all included in community dialogues about family planning, unmarried women and female adolescents may not be included as primary contraception users themselves, if social norms do not approve of their sexual activity. Our study shows that the HEP as administered in this community may have worked because of these approaches that appear to be effective. Other studies could use this type of qualitative examination to understand potentially amenable changes in attitudes and behaviors within a community.

Clearly, as shown by impact evaluations and corroborated by this study, HEWs are an effective vehicle to transfer information and ideas. The extent to which HEWs can also be used to push a more controversial public health agenda – to provide and promote access to information, education, and contraception among unmarried women and adolescents – remains to be seen. Changing social norms is a difficult endeavor and understanding where to begin and which subsequent step to take is critical. Focusing efforts on acceptance of family planning for spacing among married women can be an effective initial approach.

Appendix

Appendix #1: Interview and Focus Group Count

Total Interviews and Focus Group Participants (*n* = 59).

Key Informant Interviews (HEWs, religious leaders, teachers) (*n* = 8).

Five Focus Groups (adolescent boys, adolescent girls (2), men, women) (*n* = 46).

Life History Interviews (married women with and without children) (n = 5).

Abbreviations

DHS: Demographic health survey; HDA: Health development army; HEP: Health extension program; HEW: Health extension worker

Acknowledgements

We would like to thank our research partners at Jimma University in Ethiopia for their assistance with data collection and the overall support that they provided us in undertaking the study.

Funding

The study was funded by the Bill & Melinda Gates Foundation. They provided all funding and the authors carried out the research.

Authors' contributions

WM, RR, & ME contributed to the initiation of the study and design. RR, ME, WM & HS participated in organizing the data collection process, and RR and ME accompanied data collectors. ES, RR & BB contributed to the analysis and interpretation of the results. ES wrote the manuscript. BB, RR, HS, WM, & ME provided critical revision. All authors read and approved the final manuscript.

Competing interests

The authors declare that they have no competing interests.

Author details

[1]Department of Prevention and Community Health, The George Washington University, Milken Institute School of Public Health, 950 New Hampshire, Washington, DC, USA. [2]Department of Global Health, The George Washington University, Milken Institute School of Public Health, 950 New Hampshire, Washington, DC, USA.

References

1. Ethiopia Demographic and Health Survey. Key Indicators. Central Statistical Agency. Addis Ababa. October, 2016. https://dhsprogram.com/pubs/pdf/FR328/FR328.pdf
2. Ethiopia Mini Demographic Health Survey DHS, 2014. Central statistical agency. Addis Ababa. August 2014. https://www.unicef.org/ethiopia/Mini_DHS_2014__Final_Report.pdf
3. Ethiopia Demographic Health Survey DHS, 2011. Central statistical agency. Addis Ababa. March 2011. https://dhsprogram.com/pubs/pdf/FR255/FR255.pdf
4. Ethiopia Demographic Health Survey DHS, 2005. Central statistical agency. Addis Ababa September 2006. https://www.dhsprogram.com/pubs/pdf/FR179/FR179%5B23June2011%5D.pdf.
5. Olson DJ, Piller A. Ethiopia: an emerging family planning success story. Stud Fam Plan. 2013;44(4):445–59.
6. Fetene N, Linnander E, Fekadu B, Alemu H, Omer H, Canavan M, Smith J, Berman P, Bradley E. The Ethiopian health extension program and variation

in health systems performance: what matters? PLoS One. 2016;11(5):
e0156438. https://doi.org/10.1371/journal.pone.0156438.

7. Center for National Health Development in Ethiopia (CNDHE) and Columbia
University. 2011a. Health Extension Program Evaluation: Rural Ethiopia. Part I:
Household Survey, 2005–2010. Addis Ababa, Ethiopia: CNDHE and Columbia
University.

8. Teklehaimanot HD, Teklehaimanot A. Human resource development for a
community-based health extension program: a case study from Ethiopia.
Hum Resour Health. 2013;11(1):39.

9. Lunsford SS, Fatta K, Stover KE, Shrestha R. Supporting close-to-community
providers through a community health system approach: case examples
from Ethiopia and Tanzania. Hum Resour Health. 2015;13(1) https://doi.org/
10.1186/s12960-015-0006-6.

10. Banteyerga H. Ethiopia's health extension program: improving health
through community involvement. Perspective MEDICC Review. 2011;13(3)

11. Kok MC, Kea AZ, Datiko DG, Broerse JEW, Dieleman M, Taegtmeyer M,
Tulloch O. A qualitative assessment of health extension workers
relationships with the community and health sector in Ethiopia:
opportunities for enhancing maternal health performance. Hum Resour
Health. 2015;13(1) https://doi.org/10.1186/s12960-015-0077-4.

12. Gebre-Egziabher D, Medhanyie AA, Alemayehu M, Tesfay FH. Prevalence
and predictors of implanon utilization among women of reproductive age
group in Tigray region, northern Ethiopia. Reprod Health. 2017;14(1) https://
doi.org/10.1186/s12978-017-0320-7.

13. Medhanyie et al. The role of health extension workers in improving
utilization of maternal health services in rural areas of Ethiopia: a cross
sectional study. BMC Health Serv Res. 2012;12:352.

14. Weidert K, Gessessew A, Bell S, Godefay H, Prata N. Community health
workers as social marketers of injectable contraceptives: a case study from
Ethiopia. Global Health: Science and Practice. 2017;5(1):44–56.

15. USAID. (2015). All Eyes on Ethiopia's National Health Extension Program.
Retrieved June 8, 2017, from https://2012-2017.usaid.gov/results-data/
success-stories/all-eyes-ethiopia%E2%80%99s-national-health-extension-
program-0

16. Wang, H., Tesfaye, R., N.V. Ramana, G., & Chekagn, C. T. (2016). Ethiopia health
extension Program: An Institutionalized Community Approach for Universal
Health Coverage. The World Bank. https://doi.org/10.1596/978-1-4648-0815-9.

17. UNICEF (2013). In Ethiopia, a far-reaching health worker programme has
helped reduce child mortality across the country. Retrieved June 8, 2017,
from https://www.unicef.org/infobycountry/ethiopia_70372.html

18. Cohen D, Crabtree B. "Qualitative research guidelines project." July
2006. Retrieved February 26, 2018 from http://www.qualres.org/
HomeCase-3591.html

19. Gourlay A, Mshana G, Birdthistle I, Bulugu G, Zaba B, Urassa M. Using
vignettes in qualitative research to explore barriers and facilitating factors to
the uptake of prevention of mother-to-child transmission services in rural
Tanzania: a critical analysis. BMC Med Res Methodol. 2014;14(1):21.

20. Government of Ethiopia. (2016). The Oromia National Regional State.
Retrieved from http://www.ethiopia.gov.et/web/guest/oromia-regional-state.

21. Patton, MQ. (1999). Enhancing the quality and credibility of qualitative
analysis. HSR: Health Serv Res. 34 (5) Part II. pp. 1189–1208.

22. NVivo qualitative data analysis Software; QSR International Pty Ltd. Version
11, 2015. Melbourne, Australia.

23. Bradley EH, Curry LA, Devers KJ. Qualitative data analysis for health services
research: developing taxonomy, themes, and theory. Health Serv Res. 2007;
42(4):1758–72. https://doi.org/10.1111/j.1475-6773.2006.00684.x.

24. G.M.K. Guest, E.E. Namey, Applied Thematic Analysis, SAGE Publications, Inc.,
2012, pp. 320.

25. FMOH: Health and Health Related Indicators of Ethiopia. Addis Ababa,
Ethiopia: FMOH; 2011:2000.

26. CNHDE-Center for National Health Development in Ethiopia; The earth Institute
at Columbia. Ethiopian Health Extension Program Evaluation Study, 2007-2010,
Volume-II. Health post and HEWs performance Survey. Ethiopia; 2011

27. Sarkar A, Chandra-Mouli V, Jain K, Behera J, Mishra SK, Mehra S. Community
based reproductive health interventions for young married couples in
resource-constrained settings: a systematic review. BMC Public Health. 2015;
15(1) https://doi.org/10.1186/s12889-015-2352-7.

28. Wegs C, Creanga AA, Galavotti C, Wamalwa E. Community dialogue to shift
social norms and enable family planning: an evaluation of the family
planning results initiative in Kenya. PLoS One. 2016;11(4):e0153907. https://
doi.org/10.1371/journal.pone.0153907.

29. Withers M, Dworkin SL, Zakaras JM, Onono M, Oyier B, Cohen CR, Newmann
SJ. "Women now wear trousers": men's perceptions of family planning in
the context of changing gender relations in western Kenya. Cult Health Sex.
2015;17(9):1132–46. https://doi.org/10.1080/13691058.2015.1043144.

30. Farmer DB, Berman L, Ryan G, Habumugisha L, Basinga P, Nutt C, Kamali F,
Ngizwenayo E, St Fleur J, Niyigena P, Ngabo F, Farmer P, Rich M.
Motivations and constraints to family planning: a qualitative study in
Rwanda's southern Kayonza District. Global Health: Science and Practice.
2015;3(2):242–54.

31. Tilahun M, Mengistie B, Egata G, Reda AA. Health workers' attitudes toward
sexual and reproductive health services for unmarried adolescents in
Ethiopia. Reprod Health. 2012;9(1):19.

32. Tedros, A. G.. (2012). Ethiopia's Announcement at the London Summit on
Family Planning | Bill & Melinda Gates Foundation [video file]. Retrieved July 2,
2017 from http://www.youtube.com/watch?v=N2UzkfAv4nA&feature=plcp

22

A qualitative study of safe abortion and post-abortion family planning service experiences of women attending private facilities

Suzanne Penfold[1], Susy Wendot[2], Inviolata Nafula[3] and Katharine Footman[1*]

Abstract

Background: To inform improvements in safe abortion and post-abortion family planning (PAFP) services, this study aimed to explore the pathways, decision-making, experiences and preferences of women receiving safe abortion and post-abortion family planning (PAFP) at private clinics in western Kenya.

Methods: We conducted semi-structured interviews with 22 women who had recently used a safe abortion service from a private clinic. Interviews explored abortion-seeking behaviour and decision-making, abortion experience, use and knowledge of contraception, experience of PAFP counselling, and perceived facilitators of and challenges to family planning use.

Results: Respondents discovered their pregnancies due to physical symptoms, which were confirmed using pregnancy testing kits, often purchased from pharmacies. Respondents usually discussed their abortion decision with their partner, and, sometimes, carefully-selected friends or family members. Some reported being referred to private clinics for abortion services directly from other providers. Others had more complex pathways, first seeking care from unsafe providers, trying to self-induce abortion, being turned away from alternative safe facilities that were closed or too busy, or taking time to gather financial resources to pay for care. Participants wanted to use abortion services at facilities reputed for being accessible, clean, medically safe, and offering quick, respectful, private and courteous services. Awareness of reputable clinics was gained through personal experience, and recommendations from contacts and other health providers.

Most participants had previously used contraception, with some reports of incorrect use and many reports of side effects. PAFP counselling was valued by clients, but some accounts suggested the counselling lacked comprehensive information. Many women chose contraception immediately following PAFP counselling; but others wanted to delay decision-making about contraception until the abortion was complete.

Conclusion: Women's pathways to safe abortion care can be complex, including use of multiple abortion methods, delays due to financial barriers, and challenges accessing safe providers. Improvements in community knowledge of safe abortion care and accessibility of services are needed to reduce recourse to unsafe abortion. PAFP counselling is valued by clients but quality of counselling can be improved by exploring women's contraceptive histories, including information on more contraceptive methods, and inclusion of support for women who want to delay family planning uptake until their abortion is complete.

Keywords: Induced abortion, Kenya, Qualitative research, Private

* Correspondence: Katy.Footman@mariestopes.org
[1]Marie Stopes International, 1 Conway Street, Fitzroy Square, London W1T 6LP, UK
Full list of author information is available at the end of the article

Plain English summary

Legal restrictions on abortion were reduced in Kenya in 2010, but many women still use unsafe abortion methods. We interviewed 22 women who had recently used a safe abortion service from a private clinic about their pathways to care, how they chose the facility, their abortion and post-abortion contraceptive counselling experiences, and their use and knowledge of contraception.

Respondents discovered their pregnancies due to physical symptoms, which were confirmed using pregnancy testing kits, often purchased from pharmacies. Respondents usually discussed their abortion decision with their partner, and, sometimes, carefully-selected friends or family members. Some were referred directly to the private clinics for abortion services from other providers. Others had more complex pathways, first seeking care from unsafe providers, trying to self-induce abortion, attending alternative safe facilities that were closed or too busy, or taking time to gather finances to pay for care. Respondents sought safe, accessible, clean, respectful care from facilities that were viewed as reputable from personal experiences, and from friend, family and health provider recommendations. Respondents were often experienced contraceptive users but had discontinued due to side effects. PAFP counselling was valued by respondents, and many chose contraception immediately following counselling; others delayed contraceptive decision-making until after their recovery.

In conclusion, improvements in community knowledge of safe abortion care, accessibility of services, and PAFP counselling are needed to reduce recourse to unsafe abortion and prevent unintended pregnancy. Programmes that aim to reduce unsafe abortion should account for women's complex pathways to care and influence their pathways away from unsafe methods and providers.

Background

The World Health Organization (WHO) defines unsafe abortion as a procedure for terminating an unintended pregnancy carried out either by persons lacking the necessary skills or in an environment that does not conform to minimal medical standards, or both [1]. The persons with necessary skills and minimal medical standards are defined by the evolving WHO guidelines for safe abortion and health worker roles in safe abortion care [2–4]. In Kenya in 2010 the new constitution permitted abortion when, "in the opinion of a trained health professional, there is need for emergency treatment, or the life or health of the mother is in danger" [5]. However, the Kenyan penal code has not been updated to reflect changes in the Constitution, and the national *Standards and Guidelines on Reducing Maternal Mortality*

and Morbidity from Unsafe Abortion were withdrawn in 2012 and have not been replaced [6]. The resulting confusion about the legal status of abortion restricts women's access to safe services [7], and use of unsafe abortion providers and methods is still common [8].

In 2012, an estimated 119,112 women in Kenya received care for complications of unsafe abortion [9]. The reasons for use of unsafe services include the need for secrecy, uncertainty about the law, perceived higher cost of safe providers and lack of knowledge about abortion methods and safety [10, 11]. Increasing access to high-quality safe abortion care is crucial to prevent mortality and morbidity from unsafe abortion, which was responsible for about 13% of all maternal deaths globally in 2008 [12]. To prevent use of unsafe services, women's pathways to abortion care must be better understood.

Among women who receive safe abortion services, increasing access to post-abortion family planning (PAFP) is also an important intervention to prevent subsequent unsafe abortion by preventing unintended pregnancies [12]. Contraception is widely available [13] and knowledge about contraception is high in Kenya, yet contraceptive use remains low [14]. A study in 2012 found that 49% of pregnancies in Kenya were unintended, 41% of which ended in abortion [15]. Another study in 2012 found that about 16% of women seeking post-abortion care following an unsafe abortion reported to have had a previous induced abortion [16]. Although evidence suggests that PAFP counselling can be effective in increasing women's contraceptive uptake [17], inadequate counselling has been documented in private sector clinics in Kenya [18]. There is also limited evidence on the challenges that prevent women from using contraception after an abortion, and women's preferences for PAFP counselling.

This study aimed to explore the decision-making, experiences and preferences of women who attended private clinics in Kenya for safe abortion services. The objectives of the study were (1) to understand women's pathways to and experiences of seeking a safe abortion; (2) to understand the factors influencing the decision to seek a safe abortion service; (3) to describe women's experiences of contraceptive use and PAFP counselling.

Methods

We conducted this qualitative study in February 2016 as part of an evaluation of a quality management intervention to increase PAFP counselling and uptake in nine private clinics that are supported by the Marie Stopes Kenya 'AMUA' social franchise network in Western Region, Kenya [19]. During the pre-intervention phase of the evaluation, we interviewed women who had received an abortion or post-abortion care service at one of the nine clinics using a structured questionnaire on the day of procedure. During the informed consent process for this interview, we asked respondents whether they were interested in being contacted for a semi-structured interview at a later date. Respondents who were interested in taking part in an additional, longer interview were contacted by phone, up to 3 months after their abortion procedure.

We selected respondents for semi-structured interviews from six of the nine facilities, based on the number of respondents interested in taking part in an interview at each facility, and the geographic location of facility, to ensure that we selected both urban and rural clinics. We aimed to interview five respondents from each of the six facilities. We systematically selected interested respondents using a skip pattern, calculated based on the number of respondents expressing interest in participating from each facility, to ensure that respondents were selected from across the entire 3-month time period of the pre-intervention data collection.

Participant recruitment and data collection was conducted by six trained research assistants. The research assistants were all females aged 20–35 years, with Bachelor degrees and previous experience in qualitative interviewing. Research assistants received 2 days of training on conducting qualitative research, study procedures, informed consent, in-depth interviewing, self-reflection, the interview guide, and values clarification exercises. Practice interviews were used to ensure the research assistants could interact with clients in a sensitive, neutral and non-judgemental manner. Research assistants were supervised and supported by a field supervisor who listened to the recordings to assess the quality of the interviews and provided feedback to research assistants on points for improvement before their next interview.

We conducted the semi-structured interviews face-to-face in a private location convenient to the respondent, including clinics, hired rooms, and open spaces. We obtained individual written and oral informed consent to participate in the interview from each respondent at the start of each interview. Interviews were up to 1 h long and followed a detailed topic guide. The topic guide included questions about past and current experience and knowledge of contraception, experience of being counselled on and receiving contraception on the day of the procedure, perceptions of the barriers to family planning use, abortion-seeking behaviour, knowledge of abortion providers and experience at the clinic on the day of the abortion.

Interviews were conducted in a mixture of English, Swahili, and Luo depending on the location of the interview and the preferred language of the respondent. Interviews were audio-recorded and detailed field notes were made. Interviews were transcribed verbatim by the research assistants, and were then translated by a professional translator into English.

We conducted descriptive thematic analysis using both inductive and deductive coding, with the latter based on the research questions and topic guides [20, 21]. Data were coded in Microsoft Excel. Two coders (SP and KF) reviewed the first four interviews to reach consensus on coding structure.

Results

Facility and respondent characteristics

Twenty-two women participated in an interview. Respondents were recruited from three urban and three rural facilities in different counties of the western region of Kenya. The number of respondents per facility ranged from 2 to 5 (Table 1).

Respondents were most commonly in a relationship or married age 23–26 years and had children (Table 2). An equal number had been educated to primary level and college level (*n* = 9).

Pathways to seeking a safe abortion service

Respondents discovered their pregnancies due to physical symptoms such as weight gain, tiredness and nausea or vomiting in most cases, and more rarely due to a change in menstrual cycle. Just seven respondents mentioned a late period as being a sign of the pregnancy, while one realised her periods had stopped but did not associate this with pregnancy. Most respondents confirmed their pregnancy by using a pregnancy testing kit or service, often purchased from a pharmacy. Most respondents shared the news of the pregnancy with their partner or husband, and in some cases friends or family members. Information was shared selectively, with contacts that the respondents felt would support their decision or would not judge them. A few respondents told no one about the pregnancy or abortion, with one saying that *"I knew if I communicate even to one person, that information will spread that I have aborted"* (with partner, age 29, 1 child). Those who had shared their news were often advised on whether to terminate the pregnancy by their friends or family, and while some respondents were influenced by the opinions of partners or older family members, it was more common for the decision to be that of the respondent alone, sometimes going against advice of their partners as they felt *"it's my choice to decide"* (Married, age 30, 2 children). The reasons for terminating the pregnancy were most commonly that respondents were still in education or were caring for another young child.

Some respondents reported being referred directly to the private clinics from other providers, including staff at dispensaries and chemists where they purchased the pregnancy test. However, in other cases, respondents'

Table 1 Characteristics of Study Facilities

Facility	County	Urban / rural	Profession of main provider	Number of respondents (semi-structured interview)	Total number respondents interviewed during pre-intervention phase
1	Bungoma	Urban	Doctor	5	108
2	Uasin Gishu	Rural	Nurse	5	24
3	Trans-Nzoia	Urban	Clinical Officer	2	51
4	Migori	Rural	Nurse	2	8
5	Kisumu	Urban	Nurse	5	105
6	Homa Bay	Rural	Nurse	3	21

pathways were longer and more complex. For example, a few respondents first sought abortion services through unsafe providers or tried to self-induce before accessing formal care. One respondent had tried traditional medicine (tea made from roots and bark) as a first abortion attempt, following advice from a cousin, and thought the tea had worked after her second attempt at using it (almost 2 weeks later): *"I was convinced that it has come out. But then I saw that I was feeling the way I used to feel, when it is there... ...then I decided to go to the facility"* (Married, age 29, 5 children). One respondent reported receiving a heavy massage before seeking post-abortion care

Table 2 Respondent Characteristics

Characteristic	Number (N = 22)
Marital status	
Married	8
With partner	10
Single	3
Divorced	1
Age (years)	
18–22	7
23–26	9
27–30	4
>30	2
Number of children	
0	8
1	6
2	2
>2	6
Employment	
Student	6
Unskilled	6
Skilled	5
Not working	5
Education level	
Primary	9
Secondary	4
College	9

at the clinic, while two had tried medicines and either experienced complications or found the drugs were not effective. There were also reports of delays in accessing safe services because respondents sought abortion care from a formal provider first, but were not able to access the service because the facility was closed, could not be located, or was too busy. In one case, this resulted in a respondent obtaining pills from the chemist instead.

Some respondents also struggled to obtain money and had to delay obtaining the service while they gathered funds. However, most respondents viewed the services as good value:

"What I had was little [money]... I left it with him and told him that I was going to look for the remaining... the next day I had got [the money] and came with it... It was not a lot and it was not little according to... how I wanted to get helped. I didn't see it as expensive." (single, age 21, no children)

When recounting the abortion procedure itself at the facility, most respondents seemed to be well-counselled and informed about what would happen, including being given a choice of procedure, told what the procedure would involve, how long it would take, what level of pain and bleeding to expect and what to do in case of side effects. Respondents had varying information needs, with some wishing they had been given more information and others wanting to know very little about the abortion procedure out of fear of what it involved. Most respondents were satisfied with the clinic and the service they received and women commonly recalled feeling relieved after completing the abortion. However, in a few cases clients recalled a negative experience at certain clinics, being made to feel *"guilty"* because *"he said nothing but it was just actions, no advice, no talking...you just feel like you are doing the wrong thing..."* (with partner, age 21, no children).

Factors influencing seeking a safe abortion

The most commonly-mentioned factors influencing respondents' care-seeking were concerns of quality and safety of the service. Respondents had heard about others experiencing morbidity or mortality from unsafe abortion, and had knowledge of methods (traditional and herbal medicines, drinking tea or juice, inserting herbs into the vagina, and 'pills') which they viewed as unsafe. Fear of ineffective or unsafe methods and 'fake' providers was often a direct motivation for seeking formal abortion services:

"It is better I go to a doctor where I will be safe, where even if bleed a lot, they will know how to help me. Now that is why I did not use any other methods because you hear someone else has gone and died here and actually they were trying to remove a pregnancy." (married, age 26, 2 children)

Prior experience of the clinic was an important influencing factor; either from the respondent previously using the facility for other services such as family planning, or from friends or family specifically recommending the facility. Perceptions of the safety of the procedure, cleanliness, competency and attitude of staff, speed of service and privacy; and the possibility of obtaining family planning afterwards were specific aspects of care that influenced the reputation of a clinic: *"she told me... that this place is very nice, things are done in a clean way and then I will be washed and I won't have many complications. I told her then, take me there"* (with partner, age 20, no children).

As well as safety, respondents also valued discretion, both in terms of the provider and the method: *"I told her I don't want pills for swallowing, I don't want the one where I will bleed a lot... so that now my uncle, so that he knows"* (with partner, age 20, no children). The desire to be anonymous influenced the choice of clinic in some cases, with women deliberately travelling to a facility further away from home for this reason.

Ease of availability of abortion services was important, with some respondents mentioning they had not sought an abortion at public facilities because they feared being turned away. Cost of the service was also a consideration, with some facilities having a reputation for being more affordable. For some, cost was a low consideration relative to the need to get an abortion: *"I did not consider things to do with price. I just wanted it to be terminated"* (married, age 29, 5 children).

PAFP and contraceptive experience
Most respondents were not using contraception at the time they conceived but some were using short-acting or traditional methods. Most respondents had experience of using several methods of contraception previously, most commonly injectables and condoms. There were many reports of side effects related to contraceptive use, which sometimes meant respondents stopped using

contraception: *"Norplant was good for the first three months but onwards it started giving pressure in the chest, and I decided to terminate it"* (married, age 30, 2 children). Reasons for non-use of contraception included partner opposition and concerns about side effects. Respondents were knowledgeable about a range of contraceptives, and where to obtain them, with information commonly received from friends, family, school, health clinics, the internet, radio, television, printed media and church. However, misconceptions about some contraceptives were common.

Most respondents reported receiving some counselling about PAFP on the day of procedure. For a couple of respondents, contraceptive counselling was initiated by the respondent herself rather than the provider. Most respondents said that they were open to and appreciative of the counselling. Most commonly respondents remembered being counselled on the effectiveness of different contraceptive methods. In some cases, respondents reported being told about a wide range of contraceptive methods, but for others the options mentioned were limited to short-term methods such as condoms, oral contraceptive pills and injections. Some respondents remembered the providers explaining the benefits of contraception in terms of spacing pregnancy to enable women to care for young children they have and preventing future need for abortion. Some also spoke about being reassured about side effects of different methods, although more commonly respondents wished they had received more information about this. There were also a couple of cases where women felt they were just "being told to use family planning". Three respondents reported that they received no counselling on PAFP but would have liked to have received more information, such as on how to prevent pregnancy and sexually transmitted infections, and how different contraceptive methods worked.

Of those respondents who did not take up contraception services on the day of the abortion, reasons included not being informed about contraception by the provider, being advised to seek contraception elsewhere or later, and fear of side effects resulting from their own experience or from the experiences of other people. Respondents also chose to delay contraceptive uptake because they planned to wait until after marriage, needed to discuss it with their partners to avoid "chaos in [the] house", or wanted to complete the abortion first (owing to either the pain or anxiety of the abortion, or desire to know it was complete): *"I told him I will not...use for now; let me first finish that [abortion] medicine"* (with partner, age 23, no children). Some respondents reported obtaining contraception from elsewhere up to 1 month after the abortion, while others who intended to seek contraception after leaving the facility did not as they were too busy or forgot.

There was a range of reasons behind respondents' decisions to use contraceptive services following an abortion, several of which reflected the content of the reported counselling they received. These included not wanting to have another abortion, concern about health effects of abortion and emergency contraception, having not previously used contraception and being informed for the first time by the provider, and realising the need for family planning as the respondent was young and still in school. The most common method used to prevent pregnancy post-abortion was the implant, but others included the oral contraceptive pill, injection, condoms and the intra-uterine device (IUD).

Discussion

Our study found that several barriers and facilitators shaped respondents' pathways to safe abortion care, including delays in discovering pregnancy and lack of recognition of pregnancy symptoms; use of pregnancy test kits; advice from partners and social networks; referrals from non-abortion providers; challenges accessing facilities; and financial constraints. Respondents seeking safe abortion services in private facilities were highly influenced by the reputation of safe medical care and fear of unsafe services, as the risks of unsafe abortion and commonly-used traditional methods were well-known. The clinics' reputations of being affordable and discrete were also important. Respondents valued PAFP counselling, and, in some cases, counselling reportedly addressed specific barriers to contraceptive use, such as fear of side effects. However, counselling could be more targeted to not only address the effectiveness of methods, but also the benefits of family planning and how side effects can be managed. Most respondents had experience of using several contraceptive methods, and many reported that side effects had caused them to stop or change method, which is a common issue for continuation [22]. Several respondents wished that PAFP counselling had provided information on a wider range of contraception methods and their side effects. The range of methods available may have hindered family planning use, as observed elsewhere [23]. Many respondents opted for contraception immediately post-abortion. However, some needed time to consider their options, discuss contraception with their partner, or complete the abortion process before making decisions about family planning.

This study had a number of strengths and limitations. To understand experiences of these sensitive topics, semi-structured interviews were the most appropriate technique. They were conducted by experienced, trained, female research assistants who were native speakers of the languages of the interviewees. However, it may be that some community aspects relating to abortion and

contraception were missed, and these could have been better explored through focus group discussions. The interviews were conducted within a few months of respondents having their abortions, which reduced the chance of recall error of the abortion experience, but the timing of the interviews relative to the abortion varied between 1 and 3 months, so there was potential variation in the level of recall between respondents. This study explored the views and experiences of women who sought abortion services at private clinics in Kenya, and the results are not generalizable to women seeking abortions from other types of providers.

While respondents in our study viewed medical safety of the procedures to be an important influence on where they obtained their abortion, other evidence suggests that safety does not always have the same meaning or is not always a priority for care-seeking. A study of wider community views from western Kenya found that women felt that there was no such thing as a safe abortion method, and that cost and secrecy were more important than safety [11]. As in our study, respondents in a study by Izugbara et al. reported that dependable social networks were important in identifying an abortion provider, but this was viewed as an element of the safety of the procedure, more so than clinical safety [10]. Other elements of service safety reported by Izugbara et al. include confidentiality, concealment of the abortion, being shielded from the law, and cost [10]. A study in Zambia also found that for women seeking post-abortion care from hospitals, the need to conceal the abortion had outweighed concerns about safety [24]. Discretion of the abortion service was also prioritised by many respondents in our study, and lack of clarity about the legality of abortion and stigma associated with it may increase the value placed on discrete service provision [24].

The differences in care-seeking decisions that result in use of safe and unsafe services are likely to reflect differences in respondents' backgrounds, such as access to money, levels of education, health knowledge, nature of social networks, and capacity to overcome challenges such as stigma and lack of accessible services. The study of community views in western Kenya found that the costs of safe providers prohibited their use [11]. Although this was not the case in our study, we note that we only interviewed women for whom finance was not an ultimate barrier to care. It is likely that these different views of cost may reflect higher levels of knowledge of the health system and socio-economic status among the respondents in our study. However, we also note that the socio-demographic characteristics of the respondents in the Izugbara et al. study do not appear to be substantially different from those in our study, suggesting that there may also be an element of luck in what advice is received and by whom at the exact moment a woman is seeking an abortion, particularly in the context where there is a lack of accurate information available, and there are large numbers of options available, many of which are unsafe.

The study findings highlight potential opportunities for programmes to influence women's abortion seeking pathways to reduce recourse to unsafe abortion. Abortion pathways were complex in some cases, with multiple options being tried or used before finally accessing a safe service, as previously noted in other studies [25, 26]. Improving awareness of pregnancy symptoms, such as missed periods, may reduce delays in care-seeking. Ensuring pregnancy test kits are widely available and have links to a source of support for pregnancy crisis counselling, for example through a hotline or pharmacy referrals to clinic-based care, may increase awareness of safe abortion methods at earlier gestational ages [27]. Referrals facilitated respondents' access to safe services in some cases, and strengthening referral networks from a range of non-abortion and informal providers could also help to reduce delays in care-seeking and promote safe service use. Social networks played a key role in respondents' pathways, with clinic recommendations often coming from friends or family. Husbands and partners were most commonly confided in about the need for abortion, so increasing men's awareness of the risks of unsafe abortion and the availability of safe options may also influence women's awareness and use of safe methods. In some cases, respondents attempted to access safe services but found that clinics were not open or were too busy, so there is a need to increase the availability of safe services. As recommendations from friends influence the use of safe options, care must be woman-centred and de-stigmatising to ensure that use of safe options is replicated through word of mouth. Finally, the content of PAFP counselling should take women's contraceptive preferences and previous experience into account, include information on a wide range of methods, reassure women on how to deal with side effects, and address common misconceptions [28]. PAFP counselling should acknowledge that women may not be ready to make a decision on the day of the abortion procedure, and find ways to support women after they leave the clinic, either through mobile technologies or in-person support.

Conclusion and recommendations

Unsafe abortion is common in Kenya. Our study of the pathways and experiences of women using safe providers in western Kenya highlights the opportunities to reduce use of unsafe options and ensure women access safe options. These include reducing delays in discovery of pregnancy through improved education on pregnancy symptoms; ensuring pregnancy test kits have referral links to pregnancy crisis counselling; improving community knowledge of abortion safety and options due to the important role of advice from social networks, and particularly men due to the important role of husbands and partners; building referral networks from non-abortion and informal providers to improving referrals to safe providers; and improving the accessibility and availability of safe providers.

PAFP counselling is valued by clients and can improve access to information and clarify misconceptions, but improvements in the quality and content of counselling may further facilitate contraceptive use. While PAFP counselling should prioritise method provision immediately after an abortion to maximise protection and reduce incidental costs for repeat facility visits, it should also include steps to follow-up and support women who want to use family planning at a later date.

Abbreviations
IDI: In-depth interview; IUD: Intra-uterine device; KEMRI: Kenya Medical Research Institute; MSI: Marie Stopes International; PAFP: Post-abortion family planning

Acknowledgements
We thank the women who participated in the interviews for this study.

Funding
This study was funded by the Strengthening Evidence for Programming on Unintended Pregnancy (STEP-UP) Research Consortium, which is funded by UKaid from the Department for International Development.

Authors' contributions
KF, SW and IN conceived the methodology for the study, applied for ethical approvals for the study and managed implementation of the study. SP conducted data analysis and SP and KF wrote the first draft of the manuscript. All authors reviewed and contributed to the manuscript. All authors read and approved the final manuscript.

Competing interests
The authors declare that they have no competing interests.

Author details
[1]Marie Stopes International, 1 Conway Street, Fitzroy Square, London W1T 6LP, UK. [2]Marie Stopes Kenya, Kindaruma Road, P.O. Box 59328-00200, Nairobi, Kenya. [3]UCSF-Global programs, Morning Side Office Park, Ngong Road, P.O Box 40821-00100, Nairobi, Kenya.

References

1. World Health Organization. The prevention and management of unsafe abortion, Report of a technical working group. Geneva: World Health Organization; 1992.
2. Ganatra B, Tuncalp O, Johnston HB, Johnson BR Jr, Gulmezoglu AM, Temmerman M. From concept to measurement: operationalizing WHO's definition of unsafe abortion. Bull World Health Organ. 2014;92(3):155.
3. World Health Organization. Health worker roles in providing safe abortion care and post-abortion contraception. Geneva:World Health Organisation; 2015.
4. World Health Organization. Safe abortion: technical and policy guidance for health systems. Geneva:World Health Organisation; 2012.
5. Kenya's Abortion Provisions, Constitution of Kenya (2010), Article 26(4) The Penal Code, Laws of Kenya, Cap. 63, Revised Edition (2009), Articles 158–160, 228 and 240 [https://www.reproductiverights.org/world-abortion-laws/kenyas-abortion-provisions#constitution]. Accessed 18 Apr 18
6. Finden A. The law, trials and imprisonment for abortion in Kenya. In: Women's right to safe abortion; 2017.
7. Center for Reproductive Rights. Kenyan Women Denied Safe, Legal Abortion Services. In: Center for Reproductive Rights; 2015. https://www.reproductiverights.org/press-room/kenyan-women-denied-safe-legal-abortion-services. Accessed 18 Apr 18.
8. Hussain R. Abortion and unintended pregnancy in Kenya. New York: Guttmacher Institute; 2012.
9. African Population and Health Research Center, Ministry of Health K, Ipas, Guttmacher Institute. Incidence and complications of unsafe abortion in Kenya. Key findings of a National Study. Nairobi: African Population and Health Research Center, Ministry of Health, Kenya, Ipas, and Guttmacher Institute; 2013.
10. Izugbara CO, Egesa C, Okelo R. 'High profile health facilities can add to your trouble': women, stigma and un/safe abortion in Kenya. Soc Sci Med. 2015; 141:9–18.
11. Marlow HM, Wamugi S, Yegon E, Fetters T, Wanaswa L, Msipa-Ndebele S. Women's perceptions about abortion in their communities: perspectives from western Kenya. Reprod Health Matters. 2014;22:149–58
12. WHO. Unsafe abortion. Global and regional estimates of the incidence of unsafe abortion and associated mortality in 2008. Geneva: World Health Organization; 2011.
13. National Coordinating Agency for Population and Development, Ministry of Medical Services, Ministry of Public Health and Sanitation, Statistics KNBo, Macro I. Kenya service provision assessment survey 2010. Nairobi:World Health Organisation; 2011.
14. Kenya National Bureau of Statistics, Ministry of Health, National AIDS Control Council, Kenya Medical Research Institute, National Council for Population and Development, ICF International. Kenya demographic and health survey 2014. Nairobi:World Health Organisation; 2015.
15. Mohamed SF, Izugbara C, Moore AM, Mutua M, Kimani-Murage EW, Ziraba AK, Bankole A, Singh SD, Egesa C. The estimated incidence of induced abortion in Kenya: a cross-sectional study. BMC Pregnancy Childbirth. 2015; 15(1):185.
16. Maina BW, Mutua MM, Sidze EM. Factors associated with repeat induced abortion in Kenya. BMC Public Health. 2015;15:1048.
17. Tripney J, Kwan I, Bird KS. Postabortion family planning counseling and services for women in low-income countries: a systematic review. Contraception. 2013;87(1):17–25.
18. Wilson L, Obare F, Ikiugu E, Akora A, Njunguru J, Njuma M, Reiss K, Birungi H. Availability, use and quality of care for medical abortion services in private facilities in Kenya. Nairobi: Population Council and Marie Stopes International; 2015.
19. Wendot S, Scott R, Nafula I, Theuri I, Footman K. Evaluating the impact of a quality management intervention on post-abortion contraceptive uptake in private sector clinics in Western Kenya: a pre- and post-intervention study (in press). BMC Public Health. 2017;
20. Braun V, Clarke V. Using thematic analysis in psychology. Qual Res Psychol. 2006;3(2):77–101.
21. Sandelowski M. Qualitative analysis: what it is and how to begin. Res Nurs Health. 1995;18(4):371–5.
22. Bradley S, Schwant H, Khan S. Levels, trends, and reasons for contraceptive discontinuation. Calverton: ICF Macro; 2009.
23. Curtis C, Huber D, Moss-Knight T. Postabortion family planning: addressing the cycle of repeat unintended pregnancy and abortion. Int Perspect Sex Reprod Health. 2010;36(1):44–8.
24. Coast E, Murray SF. "These things are dangerous": understanding induced abortion trajectories in urban Zambia. Soc Sci Med. 2016;153:201–9.
25. Kalyanwala S, Zavier AJ, Jejeebhoy S, Kumar R. Abortion experiences of unmarried young women in India: evidence from a facility-based study in Bihar and Jharkhand. Int Perspect Sex Reprod Health. 2010;36(2):62–71.
26. Reichwein B, Vaid M. What obstacles do rural Indian women face when attempting to end an unwanted pregnancy? In: MSI research brief series 2013/001. London: Marie Stopes International; 2013.
27. Morroni C, Moodley J. The role of urine pregnancy testing in facilitating access to antenatal care and abortion services in South Africa: a cross-sectional study. BMC Pregnancy Childbirth. 2006;6:26.
28. Ochako R, Mbondo M, Aloo S, Kaimenyi S, Thompson R, Temmerman M, Kays M. Barriers to modern contraceptive methods uptake among young women in Kenya: a qualitative study. BMC Public Health. 2015;15:118.

23

Ambiguities in Washington State hospital policies, irrespective of Catholic affiliation, regarding abortion and contraception service provision

Hilary M Schwandt*[iD], Bethany Sparkle and Moriah Post-Kinney

Abstract

Background: In 2014, the governor of Washington State mandated that all hospitals publically post a reproductive health policy amidst concerns about the lack of clarity among the public how hospitals handled various aspects of reproductive health care.

Methods: The objective of this study is to assess the clarity of abortion and contraception service provision in the hospital reproductive health policies for the public in Washington State. All Washington State hospital reproductive health policies ($n = 88$) were analyzed in 2016 using content analysis. Results were stratified by Catholic religious affiliation of the hospital.

Results: There were more similarities than differences between the non-Catholic and Catholic hospital reproductive health policies; however, there were a few differences. Non-Catholic hospitals were more likely than Catholic hospitals to use legal language (except for emergency contraception), include conscientious clause for providers (44% vs. 0%), and were less likely to specify that emergency contraception use was available for sexual assault victims only (16% vs 54%). Most hospital reproductive health policies, regardless of Catholic affiliation, provided more confusion than clarity in terms of abortion and contraception service provision.

Conclusions: The impact of Catholic, and non-Catholic, affiliated hospital care on patients who need abortion and contraceptive services is concerning. Given the difficulties in meeting the goals of increased transparency for the public through hospital policy language, the government should instead mandate hospitals use a standardized checklist. Additionally, patients are in dire need of positive rights to information about and services to avoid the potential gap in care that the negative rights afforded to providers and facilities to opt-out of providing abortion and contraceptive services have created.

Keywords: Washington State, Reproductive health policy, Hospital, Catholic-affiliated hospital, Abortion, Contraception

Plain English summary

In 2014, the governor of Washington State mandated that all Washington State hospitals publically post their hospital's reproductive health policy. The public was concerned about the lack of clarity on how hospitals handled various aspects of reproductive health care – especially given the high, and growing, number of Catholic affiliated hospitals in the state. The objective of this study is to assess the clarity of abortion and contraception service provision in those hospital reproductive health policies for the public in Washington State. All Washington State hospital reproductive health policies ($n = 88$) were analyzed in 2016. Results were examined according to Catholic affiliation of the hospital. Most hospital reproductive health policies, regardless of Catholic affiliation, provided more confusion than clarity in terms of abortion and contraceptive service provision. The impact of Catholic, and non-Catholic, affiliated hospital care for abortion and contraceptive service provision is concerning. Given the difficulties in meeting

* Correspondence: Hilary.schwandt@wwu.edu
Fairhaven College, Western Washington University, 516 High Street, MS 9118, Bellingham, WA 98225, USA

the goals of increased abortion and contraceptive health-care guideline transparency for the public through hospital policy language, the authors recommend use of a standardized checklist by hospitals to convey abortion and contraceptive service provision. The authors also recommend that patients have more positive rights to information and services to counter balance the negative rights afforded to providers to op-out of providing abortion and contraceptive services.

Background

Over the past fifteen years the number of Catholic hospitals in the US has grown by 22%. Ten of the top 25 health systems in the US are Catholic, furthermore, one in six beds are now in Catholic hospitals [1]. The historically non-religious Washington State, deemed a state with a supportive abortion policy environment [2], has been particularly impacted by this shift, where 34% of the hospitals and 40% of the hospital beds are located in Catholic affiliated hospitals – greater than the national average [1]. This trend of increasing hospital care falling under Catholic jurisdiction is predicted to continue [3].

Reproductive health is an area of concern with Catholic dominance in healthcare. Staff in Catholic health institutions are required to abide by what are known as the "Ethical and Religious Directives for Catholic Health Care Services" (ERDs) [4]. The ERDs declare abortion is allowed only if there is no alternative option to save the mother's life, as well as a ban on all sterilizations and contraception used solely to prevent conception. The interpretation of the ERDs, and therefore care provided, differs by hospital and local bishop. This has been shown to be particularly relevant after hospital mergers [5]. In contrast to the ERDs, the American College of Obstetricians suggests abortions be obtained in a timely and unbiased manner [6]. Physicians at Catholic hospitals report hospital ethics committees deciding against their best judgement in the case of a fetal heart beat – despite the fact that the fetus is nonviable, or continuation of the pregnancy is life-threatening [7]. As a result of these interferences in reproductive medical care, there have been a few high-profile cases of mis-management of miscarriages due to decisions impacted by the ERDs [1].

Obstetrician-gynecologists report disagreeing with a ban on sterilization [8]. Female sterilization is the safest for women immediately following a delivery, for either vaginal or Caesarean births [9]. In general, restrictions on contraceptive access, including sterilization, at Catholic hospitals have led to an increase in subsequent pregnancies [10]. Lack of access to timely abortion and contraceptive services can place undue hardships on patients with less financial resources [5, 8].

Women are often unaware that the hospital they attend for reproductive health care is Catholic. A recent study found that women indicating they attend a Catholic hospital for reproductive health care were nearly six times more likely to misidentify the hospital as religiously affiliated as compared to women who attend non-Catholic hospitals [11]. Women are also unaware that Catholic affiliation of hospitals affects the contraception and abortion care they can receive. A study in Colorado examined reproductive aged women's perceptions about contraceptive and abortive care provision by hospital type, Catholic affiliated and secular, and found no difference in women's expectations of contraceptive and abortive service provision at the two facilities except for advice about natural family planning methods [12]. The ERDs are publicly available online for those who know to look for them; however, within hospitals they are provided only as an internal document and are not posted publicly on hospital websites. As a result, women are likely unaware of how their reproductive health care is limited when attending a Catholic affiliated hospital, nor will they be informed of these constraints while services are being offered.

Research shows restrictions on abortion and contraceptive service provision is not limited to Catholic affiliated health facilities. The number of facilities, and providers, offering abortion services in the USA [13], and specifically Washington State [14] has been decreasing. Perhaps in a correlated way, the abortion rate has been decreasing while the fertility rate has been increasing in Washington State [15]. Research on emergency contraception (EC) availability in hospital emergency departments in the USA found a similarly high percentage of Catholic and non-Catholic hospitals did not have EC available – and among those without EC available, only half offered referrals for EC. Unfortunately, most of the referrals were ineffective upon follow-up. Slightly more Catholic hospitals said they would provide EC only in cases of sexual assault than non-Catholic hospitals, but in both cases less than a quarter of the sample fell into this category [16]. Abortion and contraceptive services may be constrained at all types of hospitals – not just Catholic ones.

In January of 2014, the Washington State Department of Health via a mandate from the governor, required all Washington State hospitals to publicly post on the Department of Health website their current Reproductive Health policies (WAC 246–320-141) with the aim of increasing the public's understanding of each hospital's policy on their specific provision of reproductive health care. This study aims to discern whether the reproductive health policies posted provide clarity to the public about the provision of reproductive health care affected by the ERDs, specifically abortion and contraception, at hospitals in Washington State and whether clarity about service provision differs by Catholic affiliation of the hospital.

Methods

The reproductive health policies for all hospitals providing reproductive health care in Washington State were analyzed for clarity using content analysis on selected reproductive health areas impacted by the ERDs from May to July of 2016 [17]. The reproductive health areas analyzed in the policies: reproductive health, abortion, contraception, and emergency contraception, were selected based upon divergence in recommended care between Catholic doctrine via the ERDs and best health practices as outlined by medical experts.

Hospital reproductive health policy text was coded as reproductive health when language existed in the policy that explicitly stated reproductive health or was relating to the broad topic of reproductive health (1 = reproductive health theme present, 0 = reproductive health theme absent), this did not include specific types of reproductive health service provision. If the reproductive health theme was indicated as present, it was further analyzed whether reproductive health was framed in terms of legal language or not (1 = reproductive health in terms of the law, 0 = reproductive health not in terms of the law).

For abortion – any text relating to communication about, or services provided related to a direct or indirect termination of pregnancy, as well as pre-care and immediate follow-up care, was coded as abortion (1 = abortion theme present, 0 = abortion theme absent). If abortion was coded as present in a policy, further subcategories of abortion were assessed. The subcategories included abortion provision (1 = abortions provided, 0 = abortions not provided); abortion type provided - whether medical and elective abortions were provided (1), provision extended to medical abortion only (2), referrals provided (3), and whether what types of abortions provided were unclear (4); whether provision of abortion was presented in terms of the law (1 = abortion legal language, 0 = no abortion legal language); and whether the option provided for health care providers to opt out of abortion provision was included (1 = provider opt out option for abortion included, 0 = provider opt out option for abortion not included).

Any mention or discussion of provision of methods designed for the prevention of pregnancy were coded as contraception (1 = contraceptive services mentioned, 0 = contraceptive services not mentioned). If contraceptive services was coded as mentioned in a policy, whether contraceptive services were provided (1 = contraceptive services provided, 0 = contraceptive services not provided), contraceptive service provision was clearly stated or not (1 = clear contraceptive service provision, 0 = unclear contraceptive service provision), and whether contraceptive service provision was presented in terms of legal language (1 = contraception provision described in terms of legal language, 0 = contraceptive provision not described in terms of legal language) was also assessed as subcategories of contraceptive services.

For emergency contraception – any policy language about the discussion and provision of emergency contraception was coded as such (1 = emergency contraception included; 0 = emergency contraception not included). Among policies that included any mention of emergency contraception, two subcategories were also assessed – (1) whether emergency contraception provision was explained in terms of legal language (1 = emergency contraception provision in terms of legal language, 0 = emergency contraception not in terms of legal language); and (2) whether the provision of emergency contraception was mentioned in reference to sexual assault patients (1 = emergency contraception in reference to sexual assault, 0 = emergency contraception not in reference to sexual assault). All authors independently coded all policies, all inconsistencies were discussed and final decisions were made collaboratively. Direct quotes were collected to illustrate findings for each code category.

Clarity was assessed through multiple mechanisms. First, through inclusion of the term, or language that implied the term. Second through policy language indicating unambiguously directly related hospital policy and associated procedures (excluding reproductive health). Ultimately, a clear policy would include mention of each of the reproductive health terms, or language indicating the same topic as the terms, as well as language to explicitly detail the hospital procedure in terms of each code. Each hospital reproductive health policy could be coded as including all of the reproductive health areas – and associated details about policy and provision, some, or none of them.

The type of hospital organization (individual or conglomerate) and length of policy (in terms of page length) were recorded. A reproductive health term inclusion score was also created based upon a sum of the following codes (1 if present, 0 if absent): reproductive health, abortion, contraception, and emergency contraception. The correlation between the reproductive health term inclusion score and length of policy was assessed to discern whether mention of terms was more or less likely with the associated length of the policy.

For each hospital – religious affiliation and type of religion affiliation was coded. Bivariate analyses of each policy reproductive health coded term and Catholic hospital affiliation was assessed using the Chi square test statistic and an alpha value of 0.05.

Results

There were 108 hospitals listed on the Washington State Hospital Association Website [18]. On the Washington State Department of Health public reproductive health policy website [17], 98 (91%) hospitals were listed. Of the 98 hospitals, 88 (90%) hospitals had posted a reproductive health policy. Of the 88 hospitals included, 35% were part of a larger organization. Nearly a third, 30%, were religiously affiliated: 96% Catholic and 4% Seventh-Day-Adventist. Among the Catholic hospitals, 81% were part of a conglomerate.

The policy length ranged from a quarter of a page to 18 pages (mean = 2). The mean term inclusion score for non-Catholic hospitals, 1.6, was significantly less than the score, 2.2, for Catholic hospitals. The correlation between policy length and term inclusion score was (– 0.39) for non-Catholic and (–.41) Catholic affiliated hospitals, suggesting a negative relationship between policy length and inclusion of reproductive health terms.

Reproductive health care theme

Just 48% of the non-Catholic hospital's policies mentioned reproductive health compared to 73% of the Catholic hospitals, a significant difference (see Table 1). When policies did include mention of reproductive health, the statements were often vague.

"The purpose of this policy is to provide our patients with a clear summary of the commitments and expectations in these subject areas." This same hospital included this:

"… to provide access to female and male reproductive healthcare services to meet a patient's clinical needs and a patient's choice, although not every procedure is available." (Non-Catholic, Independent).

Among hospital policies that did not include any mention of reproductive health, some examples include: a general "Patient's Rights and Responsibilities" pamphlet and a 7-page forensic nurse procedure for domestic violence cases.

Reproductive health, abortion, contraception, and emergency contraception service provision in terms of the law

Non-Catholic hospital polices wrote about reproductive health (18%), abortion (24%), and contraceptive service provision (3%) in terms of legalese while none of the Catholic hospitals did, a significant difference by Catholic affiliation for both reproductive health and abortion. For emergency contraception, Catholic hospitals used legal language (19%) more so than non-Catholic hospitals (10%), but this difference is not statistically significant (see Table 1).

"It is the policy of Jefferson Healthcare to abide by RCW's 0.02.100[1] and 9.02.160[2] within the limitations of the resources and services offered at the organization." (Non-Catholic, Independent).

Without an understanding of those laws – which take time and effort to locate online, this policy would not provide much clarity for the patient about what these hospitals provide in terms of reproductive health care to patients at those hospitals. Additionally, the language of "within the limitations of the resources and services

offered" would also require insider information about the resources at that particular facility.

"Sunnyside Community Hospital will provide information to female patients in accordance with the requirements of RCW 9.02.160[2] when requested by the patient." (Non-Catholic, Independent).

A patient at this hospital would need to know about the policy in order to know what to ask, regardless, the result might be a referral to another location.

Some hospital policies would state the law, then state they didn't provide any maternity care services.

"The public hospital district complies with the Reproductive Privacy Act….The public hospital district does not provide maternity care benefits, services, or information or pregnancy termination benefits, services or information." (Non-Catholic, Independent).

The law states that provision of maternity services as a precondition for providing reproductive health services including contraceptive and abortion services. This policy states that the hospital complies with the law, since they do not offer maternity services, they do not provide contraception and abortion services.

Abortion, abortion provision, and abortion type

Very few policies explicitly named abortion. A similar percentage of non-Catholic and Catholic policies include the abortion theme (58–60%) and abortion provision (39–40%) – not statistically significant differences. Among the non-Catholic sample, 13% provide medically-indicated and elective abortions, 11% provide medically-indicated only, 5% refer out, and for 16% provision of abortion types was not stated or was unclear. All Catholic policies that included abortion provision (39%) specified only medically-indicated abortions were provided, these differences were statistically significant (see Table 1). The following are examples of clear language in terms of abortion provision:

"Within the UW Medicine integrated health system, we offer both elective and medically indicated terminations of pregnancy…" (Non-Catholic, Conglomerate).

"Elective abortion of normal pregnancy is NOT allowed in Deaconess Hospital." (Non-Catholic, Independent).

While some hospitals asserted support for women's right to abortion services, they did not always provide it. For example, one hospital included inclusive introductory language for their policy:

"This policy defines the woman's right to appropriate health care services that will enable her to go safely through pregnancy and childbirth and the freedom to decide if, when and how often to reproduce."

Yet, two sentences later this is stated:

"Grays Harbor Community Hospital does not provide medical or elective termination of pregnancies." (Non-Catholic, Independent).

Table 1 Washington State Hospital Reproductive Health Policies Term and Information Inculsion, by Catholic Affiliation, 2016

Reproductive Health*	
Catholic	73%
non-Catholic	48%
Legal Language	
Reproductive Health in terms of Legal Language*	
Catholic	0%
non-Catholic	18%
Abortion in terms of Legal Language*	
Catholic	0%
non-Catholic	24%
Contraception Service Provision in terms of Legal Language	
Catholic	0%
non-Catholic	3%
Emergency Contraception Service Provision in terms of Legal Language	
Catholic	19%
non-Catholic	10%
Abortion	
Catholic	58%
non-Catholic	60%
Abortion Provision	
Catholic	39%
non-Catholic	40%
Abortion Type*	
Catholic	
medical	39%
medical & elective	0%
referral	0%
unclear	0%
non-Catholic	
medical	11%
medical & elective	13%
referral	5%
unclear	16%
Protecting the Provider*	
Catholic	0%
non-Catholic	44%
Contraceptive Services	
Catholic	35%
non-Catholic	31%
Contraception Service Provision	
Catholic	19%
non-Catholic	16%

Table 1 Washington State Hospital Reproductive Health Policies Term and Information Inculsion, by Catholic Affiliation, 2016 (Continued)

Contraception Service Provision Clarity	
Catholic	4%
non-Catholic	6%
Emergency Contraception*	
Catholic	54%
non-Catholic	21%
Emergency Contraception Only for Sexual Assault*	
Catholic	54%
non-Catholic	16%

*$p < 0.05$

The following policy used language from the ERDs to describe their policy in terms of abortion provision:

"PeaceHealth does not allow direct abortions. Peace-Health allows the indirect termination of a pregnancy as a result of direct intervention against a maternal pathology to save the life of the mother." (Catholic, Conglomerate).

However, for a lay audience, the terms of direct vs. indirect abortion might not be understood – nor what a "direct intervention against a maternal pathology" might involve.

One hospital's entire policy was about how to handle a non-viable pregnancy. In this policy, the word abortion is never mentioned and termination of pregnancy is only mentioned once. The procedure is most often referred to as labor (Catholic, Independent).

Another hospital referred to offering termination of pregnancy due to the state law but later in the policy there were many barriers to care noted as outlined in the "pretermination" period. These processes involved at least six individuals from the hospital, paperwork on behalf of the patient and the provider, a minimum waiting period of 48 h, and a social service referral (Non-Catholic, Independent).

Another hospital clearly stated they only provide medically-indicated abortions; however, the process for providing medically-indicated abortions involved (11) hospital personnel and (13) hospital procedures (Non-Catholic, Independent).

The quote below is the entire reproductive health policy for this hospital:

"Termination of pregnancy for fetal anomalies/genetic condition is available at Yakima Valley Memorial Hospital for those patients with a confirmed diagnosis who have received genetic counseling and are making an informed decision. That is the only case in which termination is available." (Non-Catholic, Independent).

In 5% of the non-Catholic hospitals referral out for abortion was emphasized. In this example, the policy indicates they follow state policies about providing pregnancy terminations, but the language implied they would do so only through referral.

"Referral and informational services are provided to offer women and family choices regarding voluntary termination of pregnancy." (Non-Catholic, Independent).

In one hospital policy, a detailed section on abortion begins with language about providing information and transfer and ends with language about sanctions against providers who provide abortions, this is an excerpt from the following:

"All providers at Lincoln Hospital District #3 are expected to respond to any patient's questions about birth control and pregnancy-terminating procedures with openness and compassion....Any female patient wishing to receive pregnancy-terminating medication (excluding emergency contraception) or medical procedures while a patient at this hospital will be assisted in transfer to another facility...If a provider participates in termination procedures beyond what is allowed by hospital policy, Lincoln Hospital District #3 may impose sanctions on that provider." (Non-Catholic, Independent).

Protecting the provider against forced abortion provision
Only non-Catholic hospital policies (44%) included details on health providers' freedom to opt out of providing care, a statistically significant difference (see Table 1). It was common to read a non-Catholic policy that first stated the law, and then included the opt-out provision for providers, as this example shows:

"The Public Hospital District complies with the Reproductive Privacy Act...The Act contains a conscience clause acknowledging that no person may be required in any circumstance to participate in the performance of an abortion if such person objects to doing so. The Public Hospital District respects each individual's right to refuse to participate in an abortion if such person objects to doing so." (Non-Catholic, Independent).

One hospital's entire policy was about the provider's right to opt out of providing services (Non-Catholic, Independent).

The following hospital policy provides extensive detail regarding the provider opt-out option and notes that if all providers opted-out, it would be impossible to provide abortions at the facility – highlighting the tension between two laws – one that protects patient access to abortion and the other that protects providers from having to provide abortion services:

"Public hospital districts cannot perform abortions without the assistance of their medical staff and employees. The Act prohibits a public hospital district from requiring its medical staff or employees to participate in the performance of abortions. A public hospital district also is prohibited from requiring a physician by contract (including employment) to perform abortions. Physicians who refuse to perform abortions cannot be denied privileges nor can their medical staff privileges be adversely

affected. As a result, if Newport Hospital & Health Services medical staff or employees are unwilling to perform abortion services, it may be impossible for a public hospital district to provide abortion services that are substantially equivalent to the maternity care services available at its facilities." (Non-Catholic, Independent).

Contraceptive services, provision of contraceptive services, and clarity of contraceptive service provision
A similar percentage of non-Catholic and Catholic policies mention contraceptive services (31–35%), provision of contraceptive services (16–19%), and have clear language about provision (4–6%), none of which differ significantly by hospital Catholic affiliation (see Table 1). The following is an example of clear language in regards to provision of preventative services, including contraception.

"Through the primary care settings in hospital facilities, patients have access to a full array of preventative healthcare services including all forms of contraception prevention, and the prevention and treatment of sexually transmitted diseases." (Non-Catholic, Conglomerate).

In contrast, this hospital policy provides absolutely no clarity in terms of contraceptive service provision as it is unclear how the hospital responds to the law:

"The Act declares that it is the public policy of the state Washington that every individual has the fundamental right to choose or refuse birth control. The Act does not, however, impose an affirmative duty on the state or its municipal corporations, such as public hospital districts, to provide birth control or other family planning or reproductive" (Non-Catholic, Independent).

Emergency contraception
Emergency contraception (EC) was mentioned in 21%, and only in terms of sexual assault in 16%, of the non-Catholic hospital policies, while it was mentioned in 54% of Catholic policies, all of which made reference to sexual assault, both of which are significantly different by Catholic affiliation (see Table 1).

"Forks Community Hospital provides emergency contraception to victims of sexual assault only." (Non-Catholic, Independent).

Stating clearly that should a patient who doesn't indicate sexual assault request emergency contraception, they will be denied those services.

The following is the first sentence of this hospital's reproductive health policy and states that the purpose of emergency contraception is only to prevent pregnancy following sexual assault, this is just one example of a few policies making this incorrect statement:

"The purpose of PCC (post-coital contraception) is to prevent pregnancy following a sexual assault." (Non-Catholic, Independent).

This policy continues to outline the guidelines and procedures for administering emergency contraception to sexual assault victims. The entire focus of the guidelines is to determine among the population of sexual assault victims, which ones should receive emergency contraception.

Another hospital only included emergency contraception in their posted reproductive health policy. They indicated that emergency contraception information would be provided to both victims of sexual assault and those who had unprotected sex; however, only victims of sexual assault would receive the actual provision of emergency contraception (Non-Catholic, Independent).

Discussion

This research examined the content regarding abortion and contraception service provision among the posted reproductive health policies of Washington State hospitals, by hospital Catholic affiliation, in response to a call to study religious and non-religious hospital reproductive health policy transparency [11, 19]. In general, a lack of clarity about abortion and contraception service provision existed in the reproductive health policies posted by the hospitals in Washington State, regardless of Catholic affiliation, despite some of the language used to assert clarity. Overall, there were more similarities than differences between the non-Catholic and Catholic hospital reproductive health policies. The Catholic hospital policies were more likely to include reproductive health terms than the non-Catholic hospitals; however, they were less likely to indicate provision of reproductive health care – even among those areas of care mentioned. In sum, all hospital reproductive health policies, regardless of religious affiliation, lacked transparency about abortion and contraception service provision. In addition, the length of the policy was negatively correlated with inclusion of the main reproductive health terms of focus in this study.

Not all reproductive health policies included a mention of reproductive health and a few policies were policies about not providing reproductive health care.

Three percent to a quarter of the non-Catholic polies were written using the language of existing laws – whether in general or for specific issues. Nearly half of the non-Catholic reproductive health policies included a provision about provider's choice to opt-out of providing abortion care. None of the Catholic hospitals included a mention of provider opt-out, likely as it is a non-issue for facilities not performing abortions.

The most common subject included in the non-Catholic policies was abortion – yet, the term abortion was rarely used. Despite the common inclusion of the theme of abortion, just 24% clearly indicated the type of abortion provided. Emergency contraception was included in about a fifth of the non-Catholic policies. In the Catholic policies, 54% mention emergency contraception – and all were in relation to its use for sexual assault victims exclusively. In sum, the impetus for requiring hospitals in Washington State to publicly post their reproductive health policies to increase transparency in provision of abortion and contraception services was not met based upon the facts that the mere mention of important terms/themes never met 100% (21–73%) and the inclusion of details about provision of care was even lower (4–40%).

Reproductive health care is vast and encompasses many aspects of medical care. A policy on all types of reproductive health services provided by a hospital facility would be lengthy. As a result of this issue and the desire to increase transparency in types of reproductive care provided – standardized checklists including reproductive health care that differs from the standard of care is what should be included in a transparent reproductive health policy. Reproductive health procedures that potentially fall into this category include: abortion, contraception, sterilization, emergency contraception, ectopic pregnancy, and LGBTQI care – as well as others. For each of these categories, the checklist should make it clear what the organization does and does not provide [19] – especially as it differs from the medical guidelines [6]. See Table 2 as a recommended checklist template for abortion and contraceptive service provision for hospitals.

Table 2 Abortion and Contraception Service Provision Checklist for Hospitals

Services Provided and Available to all Patients 24/7	YES	REFERRAL	NO	UNSURE	Comments
Abortion Provision					
Medically-indicated abortions					
Elective abortions					
Contraceptive Method Provision, for Any Reason, Including Pregnancy Prevention					
Modern Methods (condoms, pill, injectable, implant, IUD)					
Sterilization (vasectomy and tubal ligation)					
Emergency Contraception, for victims of sexual assault					
Emergency Contraception, irrespective of sexual assault					

If providers are uncomfortable with a procedure, they do not have to provide it. Due to this right, if a patient needs services but all of the providers opt-out of providing the service, at this time the patient can't receive that service at that facility. Hospitals, and providers, are protected from discomfort in terms of abortion provision; however, there is an absence of protection for the individual patient in need of care [20]. Provider protections to not provide services have recently gained momentum. In 2018, the federal department of Health and Human Services created a Conscientious and Religious Freedom Division as well as released a new rule to strengthen provider's ability to refuse to provide services that are against their beliefs. The World Health Organization notes that providers are allowed conscientious objection to abortion provision – but that they have a duty to refer those patients to a provider, or facility, that will provide those services and in the absence of those options, and if it is not possible to ensure a referral that the provider must provide the abortion to avoid undue harm to the patient [21].

"Americans should be able to count on receiving care that meets their needs and is based on the best scientific knowledge--yet there is strong evidence that this frequently is not the case. Health care harms patients too frequently and routinely fails to deliver its potential benefits." [20]. The Institute of Medicine highlights that care should be safe, patient-centered, and timely as core needs for health care: "The patient is the source of control. Patients should be given the necessary information and opportunity to exercise the degree of control they choose over health care decisions that affect them. The system should make available to patients and their families information that enables them to make informed decisions..." [20]. It is clear that these ideals are currently not being met in abortion and contraceptive care at hospitals in Washington State, regardless of religious affiliation.

Research has shown that hospital reproductive health policies are often unclear to those providing the services as well [22]. Therefore, hospitals publicly posting transparent abortion and contraceptive service standardized checklists is just one necessary step for both providers and patients– but so is abundant patient education and awareness at the population level, during patient encounters, and in a pre-emptive manner by hospitals.

Throughout this research it was clear that some policies were really unique, and often avoided addressing all, or any, abortion and contraceptive service provision policy, while others were notable only for their similarity to the others – while remaining ambiguous. This pattern observed makes one wonder about the reach of religious healthcare on other healthcare – as it is clear that institutions look to each other for guidance.

The limitations of this research are that the content analysis of the reproductive health policies was limited to the posted reproductive health policies. Efforts were not made to find clarification to the policies by further research into the hospitals themselves. Catholic affiliation was dichotomized but the relationship between Catholic affiliation and hospital care falls along a spectrum. There were aspects of reproductive health in the hospital polices that were not included in the analysis, most often due to lack of attention to the issue, some examples include: ectopic pregnancy, sterilization, labor and delivery, sexually transmitted infections, infertility, genetic testing, and domestic violence.

Despite the limitations, this research did have a few strengths. Three researchers collaborated to create the content analysis plan. Coding was implemented independently by all three researchers – and all issues that arose during the analysis were discussed by all three and resolved in an agreeable manner. Additionally, the quantitative findings were illustrated through qualitative selection of illustrative quotes.

Future research should continue to find reasons for restrictions on abortion and contraceptive service provision at non-religious hospitals as well as the best ways to educate the public about these restrictions. It would also be interesting to know how this knowledge affects care-seeking behavior; however, it is also true that various options for care are not available to everyone.

Conclusion

In sum, the current reproductive health policies among Washington State hospitals rarely provide clarity in terms of abortion and contraception service provision for the people of Washington State – regardless of Catholic affiliation of the hospital. Public posting of a comprehensive reproductive health policy would not achieve clarity given the breadth of hospital reproductive health services. As a result, the best way to increase transparency about abortion and contraceptive service provision policy would be to require hospitals to publically post responses to a standardized checklist (see Table 2). More efforts are needed to educate the public, generally, and in patient and provider encounters about abortion and contraception service provision options. The same level of protection provided for hospitals and providers to not offer abortion and contraceptive services needs to be afforded to individual patients in the arena of receiving abortion and contraception services. It is vital that patient rights to information about contraception and abortion service provision, at all health facilities offering reproductive healthcare, regardless of religious affiliation, be rectified immediately.

Endnotes

[1]The legal language of RCW 9.02.100 is as follows: The sovereign people hereby declare that every individual

possesses a fundamental right of privacy with respect to personal reproductive decisions.Accordingly, it is the public policy of the state of Washington that:(1) Every individual has the fundamental right to choose or refuse birth control;(2) Every woman has the fundamental right to choose or refuse to have an abortion, except as specifically limited by RCW 9.02.100 through 9.02.170 and 9.02.900 through 9.02.902;(3) Except as specifically permitted by RCW 9.02.100 through 9.02.170 and 9.02.900 through 9.02.902, the state shall not deny or interfere with a woman's fundamental right to choose or refuse to have an abortion; and(4) The state shall not discriminate against the exercise of these rights in the regulation or provision of benefits, facilities, services, or information.

[2]The legal language of RCW 9.02.160 is as follows: If the state provides, directly or by contract, maternity care benefits, services, or information to women through any program administered or funded in whole or in part by the state, the state shall also provide women otherwise eligible for any such program with substantially equivalent benefits, services, or information to permit them to voluntarily terminate their pregnancies.

Acknowledgements
We would like to thank Mary Kay Barbieri for alerting us to this area of research and supporting us from start until completion. We would also like to thank Lori Freedman and Debra Stuhlberg for providing us with early mentoring, support, and confidence in our work. Finally, we would like to thank all of the people at ACLU, PP, NARAL, and others who worked so hard to make this regulation a reality, and who are still working towards reproductive justice in Washington State and beyond.

Funding
This research did not receive any specific grant from funding agencies in the public, commercial, or not-for-profit sectors.

Author's contributions
HMS, BS, MPK conceived, designed, and analyzed the data. All 3 authors wrote up the manuscript, read, and approved of the final manuscript.

Competing interests
The authors declare that they have no competing interests.

References
1. ACLU. Health Care Denied: Patients and Physicians Speak Out About Catholic Hospitals and the Threat to Women's Health and Lives.; 2016. https://www.aclu.org/report/report-health-care-denied?redirect=report/health-care-denied.
2. Jones RK, Ingerick M, Jerman J. Differences in abortion service delivery in hostile, middle-ground, and supportive states in 2014. Womens Health Issues. 2018;28(3):212 8. https://doi.org/10.1016/j.whi.2017.12.003
3. ACLU and MergerWatch. Miscarriage of Medicine: The Growth of Catholic Hospitals and the Threat to Reproductive Health Care.; 2013. https://www.aclu.org/report/miscarriage-medicine.
4. US Conference of Catholic Bishops. Ethical and Religious Directives for Catholic Health Care Services, Fourth.; 2001. http://www.usccb.org/issues-and-action/human-life-and-dignity/health-care/upload/Ethical-Religious-Directives-Catholic-Health-Care-Services-fifth-edition-2009.pdf. Accessed 12 Aug 2016.
5. Donovan P. Hospital mergers and reproductive health care. Fam Plan Perspect. 1996;28(6):281–4.
6. American College of Obstetricians and Gynecologists. Abortion policy.2014. https://www.acog.org/-/media/Statements-of-Policy/Public/sop069.pdf?dmc=1&ts=20160429T1625032644.
7. Freedman LR, Landy U, Steinauer J. When There's a heartbeat: miscarriage Management in Catholic-Owned Hospitals. Am J Public Health. 2008;98(10):1774-8.
8. Stulberg DB, Hoffman Y, Dahlquist IH, Freedman LR. Tubal ligation in Catholic hospitals: a qualitative study of Ob–gyns' experiences. Contraception. 2014;90(4):422–8. https://doi.org/10.1016/j.contraception.2014.04.015.
9. Chi I-C, Gates D, Thapa S. Performing tubal sterilizations during Women's postpartum hospitalization: a review of the United States and international experiences. Obstet Gynecol Surv. 1992;47(2):71–9.
10. Guiahi M, McNulty M, Garbe G, Edwards S, Kenton K. Changing depot medroxyprogesterone acetate access at a faith-based institution. Contraception. 2011;84(3):280–4. https://doi.org/10.1016/j.contraception.2010.12.003.
11. Wascher JM, Hebert LE, Freedman LR, Stulberg DB. Do women know whether their hospital is Catholic? Results from a national survey. Contraception. 2018. https://doi.org/10.1016/j.contraception.2018.05.017.
12. Guiahi M, Sheeder J, Teal S. Are women aware of religious restrictions on reproductive health at Catholic hospitals? A survey of women's expectations and preferences for family planning care. Contraception. 2014;90(4):429–34. https://doi.org/10.1016/j.contraception.2014.06.035.
13. Jones RK, Jerman J. Abortion incidence and service availability in the United States, 2014: abortion incidence and service availability in the United States, 2014. Perspect Sex Reprod Health. 2017;49(1):17–27. https://doi.org/10.1363/psrh.12015.
14. Dobie SA, Hart LG, Glusker A, Madigan D, Larson EH, Rosenblatt RA. Abortion Services in Rural Washington State, 1983-1984 to 1993-1994: availability and outcomes. Fam Plan Perspect. 1999;31(5):241. https://doi.org/10.2307/2991572.
15. Glusker AI, Dobie SA, Madigan D, Rosenblatt RA, Larson EH. Differences in fertility patterns between urban and rural women in Washington state, 1983–1984 to 1993–1994. Women Health. 2000;31(1):55–70. https://doi.org/10.1300/J013v31n01_04.
16. Harrison T. Availability of emergency contraception: a survey of hospital emergency department staff. Ann Emerg Med. 2005;46(2):105–10. https://doi.org/10.1016/j.annemergmed.2005.01.017.
17. Washington State Department of Health. Washington state hospital policies. 2016. http://www.doh.wa.gov/DataandStatisticalReports/HealthcareinWashington/HospitalandPatientData/HospitalPolicies.
18. Washington State Hospital Association. Washington state hospital listing. 2016. http://www.wsha.org/our-members/member-listing/.
19. Freedman LR, Stulberg DB. The research consortium on religious healthcare institutions: studying the impact of religious restrictions on women's reproductive health. Contraception. 2016;94(1):6–10. https://doi.org/10.1016/j.contraception.2016.03.015.
20. Crossing the Quality Chasm. A new health system for the 21st century: Institute of Medicine; 2000. https://www.nap.edu/read/10027/chapter/1#ii. Accessed 12 Sept 2018.
21. World Health Organization. Safe Abortion: Technical and Policy Guidance for Health Systems.; 2012. http://apps.who.int/iris/bitstream/10665/70914/1/9789241548434_eng.pdf. Accessed 12 Sept 2018.
22. Stulberg DB, Dude AM, Dahlquist I, Curlin FA. Obstetrician-gynecologists, religious institutions, and conflicts regarding patient-care policies. Am J Obstet Gynecol. 2012;207(1):73.e1–5. https://doi.org/10.1016/j.ajog.2012.04.023.

24

Early pregnancy loss in Belagavi, Karnataka, India 2014–2017: a prospective population-based observational study in a low-resource setting

Sangappa M. Dhaded[1*], Manjunath S. Somannavar[1], Jane P. Jacob[2], Elizabeth M. McClure[3], Sunil S. Vernekar[1], S. Yogesh Kumar[1], Avinash Kavi[1], Umesh Y. Ramadurg[1], Janet L. Moore[3], Dennis P. Wallace[3], Richard J. Derman[2], Robert L. Goldenberg[4] and Shivaprasad S. Goudar[1]

From 2nd International Conference on Maternal and Newborn Health: Translating Research Evidence to Practice
Belagavi, India. 26-27 March 2018

Abstract

Background: The prevalence of early pregnancy loss through miscarriage and medically terminated pregnancy (MTP) is largely unknown due to lack of early registration of pregnancies in most regions, and especially in low- and middle-income countries. Understanding the rates of early pregnancy loss as well as the characteristics of pregnant women who experience miscarriage or MTP can assist in better planning of reproductive health needs of women.

Methods: A prospective, population-based study was conducted in Belagavi District, south India. Using an active surveillance system of women of childbearing age, all women were enrolled as soon as possible during pregnancy. We evaluated rates and risk factors of miscarriage and MTP between 6 and 20 weeks gestation as well as rates of stillbirth and neonatal death. A hypothetical cohort of 1000 women pregnant at 6 weeks was created to demonstrate the impact of miscarriage and MTP on pregnancy outcome.

Results: A total of 30,166 women enrolled from 2014 to 2017 were included in this analysis. The rate of miscarriage per 1000 ongoing pregnancies between 6 and 8 weeks was 115.3, between 8 and 12 weeks the miscarriage rate was 101.9 per 1000 ongoing pregnancies and between 12 and 20 weeks the miscarriage rate was 60.3 per 1000 ongoing pregnancies. For those periods, the MTP rate was 40.2, 45.4, and 48.3 per 1000 ongoing pregnancies respectively. The stillbirth rate was 26/1000 and the neonatal mortality rate was 24/1000. The majority of miscarriages (96.6%) were unattended and occurred at home. The majority of MTPs occurred in a hospital and with a physician in attendance (69.6%), while 20.7% of MTPs occurred outside a health facility. Women who experienced a miscarriage were older and had a higher level of education but were less likely to be anemic than those with an ongoing pregnancy at 20 weeks. Women with MTP were older, had a higher level of education, higher parity, and higher BMI, compared to those with an ongoing pregnancy, but these results were not consistent across gestational age periods.

(Continued on next page)

* Correspondence: drdhadedsm@gmail.com
[1]Women's and Children's Health Research Unit, J N Medical College, KLE Academy of Higher Education and Research, Belagavi, Karnataka, India
Full list of author information is available at the end of the article

(Continued from previous page)

Conclusions: Of women with an ongoing pregnancy at 6 weeks, about 60% will have a living infant at 28 days of age. Two thirds of the losses will be spontaneous miscarriages and one third will be secondary to a MTP. High maternal age and education were the risk factors associated with miscarriage and MTP.

Keywords: Miscarriage, Medically terminated pregnancy, Early pregnancy loss, India

Background

Miscarriage is a public health issue throughout the world. Miscarriages, often defined as spontaneous pregnancy losses before 20 weeks gestational age, are estimated to occur in almost 1 in 3 pregnancies, many of which occur before the pregnancy is clinically recognized [1, 2]. This may be especially true in developing countries where women do not have ready access to health care providers.

Various factors have been associated with miscarriage, including the number of previous miscarriages, nutritional status, and the level of personal and community support [3]. Miscarriages may also be caused by various environmental, anatomical, and genetic factors. Exposure to certain infections can also increase the chance of a miscarriage [4]. Additionally, many studies have shown advanced maternal age to be significantly related to risk of miscarriage [3].

High rates of malnutrition and poor-nutrition, often measured by body mass index and hemoglobin levels among women in developing countries, may be contributing factors to high rates of early pregnancy loss [5]. Additionally, lack of health resources, including antenatal care, might also contribute to increased rates of miscarriage.

India, in particular, has reported high rates of miscarriage, particularly for women who have had previous miscarriages or unsafe abortions [6]. A household survey conducted in Bihar, India found that miscarriage rates were reported to be 46 per 1000 pregnancies (4.6%), but registration tended to occur later in pregnancy [6]. In contrast, an epidemiological study based in major cities throughout India found the prevalence of recurrent spontaneous miscarriages among Indian women to be as high as 32% [4]. None of these studies mentioned the gestational age at enrolment.

Another form of pregnancy loss is medically terminated pregnancy (MTP), which can be performed either in a hospital or at home, through medication or surgery. In India, MTPs can legally occur until 20 weeks of gestational age [7]. A recent study looked at abortion rates in health facilities within six states in India and found that MTPs accounted for 33% of pregnancies [8].

Thus, statistics on miscarriages and MTPs in India vary widely across the literature, partially due to difficulty in obtaining reliable early gestational age data among vulnerable, rural populations. Many of these studies include data from developed regions of India. Therefore, we do not have an accurate understanding of pregnancy outcomes in India's rural settings. Additionally, while studies on specific clinical contributors, such as nutrition and previous miscarriages exist, few population-based studies are available examining the rates of miscarriage and MTP and their association with maternal characteristics. Better understanding the impact of medical services on the pregnancies of rural woman, as well as the interplay of societal structure and personal health in the context of rural, developing regions, can help better target the complexities of miscarriages and MTP in these settings. These issues affect a large proportion of women throughout rural India, as well women in other parts of the world, and merit a nuanced and multidimensional approach.

Our study aims to identify the prevalence and characteristics of women who experience miscarriage or MTP in rural settings within Belagavi, India.

Methods

This study was conducted as part of the Global Network's Maternal Newborn Health Registry (MNHR), a population based, observational study conducted in six low-resource countries, including India [9]. The objective of the MNHR is to enrol all pregnant women residing within defined geographic areas, study clusters, which generally have 300 to 500 deliveries per year. This analysis includes data collected from pregnant women enrolled in the Belagavi MNHR clusters from 2014 to 2017.

All pregnant women residing within a study cluster, or giving birth within the cluster, were approached as early as possible during their pregnancy for inclusion in the MNHR. Following informed consent, women were followed by study staff, known as registry administrators (RAs). The RAs enrolled consenting pregnant women and completed perinatal outcome forms for each woman enrolled in the MNHR. RAs collected information on prenatal services and the health status of the mother, including age, hemoglobin level, weight, height, and previous pregnancies. Pregnancy outcomes and mode of delivery were also recorded.

The RAs attempted to register the women as early in the pregnancy as possible, using an ongoing registry of women likely to get pregnant and frequent pregnancy testing among those likely to get pregnant [10]. The data were then reviewed and cleaned by research staff and then entered in a local secure study computer where additional edits were performed. Data were then transmitted to a central data-coordinating center, RTI International, where additional edits were performed and resolved by the site.

Statistical analyses

We calculated the body mass index (BMI) from the mother's weight and height in kg/m^2 based on measurements generally taken < 12 weeks gestation. Hemoglobin measurements were taken at the first ANC visit and categorized. Miscarriages were defined as any spontaneous loss prior to 20 weeks. A medical termination included the elective termination of pregnancy whether the termination was performed medically or surgically. A stillbirth was defined as the birth of a baby at 20 weeks or more with no signs of life. The gestational age was based on ultrasound, if available, or otherwise the date of the last menstrual period. Women with a missing gestational age or enrolled at delivery were excluded.

Because women enrol in care at various times in pregnancy, and it appears that those who have an early miscarriage or MTP may not enrol at all, a modelling exercise to account for women not entering care was needed. To estimate the outcome of 1000 hypothetical pregnancies ongoing at 6 weeks, we applied the rates of miscarriage and MTP found in the ongoing pregnancies at 6 weeks to 7 weeks 6 days to the entire population of 1000 pregnancies. To estimate the outcomes of the remaining hypothetical pregnancies ongoing at 8 weeks, we applied the rates of miscarriage and MTP found in the ongoing pregnancies at 8 weeks to 11 weeks 6 days to the remaining ongoing pregnancies. To estimate the outcome of the remaining hypothetical pregnancies ongoing at 12 weeks we applied the rates of miscarriage and MTP found in the ongoing pregnancies at 12 weeks to 19 weeks 6 days to the remaining ongoing pregnancies. We also applied the rates of stillbirth and neonatal mortality to the remaining pregnancies at 20 weeks to determine the number of living infants at 28 days of age.

We were also interested in the characteristics of woman having miscarriages and MTPs. Descriptive analyses included frequency and distribution of risk factors for women having miscarriages and MTPs within each gestational age category. We analysed the individual risk relationship of each variable with the risk of miscarriage and MTP for all pregnancies terminating from 6 weeks to 19 weeks 6 days within the gestational age groups of 6 weeks to 7 weeks 6 days, 8 weeks to 11 weeks 6 days and 12 weeks to 19 weeks 6 days. For the outcome variables of miscarriage and MTP, relative risks (RR) and 95% confidence intervals (CI) were obtained from generalized linear models with a binomial distribution assumption and log link for binary outcomes accounting for a single

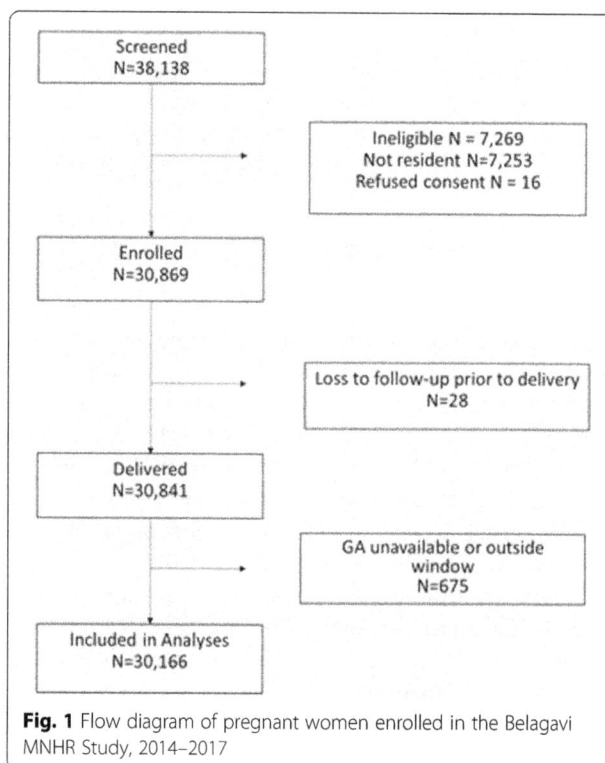

Fig. 1 Flow diagram of pregnant women enrolled in the Belagavi MNHR Study, 2014–2017

Table 1 Antenatal and obstetric care for women with a miscarriage or MTP vs those with an ongoing pregnancy at 20 weeks gestation

	Miscarriage	MTP	Ongoing pregnancy at 20 weeks GA
Enrolled, N	3598	1894	24,674
At least one ANC visit (%)	93.9	95.2	100.0
ANC visits (%)			
0	6.1	4.8	0.0
1–2	93.0	91.4	5.2
> 2	0.9	3.8	94.8
Delivery attendant (%)			
Physician	2.6	84.8	61.1
Nurse/Nurse midwife	0.7	1.2	35.8
TBA	0.1	0.7	0.4
Family/Self delivery/Other	96.6	13.2	2.7
Delivery location, N (%)			
Hospital	2.8	69.6	71.3
Clinic/Health center	0.9	9.7	24.3
Home/Other	96.3	20.7	4.4

MTP medically terminated pregnancy
ANC antenatal care
GA gestational age
TBA traditional birth attendant

Early pregnancy loss in Belagavi, Karnataka, India 2014–2017: a prospective population-based...

227

Table 2 Miscarriage and MTP rates per 1000 ongoing pregnancies among women with an ongoing pregnancy at 6, 8 and 12 weeks gestation

	Number (n/N)	Rate per 1000 ongoing pregnancies
Enrolled, N	30,166	
Enrolled by 6 weeks without loss < 6 weeks, N	2775	
Miscarriage 6,0–7,6 weeks	307/2663	115.3
MTP 6,0–7,6 weeks	112/2468	45.4
Enrolled by 8 weeks without loss < 8 weeks, N	10,452	
Miscarriage 8,0–11,6 weeks	1019/9996	101.9
MTP 8,0–11,6 weeks	456/9433	48.3
Enrolled by 12 weeks without loss < 12 weeks, N	19,200	
Miscarriage 12,0–19,6 weeks	1114/18,473	60.3
MTP 12,0–19,6 weeks	727/18,086	40.2

MTP medically terminated pregnancy
For this analysis, the denominators for miscarriage and MTP are different because in each time-period, the number of miscarriages were excluded from the denominator for MTPs, and for MTPs, the number of miscarriages were excluded from the denominator

risk factor and controlling for each of the variables as well as cluster as a random effect. All analyses were performed with SAS (Cary, NC).

Results

A total of 38,138 women were screened and of those, 30,869 (81%) were eligible and consented. Most of those who were ineligible were not residents of the catchment area (Fig. 1). Of those, 30,166 (97.8%) women had gestational age information available and were included in the analyses. Of these women, 9.2% were enrolled prior to 6 weeks gestation, 28.9% between 6 weeks and 7 weeks 6 days, 36.4% between 8 weeks and 11 weeks 6 days, 19.9% between 12 weeks and 19 weeks 6 days, and 5.6% at or after 20 weeks.

Table 1 summarizes the antenatal care (ANC) and obstetric characteristics for women with miscarriages and MTPs prior to 20 weeks and ongoing pregnancies at 20 weeks. Among women with a miscarriage, 93.9% had at least one ANC visit, while 95.2 and 100% of women with MTPs and ongoing pregnancies at 20 weeks received at least one ANC visit. Among

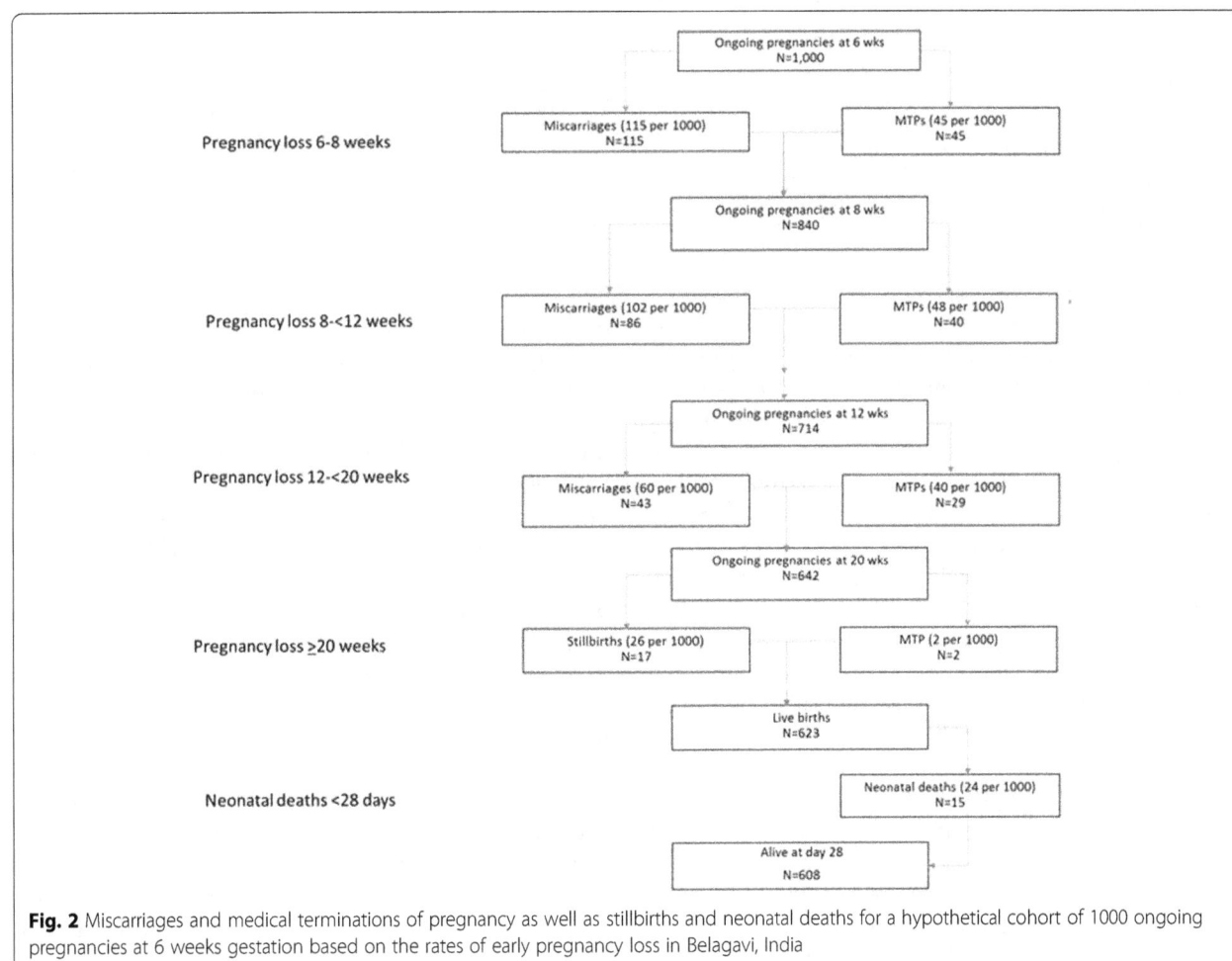

Fig. 2 Miscarriages and medical terminations of pregnancy as well as stillbirths and neonatal deaths for a hypothetical cohort of 1000 ongoing pregnancies at 6 weeks gestation based on the rates of early pregnancy loss in Belagavi, India

Table 3 Relative risk (RR) of miscarriage vs ongoing pregnancy in three gestational age groups by women's characteristics

	Miscarriage v. Ongoing 6,0–7,6 Weeks RR (95% CI)	Miscarriage v. Ongoing 8,0–11,6 Weeks RR (95% CI)	Miscarriage v. Ongoing 12,0–19,6 Weeks RR (95% CI)
Maternal age (years)			
≤ 20	1.26 (0.94, 1.69)	1.12 (0.95, 1.33)	0.94 (0.80, 1.10)
21–25	REF	REF	REF
26–30	1.11 (0.80, 1.53)	1.06 (0.90, 1.26)	1.09 (0.93, 1.29)
> 30	1.17 (0.64, 2.14)	1.42 (1.05, 1.93)	1.81 (1.37, 2.38)
Maternal education			
No formal education	0.93 (0.59, 1.46)	0.94 (0.71, 1.23)	1.12 (0.86, 1.46)
Primary	REF	REF	REF
Secondary	0.95 (0.69, 1.32)	1.10 (0.92, 1.31)	1.42 (1.20, 1.68)
University+	1.00 (0.61, 1.62)	0.89 (0.68, 1.16)	0.93 (0.68, 1.27)
Parity			
0	0.78 (0.57, 1.07)	0.73 (0.60, 0.89)	0.89 (0.75, 1.06)
1–2	REF	REF	REF
> 2	1.30 (0.88, 1.91)	1.11 (0.84, 1.48)	1.08 (0.83, 1.41)
BMI (kg/m$^{2)}$)			
Underweight, < 18.5 kg/m^2	1.00 (0.85, 1.19)	1.02 (0.96, 1.08)	1.00 (0.86, 1.17)
Normal weight, 18.5–25 kg/m^2	REF	REF	REF
Overweight /obese, > 25 kg/m^2	0.61 (0.41, 0.91)	0.89 (0.68, 1.16)	0.99 (0.77, 1.29)
Hemoglobin (gm/dl)			
Severe/Moderate, ≤ 9 g/dl	0.77 (0.61, 0.98)	0.86 (0.70, 1.06)	0.93 (0.74, 1.17)
Mild, > 9–11 g/dl	0.75 (0.61, 0.92)	0.81 (0.70, 0.93)	1.00 (0.86, 1.15)
Normal, > 11 g/dl	REF	REF	REF

BMI body mass index
REF reference group

women with a MTP, 84.8% were performed by a physician, but 13.2% occurred without a physician or nurse present. For women with pregnancies ongoing at 20 weeks, 61.1% were ultimately delivered by a physician and 2.7% were unattended. Among women having a miscarriage, 2.8% occurred within a hospital, 0.9% at a health center and 96.3% at home. For those with a MTP, 69.9% occurred at a hospital, 9.7% at a health center and 20.7% at home. Finally, among those with an ongoing pregnancy at 20 weeks, the delivery ultimately occurred in a hospital for 71.3%, at health center for 24.3 and 4.4% occurred at home.

We next estimated the rates of miscarriage and MTP per 1000 ongoing pregnancies by gestational age categories (Table 2). Among women who were enrolled by 6 weeks gestation, the rate of miscarriage between 6 weeks and 7 weeks 6 days was 115.3/1000, and the MTP rate was 45.4/1000. Among those with an ongoing pregnancy at 8 weeks, the rate of miscarriage between 8 and 11 weeks 6 days was 101.9/1000, and the rate of MTP was 48.3/1000. Finally, among those with an ongoing pregnancy at 12 weeks, the rate of miscarriage between 12 weeks

and 19 weeks 6 days was 60.3/1000 and the MTP rate was 40.2/1000.

Applying these rates to a hypothetical population of 1000 ongoing pregnancies at 6 weeks gestation (Fig. 2), we calculated that between 6 weeks to 7 weeks 6 days, there would be 115 miscarriages and 45 MTPs leaving 840 ongoing pregnancies at 8 weeks. With 840 ongoing pregnancies at 8 weeks gestation, there would then be an additional 86 miscarriages and 40 MTPs between 8 and 11 weeks 6 days gestation, leaving 714 ongoing pregnancies at 12 weeks gestation. Between 12 weeks to 19 weeks 6 days, there would be 43 miscarriages and 29 abortions leaving 642 ongoing pregnancies at 20 weeks gestation. In this population, an additional 2 MTPs were reported after 20 weeks gestation, leaving 640 pregnancies. During the study, the stillbirth rate was estimated to be 26 per 1000 and the 28-day neonatal mortality rate was 24 per 1000 (data not shown). Applying these rates to our hypothetical population, after the additional 17 stillbirths and 15 neonatal deaths were substracted from the ongoing pregnancies at 20 weeks, 608 infants would be alive at 28 days of age.

Early pregnancy loss in Belagavi, Karnataka, India 2014–2017: a prospective population-based...

229

Table 4 Relative risk (RR) of medically terminated pregnancy (MTP) vs ongoing pregnancy in 3 gestational age groups by women's characteristics

	MTP v. Ongoing 6,0–7,6 Weeks RR (95% CI)	MTP v. Ongoing 8,0–11,6 Weeks RR (95% CI)	MTP v. Ongoing 12,0–19,6 Weeks RR (95% CI)
Maternal age (years)			
≤ 20	1.24 (0.65, 2.36)	1.12 (0.78, 1.61)	0.85 (0.67, 1.08)
21–25	REF	REF	REF
26–30	2.02 (1.08, 3.77)	1.22 (0.99, 1.52)	1.15 (1.00, 1.32)
> 30	2.76 (1.34, 5.68)	2.07 (1.41, 3.05)	2.19 (1.76, 2.74)
Maternal education			
No formal education	1.02 (0.31, 3.36)	1.02 (0.59, 1.77)	1.00 (0.71, 1.41)
Primary	REF	REF	REF
Secondary	1.32 (0.54, 3.26)	1.63 (1.16, 2.30)	1.35 (1.04, 1.75)
University+	1.27 (0.48, 3.41)	1.82 (1.01, 3.28)	1.52 (1.05, 2.21)
Parity			
0	0.19 (0.08, 0.45)	0.52 (0.37, 0.74)	0.98 (0.81, 1.17)
1–2	REF	REF	REF
> 2	1.22 (0.65, 2.31)	1.42 (0.97, 2.06)	1.28 (1.00, 1.63)
BMI (kg/m^2)			
Underweight, < 18.5 kg/m^2	0.65 (0.44, 0.96)	0.79 (0.63, 1.01)	1.02 (0.88, 1.18)
Normal weight, 18.5–25 kg/m^2	REF	REF	REF
Overweight and obese, > 25 kg/m^2	1.06 (0.51, 2.20)	0.81 (0.57, 1.16)	1.15 (0.95, 1.39)
Hemoglobin (gm/dl)			
Severe/Moderate, ≤ 9 g/dl	1.57 (0.87, 2.83)	0.75 (0.46, 1.24)	1.04 (0.91, 1.19)
Mild, > 9–11 g/dl	1.16 (0.76, 1.78)	0.79 (0.61, 1.01)	0.93 (0.82, 1.05)
Normal, > 11 g/dl	REF	REF	REF

BMI body mass index
REF reference group
MTP medically terminated pregnancy

We next evaluated characteristics associated with miscarriage for three categories of gestational age (6 weeks to 7 weeks 6 days, 8 weeks to 11 weeks 6 days and 12 weeks to 19 weeks 6 days). In this analysis, the characteristics of women with a miscarriage within the gestational age category were compared to those with an ongoing pregnancy. The adjusted RR and 95% CI for each group are presented (Table 3). Among women > 30 years of age, there was an increasing risk of miscarriage as the gestational age of the pregnancy increased from 6 weeks to 7 weeks 6 days, to 8 weeks to 11 weeks 6 days, and to 12 weeks to 19 weeks 6 days. Women with a secondary education appeared more likely to have a miscarriage at 12 to 19 weeks 6 days, and women with a BMI > 25 kg/m^2 appeared less likely to have a miscarriage at 6 weeks to 7 weeks 6 days. Women with hemoglobin levels < 9 g/dl were less likely to have a miscarriage at 6 weeks to 7 weeks 6 days. Those with a hemoglobin level from 9 to 11 g/dl were less likely to have a miscarriage at 6 weeks to 7 weeks 6 days and at 8 weeks to 11 weeks 6 days. Those with a hemoglobin < 9 g/dl had a lower risk of miscarriage in all gestational age groups

although only in the earliest gestational age group were the results significant. Otherwise, there were no significant differences by the gestational age of the miscarriage observed.

Among women with an MTP, ages 26–30 and > 30 were generally associated with an increased rate of MTP, as was having a secondary or university education compared to those with a primary education. Nulliparity was associated with decreased risk of MTP in the two lowest gestational age groups. Parity > 2 was associated with a higher risk of MTP but was significant only at 12 to 19 weeks 6 days. Having a BMI < 18.5 kg/m^2 was associated with a lower rate of MTP at 6 weeks to 7 weeks 6 days and nearly so at 8 weeks to 11 weeks 6 days. Otherwise, there were no significant differences for MTP by gestational age (Table 4).

Discussion

In this study, we demonstrated that of 1000 ongoing pregnancies at 6 weeks gestational age in Belagavi, India, there will only be about 600 living infants at the end of the perinatal period. Spontaneous miscarriages account for about 2/3 of the losses and MTP for about 1/3. Stillbirths and neonatal deaths account for much smaller proportions of the losses. Miscarriage and MTP were more common at 6 to 8 weeks gestational age compared to later time-periods.

We found that a number of factors were associated with miscarriage. Older women and women with a secondary education were often at an increased risk for miscarriage when compared to women who had ongoing pregnancies. Women with low parity were often at decreased risk. BMI > 25 kg/m^2 was associated with a lower risk of miscarriage at 6 weeks to 7 weeks 6 days, but not at other times. For unexplained reasons, lower hemoglobin levels were associated with a lower risk of miscarriage prior to 12 weeks.

Our results also showed that older women, those with higher education, those with higher parity were more likely to have a MTP. Women with a BMI < 18.5 kg/m^2 were less likely to have an MTP at 6 weeks to 7 weeks 6 days. Hemoglobin levels were not associated with rates of MTP in any time-period.

Our results are broadly comparable to those in other studies. A study in a low-income country which looked at the rate of miscarriages by gestational age week, had a mean age of enrolment of nearly 14 weeks, while in our study, nearly 80% of the subjects were enrolled prior to 12 weeks [11]. Many studies estimate that around 30% of pregnancies end in a miscarriage, while in our study about 28% of ongoing pregnancies at 6 weeks were estimated to end in a miscarriage. However, the gestational age of women's enrolment and the gestational age when miscarriages become stillbirths or live births in various studies make more exact comparisons impossible. The risks for miscarriage found in our study were similar to those previously reported and included older age and higher parity. The results in our study were often not consistent across the gestational periods studied while this information was not available in most other low-income country studies [3, 4].

Strengths and limitations
Because of ongoing surveillance systems of women likely to become pregnant and the frequent pregnancy testing, we believe we have captured ongoing pregnancies as early in pregnancy as possible in a low-income country study. The rates of miscarriage and MTP likely represent the actual rates of miscarriage and MTP in ongoing pregnancies in each of the time-periods studied. Nevertheless, because pregnant women present for care at various times in pregnancy, it was necessary to use available data to construct a hypothetical cohort of 1000 women with an ongoing pregnancy at 6 weeks to enable us to calculate the overall losses expected. Therefore, one of

the potential weaknesses of the study is that the rates of miscarriage and MTP in this model are estimates. However, these estimates are based on accurate population-based data of pregnancies enrolled quite early. In general, we use self-reported data and have not validated whether or when a miscarriage or MTP actually occurred. However, because we followed the women closely, we believe these data are reasonably accurate. In some of the time-periods and with certain of the characteristics, the numbers in the cells are small and the resultant confidence intervals are relatively large, thus precision may be limited. Since the gestational age data were often obtained by LMP without ultrasound confirmation, the number of women in each gestational age group may represent an approximation.

Conclusion
Of 1000 ongoing pregnancies at 6 weeks gestation, nearly 40% will be lost prior to 20 weeks gestation, two thirds to miscarriage and one third to MTP. A much smaller percentage will be lost later to stillbirth and neonatal mortality. Risk factors for miscarriage include higher maternal age and education. In this study, for reasons not obvious to us, lower haemoglobin levels appear to be related to lower rates of miscarriage. Higher maternal age, parity, and BMI were associated with MTP. These results should enable health systems to evaluate the resources necessary to provide appropriate care for all pregnant women including those having spontaneous miscarriages and undergoing MTP.

Abbreviations
ANC: Antenatal Care; BMI: Body Mass Index; MNHR: Maternal Newborn Health Registry; MTP: Medically Terminated Pregnancy

Funding
Funding for the MNHR comes from NICHD to the participating sites and to Research triangle Institute. Publication charges for this supplement were funded by the University of British Columbia PRE-EMPT (Pre-eclampsia/Eclampsia, Monitoring, Prevention and Treatment) initiative supported by the Bill & Melinda Gates Foundation Melinda.

Authors' contributions
SMD conceived of the manuscript and wrote the first draft with input from MSS, JPJ, RLG, and EMM. SMD, MSS, SSV, YK, AK, UYR, and SSG oversaw study implementation, data collection and quality monitoring. JLM, DDW and EMM performed the statistical analyses. All authors reviewed and approved the final manuscript.

Competing interests
The authors declare that they have no competing interests.

Author details
[1]Women's and Children's Health Research Unit, J N Medical College, KLE Academy of Higher Education and Research, Belagavi, Karnataka, India. [2]Thomas Jefferson University, Philadelphia, PA, USA. [3]RTI International, Durham, NC, USA. [4]Columbia University, New York, NY, USA.

References
1. Zegers-Hochschild F, Adamson GD, de Mouzon J, Ishihara O, Mansour R, Nygren K, et al. The International Committee for Monitoring Assisted Reproductive Technology (ICMART) and the World Health Organization (WHO) revised glossary on ART terminology. Hum Reprod. 2009;24:2683–7.
2. Wilcox AJ, Weinberg CR, O'Connor JF, Baird DD, Schlatterer JP, Canfield RE, et al. Incidence of early loss of pregnancy. N Engl J Med. 1988;319:189–94.
3. Pallikadavath S, Stones RW. Miscarriage in India: a population-based study. Fertil Steril. 2005;84:516–8.
4. Patki A, Chauhan N. An epidemiology study to determine the prevalence and risk factors associated with recurrent spontaneous miscarriage in India. J Obstet Gynaecol India. 2016;66:310–5.
5. Cai Y, Feng W. Famine, social disruption, and miscarriage: evidence from Chinese survey data. CSDE Working Paper 2005: No. 04–06. Seattle: University of Washington. Available at: http://csde.washington.edu/downloads/04–06.pdf. Accessed 27 Feb 2018.
6. Pokale Y, Khadke P. Risk of recurrent miscarriage in India and the effect of paternal age and maternal age. IRA-Int J Appl Sci. 2016;3:3.
7. Hirve SS. Abortion law, policy and services in India: a critical review. Reprod Health Matters. 2004;12:114–21.
8. Singh S, Shekhar C, Acharya R, Moore AM, Stillman M, Pradhan MR, et al. The incidence of abortion and unintended pregnancy in India, 2015. Lancet Global Health. 2018;6:e111–20.
9. Goudar SS, Carlo WA, McClure EM, Pasha O, Patel A, Esamai F, et al. The maternal and newborn health registry study of the global network for Women's and Children's Health Research. Int J Gynaecol Obstet. 2012;118:190–3.
10. Kodkany BS, Derman RJ, Honnungar NV, Tyagi NK, Goudar SS, Mastiholi SC, et al. Establishment of a maternal newborn health registry in the Belgaum District of Karnataka, India. Reprod Health. 2015;12 Suppl 2:S3.
11. Dellicour S, Aol G, Ouma P, Yan N, Godfrey Bigogo G, Hamel MJ, et al. Weekly miscarriage rates in a community-based prospective cohort study in rural western Kenya. BMJ Open. 2016;6:e011088. https://doi.org/10.1136/bmjopen-2016-011088.

25

Developing a model for integrating sexual and reproductive health services with HIV prevention and care

Cecilia Milford[1]* ⓘ, Fiona Scorgie[2], Letitia Rambally Greener[1,2], Zonke Mabude[1], Mags Beksinska[1], Abigail Harrison[3] and Jennifer Smit[1]

Abstract

Background: There are few rigorous studies evaluating the benefits of vertical versus integrated delivery of healthcare services, and limited published studies describing conceptual models of integration at service-delivery level in public healthcare facilities. This article seeks to fill this gap, by describing the development of a district-based model for integrating sexual and reproductive health (SRH) and HIV services in KwaZulu-Natal, South Africa.

Methods: Baseline data were collected from seven urban public healthcare facilities through client and provider interviews, and a facility inventory was completed to assess current service integration practices. Feedback sessions were held with health providers from participating facilities to share data collected and explore appropriate integration scenarios. A conceptual model of potential service integration was then designed, and subsequently implemented and evaluated in the research sites.

Results: Key principles of the model included a focus on health system strengthening and strong community input and involvement. The model was designed primarily to support the integration of family planning into HIV services, and included measures to improve client and commodity monitoring; capacity building through training and mentorship; and a 'health navigation' strategy to strengthen referrals within and between public healthcare facilities. Endline evaluation data were collected in the same facilities following implementation of the model.

Conclusions: This manuscript demonstrates the utility of the conceptual model. It shows that service integration can be accomplished in a phased manner with support of community and healthcare providers. In addition, local context must be taken into account and the components of the model should be flexible to suit the needs of the health system.

Keywords: Integration, Reproductive health, HIV, Family planning, South Africa

Plain English summary

There are few studies evaluating the benefits of vertical versus integrated delivery of healthcare services, and limited studies describing conceptual models of health service integration in public healthcare facilities. We describe the development of a district-based model for integrating sexual and reproductive health (SRH) and HIV services in KwaZulu-Natal, South Africa.

Before the development of the model, baseline data were collected from seven urban public healthcare facilities using client and provider interviews, and a facility inventory was completed to assess how existing services were being integrated, if at all. Feedback sessions were held with healthcare providers from participating facilities to explore possible scenarios for integrating services that could work in their settings. A conceptual model of service integration was then designed, implemented and evaluated in the research sites.

* Correspondence: cmilford@mru.ac.za
[1]MatCH Research Unit (MRU), Department of Obstetrics and Gynaecology, Faculty of Health Sciences, University of Witwatersrand, Durban, South Africa
Full list of author information is available at the end of the article

Key principles of the model included a focus on health system strengthening and strong community input and involvement. The model was designed primarily to support the integration of family planning into HIV services and included strategies to improve the monitoring of patients seen and commodities used (such as female condoms or contraceptive pills); capacity building of staff through training and mentorship; and a 'health navigation' strategy to strengthen referrals within and between healthcare facilities. Endline evaluation data were collected in the same facilities following implementation of the model.

The utility of the integration model we developed is explored in the manuscript. We show that service integration can be accomplished in a phased manner with the support of community members and healthcare providers. In addition, local context must be taken into account and any model used to guide integration of healthcare services should be flexible to suit the needs of the health system.

Background

There has been a renewed focus on integrated health services in South Africa in the last 20 years [1]. This is largely in response to a growing unease about the verticalisation of HIV services, which resulted partially from the single-disease funding approach to HIV [2, 3]. Integration has also received attention thanks to an increasing desire to meet the sexual and reproductive health (SRH) needs of people living with HIV (PLHIV) [1, 4, 5]. More recently research demonstrating the teratogenic effect of Dolutegravir (first line antiretroviral regimen) on babies [6] has highlighted the need for integrated family planning and HIV services.

South Africa is a country where service integration in the fields of HIV and SRH is critically important. It has one of the largest populations of PLHIV globally, with a national HIV prevalence of almost 18% (in adults aged 15–49 years), in 2017 [7, 8]. The 'rollout' of anti-retroviral therapy (ART) was initiated by the South African government in 2005, and as of 2017, approximately 4.4 million South Africans were on ART [8]. While providing ART on this scale is challenging for the health system, and numbers on treatment still fall short of the UNAIDS 90–90–90 targets [8], remarkable success has been achieved in initiating clients on treatment. This initiation of treatment is affected by clients' ability to reach health services and, once there, to negotiate a complex range of visits and medical tests. In some settings, multiple 'stops' within one facility are required, and some clients must move repeatedly between locations which may be situated some distance apart within the facility. In addition to HIV services, these clients need to utilise SRH services, which are often not matched to their particular needs and may not necessarily be offered within HIV clinics at primary healthcare

facilities. Furthermore, clients accessing SRH services in health facilities are known to be at high risk of HIV acquisition, and therefore need to be offered integrated HIV services [1, 9].

National and international funding focus on HIV prevention and treatment was partly responsible for the verticalisation of services in South Africa, and resulted in a diversion of attention from (and neglect of) provision of comprehensive SRH services [10]. Consequently, family planning (FP) services have suffered, the range of available and accessible methods narrowed, and uptake and continuation of contraception remains a challenge. Despite recent introduction of the implant and retraining on the intrauterine device (IUD) in the public sector (post implementation of this study), unmet need for FP in South Africa continues to be high, at 18% (in married and sexually active unmarried women), in 2016 [11]. In addition, data from the 2012 South African National HIV Prevalence, Incidence and Behaviour Survey, demonstrated that two thirds (66.5%) of women (15–49 years) who had reported a pregnancy in the previous 5 years, had not intended becoming pregnant [12].

Despite the release and roll out of a national contraceptive policy and guidelines promoting contraceptive-HIV integration in 2014 [13–15], and a renewed emphasis on integrating services at facility level in South Africa, little progress has been made with SRH and HIV integration in practice. Adoption and implementation of these guidelines has been slow, and there has been limited development of policy on HIV-SRH service integration more broadly [14]. As a result, individual effort to integrate services at district or facility level may be ad hoc or relatively uncoordinated. Furthermore, there is a lack of indicators or agreed upon ways to measure integration [16–18]. In KwaZulu-Natal Province more specifically, the public healthcare services have been politically divided (District and Municipal systems), each with different administrations and budgets, which creates further challenges in service provision and integration.

Systematic reviews [17–20] demonstrate that integrating SRH and HIV services could yield a number of benefits, including increasing uptake of contraception, condom use, HIV testing, and services for prevention of mother-to-child transmission of HIV (PMTCT), along with more rapid ART initiation. However, some integration interventions have not been sufficiently evaluated [18, 20] and health, stigma and cost outcomes are not adequately reported on [19]. Furthermore, there remains little consensus on how to operationalise and best integrate these services [1].

In this manuscript we report on the development of a district-based model to provide comprehensive and integrated SRH and HIV services appropriate to the local context. At the time of this research, health services (including FP, HIV and other SRH services) in South Africa were being offered independently of one another, with few formal linkages between services. Although systems for referral are improving, even in healthcare settings that are under-resourced (often paper-based systems), under-staffed and highly burdened, tracking clients who are referred out of a facility is difficult, and missed opportunities for reaching clients with comprehensive SRH and HIV services continue to occur.

Study aim and setting

Our aim was to improve uptake of services, but also to provide input to emerging South African policy on integrated services, by generating empirical evidence on the effectiveness and feasibility of an integration model in this setting. Working in an urban district, the eThekwini District in KwaZulu-Natal Province, South Africa, the study was located in seven healthcare facilities, including five primary healthcare clinics, a community health centre and a District level hospital. We aimed to reach young women in particular, who are at highest risk of HIV acquisition and have many unmet FP and SRH needs. KwaZulu-Natal had an HIV prevalence of 18.1% in 2017 [8], and women (15-49 years) in the province have continued high levels of unmet FP need (20.1% in 2016) [11]. We sought to explore innovative community-orientated strategies to reach this group and improve their access to SRH services.

In this manuscript we describe work done to inform the development of the integration model (study design), report briefly on baseline data used to inform the model (key findings from baseline research), describe the development and key components of the model (discussion: designing the model), and reflect on the main implementing challenges experienced and lessons learned for future SRH services integration (implementation successes, challenges and lessons learned).

Endline process evaluation data are discussed only where relevant to our reflections on the effectiveness of the model, but are reported on in more detail elsewhere [21]. Activities encapsulated within the integration model drew on simple, tried-and-tested methods as well as novel and innovative approaches to health systems strengthening, often adapted from contexts outside of HIV and SRH service provision.

Methods
Study design
Part 1

Key informant interviews ($n = 21$) were held in 2008 with individuals representing non-governmental organisations (NGOs), academia and the Department of Health (DoH) [22], to gather baseline data on understandings of 'integration', perceptions of current integration practices in South Africa, and pressing integration needs. Individuals with knowledge and experience of integrating SRH and HIV services in South Africa were purposively selected. Thereafter, snowball sampling was used to ensure information-rich cases were sampled and appropriate data were collected [22]. These data were qualitatively analysed using NVivo (QSR International).

Part 2

Key informant interviews were followed by baseline research comprising facility audits and interviews with healthcare providers and clients. More specifically, four focus group discussions (FGDs) were held with healthcare providers ($n = 43$), and a cross sectional survey was conducted with providers ($n = 46$), to explore current integration practices, and challenges and experiences with these. Healthcare providers were purposively selected to represent different categories of providers working in HIV and SRH services in all the participating facilities. In the FGDs, healthcare providers were grouped together according to senior management, nurses and doctors, and enrolled nurses and counsellors, to allow participants to speak freely [21]. Providers who participated in the baseline cross-sectional survey were from antenatal, FP, primary healthcare (PHC), HIV counselling and testing (HCT) and sexually transmitted infection (STI) services. Of all baseline survey participants, 89% were female, their mean age was 43.7 years, and their mean years of working were 18.3 years [21].

An exit interview in the form of a cross-sectional survey was conducted with clients ($n = 269$) accessing HIV or reproductive health related services (including HCT, antenatal, perinatal, PHC, STI and FP services), at the seven participating facilities in 2009. The client sample was selected by ensuring representation of clients attending the different SRH services in the facilities. Approximately 30–40 clients were enrolled per clinic, and approximately 50 clients at the hospital, and 82% of the clients were female. Client interviews explored services accessed and experiences with and attitudes towards integrated services. This information was supplemented by facility inventories conducted within the participating facilities, which enabled better understanding of the SRH, FP and HIV services offered at these facilities, and the extent to which these services were already integrated.

Part 3

Results from the baseline data (Parts 1 and 2) were explored, and used to inform the development of an integration model that responded to the needs and challenges specific to the context within which we were working. Specific integration gaps and challenges, as well as current practices that were identified by clients, providers and key stakeholders were focused on in order to develop a model that could be tailored to the specific healthcare facilities we were working in. This draft model was presented to different working groups which were established for the duration of the project. The purpose of the working groups was to inform the process of developing the integration model and to support its implementation. The groups included a District Working Forum (DWF), comprising operations and nursing service managers and nursing staff from the seven facilities. The DWF met twice a year throughout the project period and reviewed the proposed integration model, provided input to model development and implementation, assessed overall progress, and offered experiential advice and support. A Scientific Advisory Board (SAB), including academics, integration experts and managers in the local and municipal DoH, and a Community Advisory Board (CAB), which comprised of community health workers, NGO personnel, and other community role-players who represented the communities served by the health systems, also provided ongoing input to the model development and implementation process. In addition, the study team met regularly throughout the project with healthcare providers at the participating facilities to elicit input and provide iterative feedback on the integration model. Due to the frequent and interactive meetings with the groups, real time feedback was incorporated into development of the model.

Part 4

Following the implementation of the model, endline process evaluation data were collected (in 2011) via a cross sectional survey with providers ($n = 44$) and clients ($n = 300$), and facility inventories were conducted within participating facilities. Providers and clients who participated in the endline were sampled in the same way as for the baseline survey. Data were collected on the same parameters at baseline and endline to determine explore changes in data and determine usefulness and success of the model (and are reported elsewhere). Cross-sectional data were entered into SPSS versions 24 and 25, and descriptive statistics were calculated. Where necessary Pearson's Chi-square and Fisher's Exact Test were used to determine significance of change in variables over time.

This manuscript focuses on Part 3 – the development of an integration model, based on initial findings from the baseline research (as described in Parts 1 and 2).

Study approvals and support

The study was approved by the University of the Witwatersrand's Human Research Ethics Committee (M080624). The University of KwaZulu-Natal's Biomedical Research Ethics Committee provided reciprocity approval. Provincial, District and Municipal DoH approval were obtained, along with site support from each of the participating healthcare facilities.

Results

This manuscript describes the development of the integration model, based on initial findings from baseline research. Key baseline findings are presented here as they pertain to the model development, and more detailed evaluations, comparing baseline and endline results are reported elsewhere[1] [21].

Key findings from baseline research

Information elucidated from those involved both in providing and receiving services in the study facilities proved to be essential in orientating the model development process.[2] Client survey data demonstrated that although clients were able to access the SRH services they required, they expressed some frustration with long waiting times – where almost a quarter (24.1%) at baseline did not agree that the waiting time was reasonable. Little integration of services appeared to be happening, and SRH services received by clients were not comprehensive. Few clients who had accessed the clinic for FP services on the day of the interview were offered other SRH or HIV services by a provider. Less than a third (29.7%) attending FP services had been offered HCT services on that day or at previous FP visits. However, communication about male condoms and dual protection was common, irrespective of the reason for the clinic visit. More than a third (34.1%) of clients reported having queued more than once in a single day for separate services at the same facility.

Clients indicated a preference for seeing the same provider on returning clinic visits, more than three quarters (77.3%) specified that if given a choice, they would like to see the same provider at each visit, suggesting that continuity of care is an important consideration when designing integrated services. This preference was also about the availability of a 'one-stop shop' for accessing PHC, HIV and FP services within the same facility, believed to result in shorter waiting times. Both healthcare providers and key informants expressed favourable attitudes towards the integration of HIV and FP services [21, 22], and some believed it would be more convenient for clients to access all the services they needed from the same provider [21]. Providers and key informants also wanted greater involvement of the community in service integration (including peer support systems), implying a potential extension of integration programmes beyond health facilities themselves.

Health providers expressed some concerns about the feasibility of integrating services, fearing an increase in workload and consultation times, making it difficult for them to see all clients coming to the facility in a single day [21]. An additional challenge anticipated by providers was the translation of new policies and guidelines into practice due to numerous operational barriers, such as shortage of resources – infrastructural, human and financial [21]. Perhaps because of these concerns, key informants stressed that integration of services should be flexible and tailored to specific contexts.

Discussion: Designing the model

Our challenge was to design a model of integration that could meet the needs and challenges of this setting, but also be feasible, practical and affordable for the participating facilities. Based on key informant opinion [22] and a review of the integration literature, it was clear that our model needed to allow for internal variation between sites, and it also had to be relevant to the context of the broader health system. Our approach, therefore contained broad generic components, allowing for some adaptation at sites, recognising that "one size *doesn't* fit all" [23].

In addition to a lack of agreed upon indicators to measure integration [16–18], another reason why it is difficult to evaluate the merits and drawbacks of integration efforts across different settings is that "integration" itself has been conceptualised in many different ways [10, 24]. Some have described it as a "spectrum" [25] or, as a "continuum rather than as two extremes of integrated/not integrated" [26]. Furthermore, integration has been characterised as "full" (multiple services offered on-site) versus "partial" (referral to off-site services) [27]. It can be facility level, provider initiated/driven, or client initiated/driven. There is a further need to identify the *direction* of integration: i.e. what new or existing services are being integrated into which existing programme or service? A WHO systematic review on linkages between SRH and HIV services, identified at least six possibilities: antenatal care clinics adding HIV services; HCT centres adding HIV services; FP clinics adding HIV services; HIV clinics adding SRH services; STI clinics adding HIV services; and PHC clinics adding HIV and/or SRH services [28].

In our study, decisions about direction of integration were informed by baseline findings that identified provision of FP and other SRH services to PLHIV as a neglected priority in this setting, which has more recently been highlighted by the teratogenic effects of Dolutegravir in early pregnancy [6]. We therefore designed a model that integrated FP into existing HIV services, and HIV into FP services, but which could ultimately be adapted to support a range of alternative configurations. Integrating FP into HIV services has numerous potential benefits. It creates opportunities for reaching men with FP information and services (for example in PHC related services), and for counselling serodiscordant couples and assessing the suitability of a contraceptive method for PLHIV, for instance in regard to potential drug interactions between contraceptive method and ART. It also allows for the promotion of dual protection and reiteration of FP messages, along

with the resupply of FP methods to HIV clients during regular repeat visits [23]. On the other hand, integrating HIV services into FP services allows for HCT and HIV services to be provided to clients accessing FP methods.

In our model, these services were integrated at both provider and facility level. In the former, one provider would offer multiple services, while the latter involved mechanisms to support internal referral, either at the same visit or a future one. Measures to maintain effective linkages between services were also included to improve coverage and continuity of care.

Some challenges emerged during model development. These centred on questions of how to ensure genuine community involvement; of building capacity without over-relying on training; and of making a difference to the quality of services in an already over-burdened health system with high staff turnover. Additional challenges became evident when reviewing the literature on potential barriers to the effectiveness of integrated programmes. At the facility- and health systems-levels, such barriers could include: a lack of clear guidelines on which service is to be integrated in which department and how; inadequate integrated training for supervisors; and stock-outs of contraceptive supplies [4]. From the perspective of clients, integration could be less effective if they perceive integrated services to involve long waiting times and inadequate privacy; and to allow insufficient time for asking questions during consultations [29]. Overall, we wanted to anticipate potential barriers such as these and pre-empt them as far as possible.

A preliminary integration model was initially presented to role-players from the SAB, DWF and CAB, and their input requested. Specifically, healthcare providers gave valuable input on what was realistic and reasonable within their facilities. The components and details of the model were adjusted based on these discussions. The final model comprised four inter-connected intervention areas, namely: capacity building; health systems strengthening; service level activities and interventions; and community input and involvement (see Fig. 1). Key expected outcomes included improvements in the practice of offering SRH and HIV services to clients – including greater efficiency, effectiveness and higher uptake of services – which in turn could facilitate recommendations for updating policies on integrated services. Each of these component intervention areas are described in more detail in the sections that follow.

1. Capacity building: Training and mentorship

Building the capacity of healthcare providers to offer integrated services was an essential component in the model. Capacity building also underpinned activities directed at health systems strengthening and interventions designed to improve the quality of individual services.

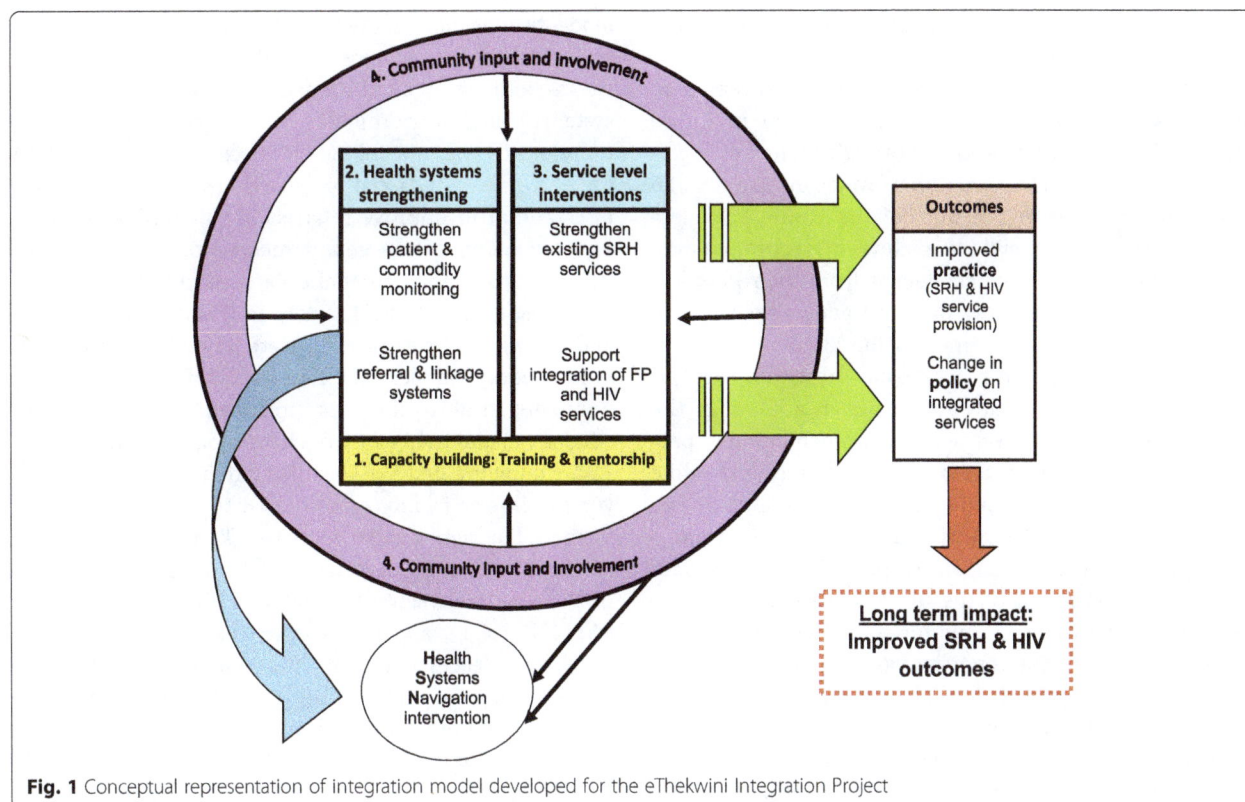

Fig. 1 Conceptual representation of integration model developed for the eThekwini Integration Project

Baseline research indicated that in many cases, only up-dates were needed on new policies or developments in the fields of HIV and SRH, rather than full training in basic material that was already familiar to providers. In each instance, HIV and SRH topics were addressed from the perspective of integrated services. Importantly, training was also provided on more 'systemic' issues, such as methods to strengthen referral systems, monitoring and evaluation (M&E) and record keeping. To increase attendance, training sessions were conducted on-site, in providers' own facilities. They also included non-clinical staff (such as clinic receptionists and security guards), along with community representatives serving on the project's CAB.

In the early stages of the project, many providers had indicated that training may have limited effect on practice in the long term, as providers return to work and seldom implement the theoretical knowledge learned during training. In anticipation of this, we conducted post-training mentorship in one facility. We used one-on-one mentorship to guide the application of new skills and knowledge, and to improve confidence to do this, once providers had returned to their posts. Support was also offered to the facility supervisor, equipping her with skills required to take ownership of the mentorship programme over time. Peer mentorship has been demonstrated as effective and feasible in capacity building for SRH and HIV service integration [30].

2. Health systems strengthening

Many of the challenges associated with implementation of integrated services stem from systemic weaknesses, where the health system itself is burdened by infrastructural, logistical, training and service management limitations [4]. While 'fixing' the health system was too ambitious, an integration model would be incomplete if it aimed only to combine services that had previously been offered vertically and did nothing to strengthen the functioning of the broader health system in which services were couched. Two key interventions were therefore included, to contribute to health systems strengthening: measures to improve client and commodity monitoring, and to improve referrals and linkages between services.

Improving information and supply chains: Client and commodity monitoring

Many challenges surround the recording of client data in public facilities in South Africa. Healthcare providers are required to enter client data by hand into multiple registers for each consultation, which is cumbersome and time consuming, and may inevitably lead to incomplete and inaccurate entries. Baseline data and planning discussions with stakeholders revealed the need for a single, streamlined register in which all client details could be captured [31]. Such a change however, was unfortunately beyond the scope of the project, as it would have required national DoH input and would have taken several years to implement.

Instead, we assessed the practice of record-keeping to identify shortcomings that could be targeted in future interventions. This involved a thorough review of registers and patient-held cards that were in use in the healthcare facilities at the time of the study. Providers were interviewed to build a picture of record-keeping overall, and to isolate the challenges from their perspective. On the basis of these data, we generated a list of recommendations to link monitoring systems more effectively with integrated practice and presented these to local and provincial health authorities in a 'State of the Art' dissemination meeting. Recommendations presented included reducing the number of registers while still capturing the same indicators that were already being recorded in a more integrated manner; formal training of healthcare providers on the practicality of the data and on understanding of the importance of the indicators being measured and monitored in clinic registers, to facilitate more reliable reporting; as well as the employment and training of dedicated data clerks to facilitate higher quality data capture.

Although we were unable to implement these recommendations as part of our model as this would have required extensive high level DoH input, which was not feasible within the study timeline, we were able to train providers to improve record-keeping practice within the existing system. In addition, regular feedback sessions were held in facilities to inform providers about client statistics in their facilities, which were generated at a provincial level, based on facility level data entry. These sessions highlighted incomplete data records and reinforced the importance and usefulness of accurate record keeping in facilities, and facilitated improvements in data record keeping.

Securing health commodities and ensuring that procurement is reliable has been identified as an often overlooked need in integration planning [28]. Based on an initial assessment of how FP commodities were being monitored in the study facilities, we designed a series of interventions to strengthen the supply chain overall and improve monitoring systems for procurement and re-supply to minimise stock-outs. Providers were trained to use these monitoring systems and were supported in their attempts to access stock from central distribution points. Support was provided to all facilities to ensure a continuous supply of contraceptives, particularly in a newly established HIV Wellness Centre linked to the antiretroviral (ARV) Clinic in one facility, which had no previous experience with stocking and ordering these commodities. In addition, a guidance note was developed to facilitate access to female condoms at facility level, and the numbers of female condoms distributed were measured throughout the project.

Innovative methods to improve referral & linkage systems

Our baseline data demonstrated that referrals at the study sites – both within and between facilities – were often unsystematic and uncoordinated, with no systems in place to monitor referral and follow-up success rates. To address these gaps, we adapted a 'Health Systems Navigation' intervention to improve referrals in this setting – a concept originating in cancer-treatment settings in the United States, but with the potential to be used in HIV service settings in southern Africa [32–34]. In this intervention, peer and other lay support workers were trained to assist clients in navigating complex HIV care and SRH services, thereby improving health outcomes (treatment initiation and/or adherence) and the quality of client experience and care.

We implemented the 'health systems navigator' intervention in one facility only (the District Hospital) in our setting. The aim was to increase client referrals within the SRH sector (FP, antenatal and postnatal care, abortion), and between designated HIV services (ART, PMTCT, HCT), and to improve clients' overall experiences when accessing healthcare. Aside from making integrated services part of routine practice, this innovation aimed to help break down community members' fears of asking for help in the health system and their reluctance to request specific SRH services owing to stigma.[3]

Navigators were trained in several roles. They gave health talks to clients in facility waiting areas and at community level events on a wide range of SRH, FP and HIV topics, while also offering information on the availability of integrated services. Navigators escorted clients to service points where needed, and actively followed up referrals afterwards to ensure that clients had successfully accessed relevant SRH and HIV services. Both clients and healthcare providers provided favourable feedback on the inclusion of health navigators in the integration model. The navigator role was structured to be comparable with the local Community Health Worker skills level and remuneration, in order to ensure operational feasibility and facilitate future sustainability should the model be scaled up.

3. Service-level interventions

With these health systems strengthening interventions in place, our focus turned to address the specific services targeted for integration. Our intention was to introduce FP services into ARV clinics, HIV Wellness Centres, Well Baby and PMTCT clinics – all of which had previously provided limited FP services to clients or none at all. This integration at service-level was kick-started by a series of training, or capacity-building, activities and consolidated through an expansion of existing SRH services.

Supporting integration of FP and HIV services

Effective integration of FP and HIV services required an element of task shifting. HIV service providers (counsellors, ARV providers, and PMTCT providers) were trained to also counsel their clients on FP needs and other SRH concerns. Furthermore, we trained FP service providers to perform HCT in sites where there were too few dedicated HIV counsellors.

Training was structured to respond to the particular needs of individual facilities, rather than offered as a generic package. In spite of this tailored, specific approach, however, many of the sessions across facilities turned out to be standard, and covered a variety of SRH and HIV topics, including: integrated female condom training; HCT and FP integration; ARV services and FP integration; expanding the FP method choice; and counseling clients on dual protection. All levels of healthcare providers were invited to participate in the training in order to facilitate integration practices both within and between healthcare facilities. Several job aids were used in this training, including female pelvic models and male condom models, the national guidelines on contraception, and information, education and communication (IEC) materials on emergency contraception, female condom use, and medical male circumcision. To ensure that an expanded method choice was being offered to clients, we also trained providers in the use of the WHO Reproductive Choices Flip-chart [35] and supplied them with copies of this tool for use during consultations. The flip-chart is designed to strengthen providers' ability to offer clients a wider selection of contraceptive methods, encourage them to choose the most acceptable contraceptive method, and address broader SRH issues.

Expanding and promoting existing SRH services
Creating and implementing the integration model offered an opportunity to push the boundaries of existing SRH services, reconfiguring old services or even introducing wholly new ones. In addition to expanding the repertoire of FP methods offered to clients, in one facility we worked with healthcare providers to facilitate promotion of emergency contraception and to make it more accessible – by extending the service over weekends, when demand was likely to be higher. By implementing this in one facility only, we were able to explore the feasibility of expanding SRH services in other sites where there is operational feasibility and provider support.

IEC messaging was an integral part of the strategy to build awareness of the full range of SRH services on offer in facilities, particularly where they had not previously been offered. We used messaging printed on t-shirts, posters and pamphlets to promote dual protection, emergency contraception, female condoms and medical male circumcision, all couched within a broader context of integrated services. Health systems navigators wore these t-shirts, which not only made them visible to clients but also helped to communicate the availability of multiple services at the facility.

4. Getting everyone on board: Engaging the community
Community input and involvement was integral to the process of intervention design. Through the CAB and DWF, sustained input was elicited from community members and key stakeholders. While the CAB drew its members largely from clinic volunteers, NGO personnel and other community role-players, the DWF comprised mostly senior facility staff. Their participation in the study extended beyond feedback sessions, however, to include involvement in a series of broader local health-promotion activities. Through these forums, we sought buy-in from facilities and DoH, and built networks and relationships with community members and health authorities on the ground, harmonising our collective efforts to improve SRH and HIV services in the district.

Training in integrated services, expanded SRH services and promotion of female condoms was offered to members of the CAB, who readily accepted this opportunity to become better equipped to play active roles in their communities and facilities. Once NGOs, identified by CAB members as being active in areas around the study sites, had been mapped, we were also able to invite members of relevant NGOs to participate in training sessions. Finally, health systems navigators linked up with local NGO representatives during community outreach activities, joining them at community events to give talks on various SRH topics and raise awareness of the newly integrated services available.

Implementation successes, challenges and lessons learned
A 'success story' from our study was the introduction of health systems navigators, which represented a possible solution to the difficulties around task-shifting and around changing scopes of practice. This component of the model demonstrated that there is strong potential for a new cadre of staff to take on multiple tasks and facilitate integrated services within South Africa's over-loaded public healthcare system. The health systems navigators active in our study facilities managed to relieve some of the nurses' workload: nurses reported that time had been freed up for them to focus on both clinical and administrative duties, making this a promising intervention that could be further developed and scaled up. The health systems navigators were utilised by nurses for activities beyond their original scope of work, including filing and other administrative tasks. Furthermore, since the conclusion of our integration study, navigators have been funded in the Province of KwaZulu-Natal by external funders (such as Pepfar), and are now working in SRH services in public healthcare facilities [34, 36].

In addition, the creation of a DWF was a particularly successful project component. Including healthcare providers from all levels of participating facilities (operational, managerial and nursing staff), enabled project buy-in and support. The regular meetings facilitated real-time contributions to the model development and implementation, and ensured that challenges could be addressed timeously if necessary.

Several obstacles made it difficult to fully implement all components of the model or to do so as originally planned. We found that – unsurprisingly – integrated service delivery takes time to establish and support. Buy-in and approvals from some partners took longer than anticipated, and required enormous investment into building relationships. We learned early on that it was essential to stagger the process of introducing new practices and not bombard facilities with activities all at once. As with any process of initiating institutional change, internal resistance must be acknowledged and accommodated, with appropriate sensitivity to the existing workloads of providers, which are often substantial.

It was sometimes difficult to get full attendance of providers at training sessions due to numerous factors such as heavy workloads, high turnover of staff and multiple commitments (such as staff meetings and district training programmes). Training was conducted on-site at hours convenient to healthcare providers and frequently rescheduled in order to address this challenge – but it remained difficult throughout implementation, and possibly diminished the impact of the intervention overall.

Despite our efforts to improve commodity monitoring and procurement, there were also frequent stock-outs, specifically of female condoms. This may have been because facilities were too busy to prioritize female condom planning, amidst competing demands on their time and other resources. Unfortunately, we also discovered that our involvement in facilitating procurement of female condoms ironically became a disincentive for facility staff to take on this task themselves.

An important lesson learned during capacity building activities was that it was important to know how flexible providers' 'scope of practice' was prior to training them. Without this, the promotion of task-shifting was virtually impossible. One example was the attempt to train enrolled nurses and nursing assistants to counsel clients on the importance of contraception and to perform HCT, but HIV and contraceptive method counseling was not considered to be part of their formal 'scope of practice', therefore they were often not confident enough to counsel clients.[4] In another example, we wanted to involve support staff (security guards, clerks, and nursing assistants) in more innovative ways and task-shift some integration responsibilities to them. Clerks in particular were identified as being under-utilised in facilities. Since we were not permitted to propose changes to job profiles in the research sites, these intentions could not be realised, although the initiative is nonetheless recommended for future integration efforts. An important outcome of this study is the finding that clerks and other healthcare facility support staff could do more, but that standard job descriptions and expectations may prevent this from happening. However, in our study, security guards were trained on services provided and were able to direct clients to these services and to condom dispensers located outside facilities, after hours.

A few interventions were clearly needed in this setting but fell outside of the project's scope or were simply not pragmatic to implement. Firstly, more substantive changes were needed in the area of client flow and consultation hours. In all facilities, clients were only seen in the mornings (on a 'first-come-first-served' basis), as healthcare providers generally used the afternoons to catch up on administrative duties. If clients had to be referred for any additional critical care, this could also only happen in the mornings. Clients consequently arrived very early in the morning in order to secure their place in the queue, and often ended up waiting several hours to be seen. The provision of additional, integrated services to clients could potentially increase the duration of each consultation, leading to even longer waiting times for clients. In our context, extending consultation times beyond the mornings would certainly have lessened waiting times – but it was not possible for several reasons. Most clients depended on public transport, which is more limited later in the day compared to early mornings in this setting. Furthermore, providers themselves were reluctant to see clients in the afternoons, even if this meant that client-flow continued to be slow with rushed consultation times. Instituting human resource-level interventions to reduce waiting times – such as enabling flexi-hours and the use of shifts – were therefore omitted from the model, even if they made sense in theory.

Secondly, we wanted to implement a patient card system to facilitate improved record-keeping and linkages between services. This method of managing client data could be used as a tool to empower women to take control of their own health. For example, patient cards could capture multiple information including HCT, HIV status and CD4 count, in addition to serving as an FP tool. However, it requires a comprehensive tracking system, and needs to be consistently used to be effective. Introducing such an intervention would have needed buy-in at a higher level, as it would have had implications for wider DoH activities across the province and beyond, but it remains an important intervention for future consideration.

Finally, we identified and drafted a plan for an adolescent SRH clinic to be offered at one site, offering specific clinic times for school-going youth, dedicated FP queues for adolescents, and similar interventions. Due to unforeseen delays with ethics application processes, this was never implemented. It was viewed as an acceptable intervention and would be critical in future integration scenarios, in order to be able to provide multiple services to this vulnerable population.

Despite the fact that this model was implemented some time ago, and that supportive integration policies have been implemented since this study was undertaken, integration in practice has been slow [1, 5, 14]. Therefore, findings from this study remain useful to inform future integration policies and practices in this this setting.

Conclusions

The project demonstrated that even a multi-faceted, complex model of integration can be implemented in low-resource, high-burden public healthcare systems, if it is done in a phased manner with buy-in and support of both community and healthcare providers. The process of design and implementation needs to take local context and facility level into account, and should be flexible to suit the needs of both the health system and the clients in order to have optimum effect. There need to be linkages between multiple health systems functions and components, including policy, financing mechanisms, supply chain management, and healthcare worker training [5]. We were able to present a draft integration strategy to stakeholders and policy makers at national, provincial and district DoH levels, that drew on empirical data from implementation of the model. Out of this experience, we made various recommendations for policy and planning. These recommendations include three key priority areas. Firstly, to develop integrated training and mentoring programmes – prioritise, revive and strengthen existing programmes, promote community training and use innovative methods (such as health systems navigation) to support this initiative. Secondly, to ensure a basic minimum package of integrated services, tailored to individual facilities, with standardised service points for integration, and integration indicators. Finally, to ensure communities are involved and engaged in integration activities, with a focus on hard to reach groups such as males and adolescents -using a bottom up approach. It is important to note that change is slow, and any suggestions for change require negotiation over time. The South African government is currently prioritising "putting integration into practice" [1], and our findings and recommendations have the potential to inform future policy and practice in this field.

Endnotes

[1]Additional analyses have been submitted for publication elsewhere.

[2]The detailed results of the baseline and endline research will be published elsewhere, and are not presented in this manuscript, which focuses solely on the integration model. Key baseline findings are highlighted here to demonstrate findings which guided the model development.

[3]The health systems navigation component will be published elsewhere.

[4]Enrolled nurses or staff nurses are limited in scope of work by the Nursing Act (Act 33 of 2005), to only provide nursing care and treatment under the supervision of a professional nurse.

Abbreviations
ART: Antiretroviral therapy; ARV: Antiretroviral; CAB: Community advisory board; DoH: Department of Health; DWF: District working forum; FP: Family planning; HCT: HIV counselling and testing; IUD: Intrauterine device; NGO: Non-governmental organisation; PLHIV: People living with HIV; PMTCT: Prevention of mother-to-child transmission of HIV; SAB: Scientific advisory board; SRH: Sexual and reproductive health

Acknowledgements
The authors are grateful to the William and Flora Hewlett Foundation for funding development and implementation of the integration model in KwaZulu-Natal province. We would also like to thank Jacqueline Pienaar, Claudia Ngoloyi, Ross Greener and Kathryn Church for valuable contributions to the study. Finally, we thank the participating healthcare facilities, providers and clients, who gave time and input to the study.

Funding
This study was funded by the William and Flora Hewlett Foundation.

Authors' contributions
CM, FS LRG, ZM, MB, AH & JS contributed to the development and assessment of the integration model. CM, LRG, MB, JS developed and implemented the baseline and endline research and analysed this data. FS prepared initial drafts of the manuscript, and CM reworked for finalisation. All authors read and contributed to draft versions of and the final manuscript.

Competing interests
The authors declare that they have no competing interests.

Author details
[1]MatCH Research Unit (MRU), Department of Obstetrics and Gynaecology, Faculty of Health Sciences, University of Witwatersrand, Durban, South Africa. [2]Wits RHI (Reproductive Health and HIV Institute), Faculty of Health Sciences, University of the Witwatersrand, Johannesburg, South Africa. [3]Department of Behavioral and Social Sciences, Brown University School of Public Health, Providence, RI, USA.

References

1. Mantell JE, Cooper D, Exner TM, Moodley J, Hoffman S, Myer L, et al. Emtonjeni-a structural intervention to integrate sexual and reproductive health into public sector HIV Care in Cape Town, South Africa: results of a phase II study. AIDS Behav. 2017;21(3):905–22.

2. Bowser D, Sparkes SP, Mitchell A, Bossert TJ, Barnighausen T, Gedik G, et al. Global Fund investments in human resources for health: innovation and missed opportunities for health systems strengthening. Health Policy Plan. 2014;29:986–97.

3. Rabkin M, El-Sadr WM, De Cock KM. The impact of HIV scale-up on health systems: a priority research agend. J Acquir Immunce Defic Syndr. 2009;52:S6–S11.

4. Church K, Mayhew SH. Integration of STI and HIV prevention, care, and treatment into family planning services: a review of the literature. Stud Fam Plan. 2009;40(3):171–86 PubMed PMID: 19852408.

5. Hope R, Kendall T, Langer A, Barnighausen T. Health systems integration of sexual and reproductive health and HIV services in Sub-Saharan Africa: A scoping study. J Acquir Immune Defic Syndr. 2014;67(Supplement 4):S259–S70.

6. Dolutegravir for HIV: a lesson in pregnancy safety research The Lancet Global Health. 2018;391(10137):2296. https://www.thelancet.com/journals/lancet/article/PIIS0140-6736(18)31265-0/fulltext.

7. Statistics South Africa. Mid year population estimates, 2017. 2017. http://www.statssa.gov.za/publications/P0302/P03022017.pdf. Accessed 1 Sep 2017.

8. HSRC. South African national HIV prevalence, incidence, behaviour and communication survey, 2017. HSRC Launch; 17 July 2018. http://www.hsrc.ac.za/uploads/pageContent/9234/FINAL%20Presentation%20for%2017%20July%20launch.pdf. Accessed 1 Aug 2018.

9. Ndhlovu L, Searle C, Miller R, Fisher A, Snyman E, Sloan N. Reproductive health services in KwaZulu-Natal, South Africa: A situation analysis study focusing on HIV/AIDS services. Horizons Program, KwaZulu-Natal Department of Health; 2003.

10. Smit JA, Church K, Milford C, Harrison AD, Beksinska ME. Key informant perspectives on policy- and service-level challenges and opportunities for delivering integrated sexual and reproductive health and HIV care in South Africa. BMC Health Serv Res. 2012;12:48.

11. Department of Health, SA Medical Research Council, DHS Program. South Africa Demographic and Health Survey 2016: Key Indicator report. Pretoria: Statistics South Africa, 2017. http://www.mrc.ac.za/sites/default/files/files/2017-05-15/SADHS2016.pdf. Accessed 28 Jun 2018.

12. Chersich MF, Wabiri N, Risher K, Shisana O, Celentano DD, Rehle T, et al. Contraception coverage and methods used among women in South Africa: a national household survey. S Afr Med J. 2017;107(4):307–14.

13. Department of Health. National Contraception and fertility planning policy and service delivery guidelines. Pretoria: Government of the Republic of South Africa; 2012. https://www.medbox.org/south-africa/national-contraception-and-fertility-planning-policy-and-service-delivery-guidelines/preview?q=. Accessed 16 Oct 2018

14. Cooper D, Mantell JE, Moodley J, Mall S. The HIV epidemic and sexual and reproductive health policy integration: views of south African policymakers. BMC Public Health. 2015;15:217.

15. Health-e News. Guidelines: national contraception, fertility planning policy. 2014. https://www.health-e.org.za/2014/05/06/guidelines-national-contraception-fertility-planning-policy/. Accessed 16 Oct 2018.

16. Church K, Warren CE, Birdthistle I, Ploubidis GB, Tomlin K, Zhou W, et al. Impact of integrated services on HIV testing: a randomised trial among Kenyan family planning clients. Stud Fam Plan. 2017;48(2):201–18.

17. Lindegren ML, Kennedy CE, Bain-Brickley D, Azman H, Creanga AA, Buler LM, et al. Integration of HIV/AIDS services with maternal, neonatal and child health, nutrition, and family planning services. Cochrane Database Syst Rev. 2012;9(10):CD010119.

18. Spaulding AB, Brickly DB, Kennedy C, Almers L, Packel L, Mirjahangir J, et al. Linking family planning with HIV/AIDS interventions: a systematic review of the evidence. AIDS. 2009;23(Suppl 1):S79-88.

19. Kennedy C, Spaulding AB, Brickley DB, Almers L, Mirjahangir J, Packel L, et al. Linking sexual and reproductive health and HIV interventions: a systematic review. J Int AIDS Soc. 2010;13:26.

20. Lisy K. Integration of HIVAIDS services with maternal, neonatal and child health, nutrition, and family planning services. Public Health Nurs. 2013; 30(5):451–3.

21. Milford C, Rambally Greener L, Beksinska M, Greener R, Mabude Z, Smit J. Provider understandings of and attitudes towards integration: implementing an HIV and sexual and reproductive health service integration model, South Africa. Afr J AIDS Res. 2018;17(2):183–92.

22. Smit JA, Church K, Milford C, Harrison AD, Beksinska ME. Key informant perspectives on policy- and service-level challenges and opportunities for delivering integrated sexual and reproductive health and HIV care in South Africa. BMC Health Serv Res. 2012;12(48):1–8.

23. WHO. Strategic Considerations for Strengthening the Linkages between Family Planning and HIV/AIDS Policies, Programs, and Services. Geneva: World Health Organization; 2009. http://www.who.int/reproductivehealth/publications/linkages/fp_hiv_strategic_considerations.pdf. Accessed 16 Oct 2018

24. Atun R, de Jongh T, Secci F, Ohiri K, Adeyi O. Integration of targeted health interventions into health systems: a conceptual framework for analysis. Health Policy Plan. 2010;25(2):104–11.

25. Coker R, Balen J, Mounier-Jack S, Shigayeva A, Lazarus JV, Rudge JW, et al. A conceptual and analytical approach to comparative analysis of country case studies: HIV and TB control programmes and health systems integration. Health Policy Plan. 2010;25(Suppl 1):i21–31.

26. WHO. Integrated Health Services - What and Why? Geneva: WHO; 2008. http://www.who.int/healthsystems/technical_brief_final.pdf. Accessed 16 Oct 2018

27. Spaulding AB, Brickley DB, Kennedy C, Almers L, Packel L, Mirjahangir J, et al. Linking family planning with HIV/AIDS interventions: a systematic review of the evidence. AIDS. 2009;23(Suppl 1):S79–88.

28. WHO, UNFPA, IPPF, UNAIDS, UCSF. Sexual and reproductive health and HIV: linkages: evidence review and recommendations. UNAIDS, 2008. http://www.who.int/hiv/pub/sti/sex_worker_implementation/swit_chpt4.pdf?ua=1. Accessed on 1 Feb 2018.

29. Maharaj P, Cleland J. Integration of sexual and reproductive health services in KwaZulu-Natal, South Africa. Health Policy Plan. 2005;20(5):310–8.

30. Ndwiga C, Abuya T, Mutemwa R, Kimani JK, Colombini M, Mayhew S, et al. Exploring experiences in peer mentoring as a strategy for capacity building in sexual reproductive health and HIV service integration in Kenya. BMC Health Serv Res. 2014;14:98.

31. Mutemwa R, Mayhew S, Colombini M, Busza J, Kivunaga J, Ndwiga C. Experiences of health care providers with integrated HIV and reproductive health services in Kenya: a qualitative study. BMC Health Serv Res. 2013;13:18.

32. Gabram SGA, Lund MJB, Gardner J, Hatchett N, Bumpers HL, Okoli J, et al. Effects of an outreach and internal navigation program on breast cancer diagnosis in an urban cancer center with a large African-American population. Cancer. 2008;113(3):603–7.

33. Bertoni K. Better access to health care through system navigation. Canadian Nurse. 2009;105(2):17–8.

34. Bassett IV, Coleman SM, Giddy J, Bogart LM, Chaisson CE, Ross D, et al. Sizanani: a randomised trial of health systems navigators to improve linkage to HIV and TB care in South Africa. J Acquir Immunce Defic Syndr. 2016;73(2):154–60.

35. World Health Organization. Reproductive choices and family planning for people living with HIV: Counselling Tool. 2012. http://apps.who.int/iris/bitstream/10665/43609/1/9241595132_eng.pdf?ua=1. Accessed 16 Oct 2018.

36. Greener L, Greener R, Beksinska M, Sithole K, Lafort Y, Smit J. Health systems navigators: Improving access to public sector HIV and sexual and reproductive health services among female sex workers in KwaZulu-Natal. 8th South Africa AIDS Conference; 13 June 2017; Durban, South Africa 2017. http://www.saaids.com/Presentations%20AIDS%202017/Tuesday,%2013%20June%202017/Hall%207/16h00-%2017h30/SA%20Aids%202017%20L%20Greener%20(DIFFER%20HSNs)_FINAL.pdf. Accessed 1 Nov 2018.

Permissions

List of Contributors

Sowmya Rajan
Global Health Innovations Center, Duke University, Durham, NC 27701, USA

Priya Nanda
Bill and Melinda Gates Foundation, New Delhi, India

Lisa M. Calhoun
Carolina Population Center, University of North Carolina at Chapel Hill, Chapel Hill, USA

Ilene S. Speizer
Carolina Population Center, University of North Carolina at Chapel Hill, Chapel Hill, USA
Gillings School of Global Public Health, University of North Carolina at Chapel Hill, Chapel Hill, USA

Adélaïde Compaoré and Halidou Tinto
Clinical Research Unit Nanoro, Institut de Recherche en Sciences de la, Santé, Direction Régionale du Centre-Ouest, Nanoro, Burkina Faso

Sabine Gies
Department of Biomedical Sciences, Prince Leopold Institute of Tropical Medicine, Antwerp, Belgium
Medical Mission Institute, Würzburg, Germany

Bernard Brabin
Liverpool School of Tropical Medicine and Institute of Infection and Global Health, University of Liverpool, Liverpool, United Kingdom; Global Child Health Group, Academic Medical Centre, University of Amsterdam, Amsterdam, The Netherlands

Loretta Brabin
Division of Cancer Sciences, Faculty of Biology, Medicine and Health, University of Manchester, Manchester, UK

Alehegn Bishaw Geremew and Abebaw Addis Gelagay
Department of Reproductive Health, Institute of Public Health, College of Medicine and Health Science, University of Gondar, 196 Gondar, Ethiopia

Telake Azale
Department of Health Education and Behavioral Sciences, Institute of Public Health, College of Medicine and Health Sciences, University of Gondar, Gondar, Ethiopia

Changchang Li
Department of Health Policy and Management, School of Public Health, Sun Yat-sen University, 74 Zhongshan Road, Guangzhou 510080, China
Guangzhou Key Laboratory of Environmental Pollution and Health Risk Assessment, School of Public Health, Sun Yat-sen University, 74 Zhongshan Road, Guangzhou 510080, China
Department of Biostatistics and Epidemiology, School of Public Health, Sun Yat-sen University, 74 Zhongshan Road, Guangzhou 510080, China

Zhijiang Liang and Qingguo Zhao
Department of Public Health, Guangdong Women and Children Hospital, 521, 523 Xing Nan Street, Guangzhou 511442, China

Michael S. Bloom
Departments of Environmental Health Sciences and Epidemiology and Biostatistics, University at Albany, State University of New York, Rensselaer, USA

Qiong Wang, Huanhuan Zhang, Suhan Wang and Cunrui Huang
Department of Health Policy and Management, School of Public Health, Sun Yat-sen University, 74 Zhongshan Road, Guangzhou 510080, China
Guangzhou Key Laboratory of Environmental Pollution and Health Risk Assessment, School of Public Health, Sun Yat-sen University, 74 Zhongshan Road, Guangzhou 510080, China

Xiaoting Shen
Center for Reproductive Medicine, The First Affiliated Hospital of Sun Yat-sen University, 74 Zhongshan Road, Guangzhou 510080, China

Weiqing Chen
Guangzhou Key Laboratory of Environmental Pollution and Health Risk Assessment, School of Public Health, Sun Yat-sen University, 74 Zhongshan Road, Guangzhou 510080, China

Yan Lin
Department of Children Health Care, Shenzhen Women and Children Hospital, Shenzhen, China

Martin C. Koch, Johannes Lermann, Simone K. Renner, Stefanie Burghaus, Janina Hackl, Ralf Dittrich, Sven Kehl, Patricia G. Oppelt, Thomas Hildebrandt, Caroline C. Hack and Stefan P. Renner
Universitätsklinikum Erlangen, Frauenklinik, Universitaetsstrasse 21-23, 91054 Erlangen, Germany

Niels van de Roemer
Valley Electronics AG, Marienstraße 16, 8003 Zurich, Switzerland

Uwe G. Pöhls
Praxis, Kaiserstraße 26, 97070 Würzburg, Germany

Falk C. Thiel
Klinik am Eichert, Frauenklinik, Eichertstraße 3, 73035 Göppingen, Germany

Hamdia M. Ahmed and Mosleh S. Kareem
College of Nursing, Hawler Medical University, Erbil, Kurdistan Region, Iraq

Nazar P. Shabila
Department of Community Medicine, Hawler Medical University, Erbil, Kurdistan Region, Iraq

Barzhang Q. Mzori
Directorate of Health, Erbil, Kurdistan Region, Iraq

Xiayun Zuo, Chaohua Lou, Ersheng Gao and Qiguo Lian
Key Laboratory of Reproduction Regulation of NPFPC, SIPPR, IRD, Fudan University, 779 Laohumin Road, Shanghai 200237, China

Iqbal H. Shah
Department of Reproductive Health and Research, World Health Organization, Geneva, Switzerland

N. C. Schmidt, M. Epiney and O. Irion
Department of Obstetrics and Gynecology, University Hospitals of Geneva, Geneva, Switzerland

V. Fargnoli
Department of Sociology, University of Geneva, Geneva, Switzerland

Marilia Arndt Mesenburg, Cesar Gomes Victora, Andrea Homsi Damaso and Mariangela Freitas da Silveira
Post-Graduate Program in Epidemiology, Federal University of Pelotas, Pelotas, Brazil

Suzzane Jacob Serruya, Rodolfo Ponce de León
Latin American Center of Perinatology, Women and Reproductive Health, Montevideo, Uruguay

Marlos Rodrigues Domingues
Post-Graduate Program in Physical Education, Federal University of Pelotas, Pelotas, Brazil

Niveen M. E. Abu-Rmeileh, Rula Ghandour, Marina Tucktuck and Mohammad Obiedallah
Institute of Community and Public Health, Birzeit University, BirzeitWest BankoPt, Palestine

José Atienza-Carrasco
Nursing Surgery Service, Hospital Costa del Sol, Málaga, Spain

Manuel Linares-Abad
School of Health Sciences, Universidad de Jaén, Jaén, Spain

María Padilla-Ruiz
Research Unit. Agencia Sanitaria Costa del Sol, Marbella, Spain
Health Services Research on Chronic Patients Network. REDISSEC, Madrid, Spain

Isabel María Morales-Gil
School of Health Sciences, Universidad de Málaga, Málaga, Spain

Frankie J. Fair, Helen Watson and Hora Soltani
Faculty of Health and Wellbeing, Sheffield Hallam University, Collegiate Crescent, Sheffield, UK

Rachel Gardner
Sheffield Maternity Services Liaison Committee and Sheffield user group charity – Forging Families, Sheffield, UK

Lucy November and Jane Sandall
Division of Women and Children's Health, Faculty of Life Sciences and Medicine, Kings College London, St Thomas' Campus, Westminster Bridge Road, London SE1 7EH, UK

Friday Okonofua
University of Medical Sciences, Ondo City, Ondo State, Nigeria
The Women's Health and Action Research Centre, WHO Implementation Research Group, Benin City, Nigeria
Centre of Excellence in Reproductive Health Innovation, University of Benin, Benin City, Nigeria

Lorretta Ntoimo
The Women's Health and Action Research Centre, WHO Implementation Research Group, Benin City, Nigeria
Department of Demography and Social Statistics, Federal University Oye-Ekiti, Oye, Ekiti State, Nigeria

Rosemary Ogu
The Women's Health and Action Research Centre, WHO Implementation Research Group, Benin City, Nigeria
Centre of Excellence in Reproductive Health Innovation, University of Benin, Benin City, Nigeria
Department of Obstetrics and Gynaecology, University of Port Harcourt, Port Harcourt, Rivers State, Nigeria

Hadiza Galadanci
Aminu Kano Teaching Hospital, Kano, Nigeria

Rukiyat Abdus-salam
Adeoyo Maternity Hospital, Ibadan, Oyo State, Nigeria

Mohammed Gana
General Hospital, Minna, Niger State, Nigeria

Ola Okike
Karshi General Hospital, Federal Capital Territory, Abuja, Nigeria

Kingsley Agholor
Central Hospital, Warri, Delta State, Nigeria

Eghe Abe
Central Hospital, Benin City, Edo State, Nigeria

Adetoye Durodola
General Hospital, Ijaye Abeokuta, Ogun State, Nigeria

Abdullahi Randawa
Ahmadu Bello University, Zaria, Kaduna State, Nigeria

Sumit Kane
KIT Royal Tropical Institute, Mauritskade 63, Amsterdam 1092 AD, The Netherlands
Nossal Institute for Global Health, Melbourne School of Population and Global Health, University of Melbourne, Level 5, 333 Exhibition Street, Melbourne, VIC 3010, Australia

Matilda Rial
Independent Consultant, Wau, Western Bahr el Ghazal, South Sudan

Maryse Kok
KIT Royal Tropical Institute, Mauritskade 63, Amsterdam 1092 AD, The Netherlands

Anthony Matere
School of Public and Environmental Health, University of Bahr el Ghazal, Wau, Western Bahr el Ghazal, South Sudan

Marjolein Dieleman
KIT Royal Tropical Institute, Mauritskade 63, Amsterdam 1092 AD, The Netherlands
Athena Institute for Research on Innovation and Communication in Health and Life Sciences, Faculty of Earth and Life Sciences, VU University Amsterdam, Amsterdam, The Netherlands

Jacqueline E. W. Broerse
Athena Institute for Research on Innovation and Communication in Health and Life Sciences, Faculty of Earth and Life Sciences, VU University Amsterdam, Amsterdam, The Netherlands

David J. Amor
Murdoch Children's Research Institute, Royal Children's Hospital, Parkville, Australia
Department of Paediatrics, The University of Melbourne, Parkville, Australia
Melbourne IVF, East Melbourne, Australia

Annabelle Kerr, Nandini Somanathan, Jan Hodgson and Sharon Lewis
Murdoch Children's Research Institute, Royal Children's Hospital, Parkville, Australia
Department of Paediatrics, The University of Melbourne, Parkville, Australia

Alison McEwen
Graduate School of Health, University of Technology, Sydney, Australia

Marianne Tome
Melbourne IVF, East Melbourne, Australia

Niouma Nestor Leno
Bureau de Stratégie et de Développement du Ministère de la Santé, Conakry, Guinea
Chair de Santé Publique de l'Université Gamal Abdel Nasser de Conakry, Conakry, Guinea

Alexandre Delamou
Chair de Santé Publique de l'Université Gamal Abdel Nasser de Conakry, Conakry, Guinea
Centre National de Formation et de Recherche en Santé Rurale de Maferinyah, Forécariah, Guinea
Department of Public Health, Institute of Tropical Medicine, Antwerpen, Belgium

Youssouf Koita
Programme National de Prise en Charge Sanitaire et de Prévention des IST/ VIH/Sida (PNPCSP) du Ministère de la Santé, Conakry, Guinea

Thierno Souleymane Diallo
Secrétariat Exécutif du Comité National de Lutte contre le Sida (SECNLS), Conakry, Guinea

Abdoulaye Kaba
Bureau de Stratégie et de Développement du Ministère de la Santé, Conakry, Guinea

Therese Delvaux, Wim Van Damme and Marie Laga
Department of Public Health, Institute of Tropical Medicine, Antwerpen, Belgium

Ahmed Zohirul Islam
Department of Population Science and Human Resource Development, University of Rajshahi, Rajshahi 6205, Bangladesh

Ritesh Mistry and Anjuli Dasika
Department of Health Behavior and Health Education, University of Michigan School of Public Health, 1415 Washington Heights, SPH I, Room 3806, Ann Arbor, MI 48109-2029, USA

Andrew D. Jones and Ujwala Kulkarni
Department of Nutritional Sciences, University of Michigan, Ann Arbor, USA

Mangesh S. Pednekar, Gauri Dhumal and Prakash C. Gupta
Healis Sekhsaria Institute for Public Health, Navi Mumbai, India

Mangala Gomare
Municipal Corporation of Greater Mumbai, Mumbai, India

Demeke Lakew Workie, Dereje Tesfaye Zike and Haile Mekonnen Fenta
Statistics Department, Science College, Bahir Dar University, Bahir Dar, Ethiopia

Mulusew Admasu Mekonnen
PMA2020/Ethiopia project and John Snow Inc (JSI) SEUHP/Ethiopia

Erica Sedlander, Jeffrey B. Bingenheimer, Mark C. Edberg, Rajiv N. Rimal and Hina Shaikh
Department of Prevention and Community Health, The George Washington University, Milken Institute School of Public Health, 950 New Hampshire, Washington, DC, USA

Wolfgang Munar
Department of Global Health, The George Washington University, Milken Institute School of Public Health, 950 New Hampshire, Washington, DC, USA

Suzanne Penfold and Katharine Footman
Marie Stopes International, 1 Conway Street, Fitzroy Square, London W1T 6LP, UK

Susy Wendot
Marie Stopes Kenya, Kindaruma Road, Nairobi, Kenya

Inviolata Nafula
UCSF-Global programs, Morning Side Office Park, Ngong Road, Nairobi, Kenya

Hilary M Schwandt, Bethany Sparkle and Moriah Post-Kinney
Fairhaven College, Western Washington University, 516 High Street, MS 9118, Bellingham, WA 98225, USA

Sangappa M. Dhaded, Manjunath S. Somannavar, Sunil S. Vernekar, S. Yogesh Kumar, Avinash Kavi, Umesh Y. Ramadurg and Shivaprasad S. Goudar
Women's and Children's Health Research Unit, J N Medical College, KLE Academy of Higher Education and Research, Belagavi, Karnataka, India

Jane P. Jacob and Richard J. Derman
Thomas Jefferson University, Philadelphia, PA, USA

Elizabeth M. McClure, Janet L. Moore and Dennis P. Wallace
RTI International, Durham, NC, USA

Robert L. Goldenberg
Columbia University, New York, NY, USA

Cecilia Milford, Zonke Mabude, Mags Beksinska and Jennifer Smit
MatCH Research Unit (MRU), Department of Obstetrics and Gynaecology, Faculty of Health Sciences, University of Witwatersrand, Durban, South Africa

Fiona Scorgie
Wits RHI (Reproductive Health and HIV Institute), Faculty of Health Sciences, University of the Witwatersrand, Johannesburg, South Africa

Letitia Rambally Greener
MatCH Research Unit (MRU), Department of Obstetrics and Gynaecology, Faculty of Health Sciences, University of Witwatersrand, Durban, South Africa Wits RHI (Reproductive Health and HIV Institute), Faculty of Health Sciences, University of the Witwatersrand, Johannesburg, South Africa

Abigail Harrison
Department of Behavioral and Social Sciences, Brown University School of Public Health, Providence, RI, USA

Index

www.ingramcontent.com/pod-product-compliance
Lightning Source LLC
Chambersburg PA
CBHW080505200326
41458CB00012B/4089